QUALITY
LONGEVITY ™

YOUR SCIENTIFIC GUIDE TO GREAT HEALTH AND LONGEVITY.

Caution
If you are taking a prescription drug or have a health problem, obtain the advice of a health practitioner who is experienced in the effects of changing how you eat and exercise.

False facts are highly injurious to the progress of science, for they often endure long.

Charles Darwin
Scientist, Naturalist and Author — 1809 to 1882

Progress is not created by contented people.

Frank Tager

Seventh Edition
Published by, and research supported by:

Advanced Health Center
34146 Selva Road, Suite 200
Monarch Beach, California, 92629.
Phone (714) 661-4001 Fax (714) 661-1666

Quality Longevity, The Quality Longevity Program,
Prime Test are trademarks of Advanced Health Center.
Copyright 1978, 1980, 1982, 1991, 1994 and 1995
by Mark Lovendale. All rights reserved.

Credits:
Photograph, outside back cover: Valentine Mayer

Printing code: 1 2 3 4 5 6 7 8 9 10 11 12

Library of Congress Catalog Card Number: 94-73781

Lovendale, Mark.
    Quality longevity.
    Includes bibliographical references.
    1. Allergy. 2. Heart disease. 3. Diet therapy.
4. Blood tests. 5. Longevity. I. Title.

ISBN 0-945196-22-9

I am sick of diseases, I want to know origins and processes ... If we are to prevent disease it is to the beginning of the chain of accumulating stresses that we must look.

Clifford Allbutt
Medical Historian and Author — 1836 to 1925

THE QUALITY LONGEVITY PROGRAM™

This program will help you understand the latest breakthroughs in health care and longevity. Within a month, the knowledge you gain will enable you to improve your health dramatically.

The 1988 Surgeon General's report states that diet-caused diseases account for 68 percent of all deaths in the United States. This means that choosing the wrong foods is killing more Americans than infectious diseases, smoking, alcohol, drugs, accidents, traditional medical procedures, stress and the aging process — *combined*. And that is just the beginning. Most people are unknowingly tearing down their health faster than it can be repaired by any amount of doctors, drugs and money. Virtually no one gets to die of old age.

The solution lies in replacing damaging behavior with preventive behavior. A basic principle of preventive care is to avoid foods, chemicals or other items which cause health problems.

Recent research has shown that delayed food and chemical allergies are the most often missed diagnosis in medicine today. Delayed allergies are very different from the acute type of allergies which are understood and treated by traditional allergists. A delayed allergic reaction may take hours or days to show up and can cause a broad range of both common and unusual symptoms.

Over the last few years, extensive research has revealed a better way of testing for delayed food and chemical allergies. It is now possible to find the underlying cause of many common ailments from a small blood sample. This improved approach is called the Prime Test.™

The Prime Test reveals an offending substances by combining a small amount of a person's white blood cells with a microscopic amount of each food and chemical. If the cells stay healthy, active and alive, the item is not likely to cause symptoms. However, if the white blood cells wrinkle, burst open and die, a food or chemical has been found which is often the underlying cause of many health problems. Many symptoms have been eliminated by avoiding the foods and chemicals which damage people's white blood cells.

The Prime Test makes it possible to have a new type of nutritional counseling — one which helps people become free of their symptoms.

Discovering your health-building foods as well as your health-damaging foods and chemicals by using the Prime Test is a primary step toward removing the cause of a broad range of symptoms. It is also important to select foods low in fat, moderate in protein and high in complex carbohydrates to become free of additional symptoms. It is now possible to enjoy good health without symptoms reoccurring, and fully live a much longer life.

A clean environment, in combination with aerobic and strength exercise, is necessary to regain and maintain health. In conjunction with eating your compatible foods, it is important to support your health by fulfilling your unique needs with compatible vitamins, minerals and specialized supplements which do not cause allergic reactions.

The Quality Longevity Program brings together, for the first time, the beneficial parts of the best health programs. The combined effect of these breakthroughs enables you to remove the causes of most health problems and thereby free yourself from most symptoms while significantly exceeding normal levels of health and longevity.

The Quality Longevity Program is the leading edge of health care. You are starting on a path of discovery that will continually give you rewards, and add enjoyable years to your life.

The doctor of the future will give no medicine,
but will interest his patient in the care
of the human frame, in diet, and in the
cause and prevention of disease.

Thomas A. Edison
Inventor — 1847 to 1931

Guarantee

The Quality Longevity Program comes with a symptom back guarantee. If you go back to your old way of eating, your old symptoms will come back, or you may develop new symptoms. This sometimes happens in minutes, sometimes in months, sometimes every time you eat an allergy-causing food or chemical, and sometimes only occasionally.

Use the memory of your symptoms to help you continue eating your compatible foods. Symptoms which cause us discomfort are helpful if we understand their cause, for they show us the importance of changing old habits.

What you learn from this book will enable you to be much healthier for the rest of your life, even if you slip back from time to time. You will experience the value of removing the causes of your symptoms, rather than just treating them. Treating symptoms with over-the-counter medications, prescription drugs, surgery or allergy injections does not solve the health problems because most of the damage to your body goes on even if you treat or block out the symptom.

It is hard to visualize what it would be like to be more than 100 years old, feel fine and be full of energy because no one has seen anyone who has used the principles in this book for an extended length of time. By starting now, you have the chance of experiencing your full potential.

If I'd known I was going to live this long,
I'd have taken better care of myself.

Eubie Blake
Jazz Musician — 1883 to 1983

CONTENTS

Introduction

You are starting on a path of discovery which will guide you to great health and give you freedom from disease never before possible. The more you take advantage of the breakthroughs presented in *Quality Longevity,* the better your health will be and the sooner you will become free from your symptoms.

The awareness you gain by carefully following The Quality Longevity Program for one month will help you enjoy the rest of your life more, and you will have more life to enjoy.

Our immune system is a vital factor in how we feel and how long we live. A central part of this system is the role our white blood cells play in keeping our bodies and minds healthy. If our white blood cells react to some of the foods and chemicals we consume, the cells become damaged or destroyed. This immune reaction causes numerous ailments throughout the body and accelerates the aging process.

By avoiding the reactions which kill our white blood cells, we can become free of most chronic ailments and rejuvenate our immune systems.

When other mammals eat foods compatible with their bodies, they are free of most chronic ailments and live about 9 times their age at the start of puberty. Humans start puberty around 13 years old. By multiplying 9 times 13 we get 117; thus, we can expect over 100 years of healthy life when we eat foods compatible with our bodies.

The full health potential of The Quality Longevity Program is not known because no large group of people has combined all these approaches for maximizing health and longevity for a sufficient period of time. However, there are several remote groups which are free of most degenerative ailments, and they have one thing in common — the people consume around 10 percent of their calories from fat.

One of the groups close to this level of fat intake lives in Vilcabamba, Ecuador. Its members eat foods which have an average caloric content of 12 percent fat, and more of them live longer than do people in any other group in the world. According to their church baptismal records, 1,100 people out of 100,000 live to be 100 years old.

As fat consumption goes up, the longevity rate goes down. On the Black Sea coast of Russia, there is a group of people who eat foods which have an average caloric content of about 25 percent fat. Their record keeping is questionable; however, the indication is that 600 out of 100,000 people live to be 100 years old.

In the Hunza area of Pakistan, people also eat foods with an average caloric content of around 25 percent fat. Accurate birth records were not kept, but their longevity rate appears to be similar to the Black Sea region of Russia.

Studies of these groups indicate that when people eat 12 percent of their calories in fat instead of 25 percent, the chance of living to be 100 years old almost doubles.

In Europe and the United States, people eat meals which are 30 to 45 percent fat, and daily consume more than 250 milligrams of cholesterol. At these high levels, only 3 out of 100,000 people live to be 100 years old.

There are other important factors for obtaining improved longevity besides low fat diets; however, high-fat, high-cholesterol diets are a major reason only 3 out of 100,000 people live to be 100 in the United States compared to 1,100 out of 100,000 in Ecuador.

The oldest person to have ever lived, who's age has been verified by several documents, is still alive as of January, 1995. Her name is Jeanne Calment and on the 21st of February, 1995 she will be 120 years old. This Frenchwoman is happy and alert and has lived her life in fairly good health. She accomplished her record age without any of the breakthroughs that are presented in *Quality Longevity.* By starting now you may be the one who sets a new world record and accomplishes it in great health.

Research done on several different types of animals demonstrates that eating fewer calories creates better health and longer life. Because fat is such a concentrated source of calories, when you accurately reduce fat in the diet the total number of calories goes down dramatically.

When you hear of people who died in their sixties, seventies, eighties or nineties of a heart attack, stroke, cancer or another degenerative ailment, the most common cause of their death was a lifetime of eating the wrong foods. They did not get to die of old age or natural causes.

Most people have been unknowingly eating meals containing damaging foods and thus have had health problems for most of their lives. They suffer unnecessarily and kill themselves long before their natural time by hanging onto their old way of eating.

Taking advantage of the information in *Quality Longevity* enables you to avoid the errors of the past and live a longer life at a much higher level of health.

In the final analysis, it is important to feel good every day while living your maximum possible life span. The Quality Longevity Program makes this possible for the first time. How healthy you will be is now up to you. The choice is yours.

Update

Scientific and medical studies done since *Quality Longevity* was first published in 1980 have confirmed its four basic fundamentals. The fundamentals are: first — delayed food and chemical allergies are the major cause of most people's chronic health problems; second — a very low-fat, very low-cholesterol, moderate-protein, moderate-calorie, high-complex-carbohydrate diet will prevent and reverse most degenerative diseases; third — aerobic and resistance exercise are essential for achieving health and fully enjoying life; fourth — an individualized program of supplements that do not cause allergic reactions is important for strengthening the body and replacing deficiencies.

In 1980, these fundamentals were brought together for the first time in *Quality Longevity*. This unique combination has withstood the test of time.

Warning

Be sure you use the information in this book with the guidance of a specially trained doctor who understands delayed food and chemical allergies and related addictions. Most traditional allergists do not believe delayed food allergies exist and often try to talk people out of obtaining blood tests for delayed food allergies and the necessary counseling.

Unless we put medical freedom into the Constitution, the time will come when medicine will organize itself into an undercover dictatorship. To restrict the art of healing to one class of men and deny equal privileges to others, will constitute the Bastille of medical science. All such laws are un-American and despotic.

Benjamin Rush
A Founding Father of the United States, Physician, Author Surgeon General of the Continental Army and Signer of the Declaration of Independence — 1745 to 1813

The Potential of The Quality Longevity Program

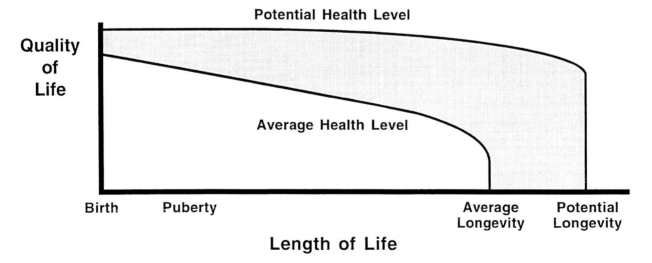

The area above the Average Health Level indicates the potential improvement available to you by taking advantage of The Quality Longevity Program.

The goal is to achieve as high a level of health as you can and stay there as long as possible. Move your level of health to the top line and then far to the right.

Possibilities

Americans spend over 900 billion dollars a year trying to become free of their symptoms, with little success. We are told we have bought the best health care system in the world, but most people are now aware something is terribly wrong.

This comprehensive preventive care program takes advantage of the breakthroughs related to delayed food and chemical allergies and the scientifically valid levels of the major nutrients. Thus, it is the major step toward solving the health problems in America and the world.

Many of the most health-damaging foods and chemicals are also damaging to the environment. The Quality Longevity Program gives you powerful information which enables you to look and feel better while you improve your health and add enjoyable years to your life.

All truth passes through three stages.
First, it is ridiculed.
Second, it is violently opposed.
Third, it is accepted as being self-evident.

Schopenhauer
German Philosopher — 1788 to 1860

Acknowledgments

No person has accomplished more in the twentieth century to develop an accurate understanding of the underlying cause of chronic ailments than Theron G. Randolph, MD.

While studying the progress of a large group of his patients, I saw a wide range of chronic ailments clear up and go away when his patients avoided their delayed food and chemical allergies. To see the ailments brought back by reintroducing the allergic food or chemical was very convincing. When the item was once again avoided, the symptoms went away again. This is something the traditional medical approach of treating symptoms is unable to do.

What I learned from Dr. Randolph about delayed allergies changed my life in two important ways. First, the knowledge enabled me to make many improvements in my health and enjoyment of life. Second, sharing this breakthrough is so personally rewarding that I changed my career and started helping people become healthy.

I found that more than nine out of ten people had some recurring health problem which was causing them problems. I was delighted to find that discovering and removing delayed food and chemical allergies enabled most people to become free of their symptoms.

I began helping Dr. Randolph communicate his numerous breakthroughs to health professionals and people with health problems.

I am grateful to Dr. Randolph for his articulate answers to my questions since 1973.

The courageous doctors who are using the awareness of delayed food and chemical allergies are to be congratulated for providing the best preventive and curative care long before traditional doctors change their ways.

A long habit of not thinking a thing wrong, gives it a superficial appearance of being right, and raises a formidable defence of custom.

Thomas Paine
A Founding Father of the United States, inspiration for the Declaration of Independence and Author — 1737 to 1809

The next major piece of the health puzzle came to me from Nathan Pritikin. In 1976 I went to a medical conference and heard one of his first lectures in which he explained the underlying causes of degenerative diseases.

I followed the progress of numerous people going through his center and saw them become free of their degenerative disease symptoms. I began to enroll doctors and the public in this important part of preventive care.

Nathan's generosity with his time and vast knowledge further improved my health and empowered me to help others to become healthy.

The Quality Longevity Program has been supported and spread by those who have decided to take advantage of this unique combination of health approaches. Thank you all, with special appreciation to Stephen White, Mark Matulis, Gordon V. Brown, Ken Stone, Linda Tombolato, Robert Pottenger, Jr, MD, Ken Aubuchon, Mark Reilly, Robert Oppenheimer, John Lloyd, Ali McDaniel and Paul Davies for your support.

Chapter 1

Freedom from Delayed Food and Chemical Allergies

The ancient Greeks discovered that some people had reactions to foods and the reactions caused a broad range of health problems. In the past it was difficult to find out which foods were causing the ailments until it was discovered that these delayed allergic reactions also damage and kill white blood cells. Delayed allergic reactions can cause symptoms minutes or days after exposure and cause symptoms anywhere in the body or in the brain.

These delayed allergic reactions can cause a wide range of problems at any location in your body. Most people are relieved to discover that they do not have several different ailments, but a single problem causing numerous symptoms. Some people are surprised by the number of foods which are damaging them. However, they become enthusiastic when they use the information you are about to read and become healthier than ever before.

White blood cells are the first line of defense against infectious diseases and cancer cells. Without them we would not survive for a week. Everyone's health is improved by having healthy white blood cells. Many ailments are caused entirely or in part by delayed allergic reactions that damage and kill our white blood cells.

When white blood cells are damaged or killed by delayed allergic reactions, it is called a cytotoxic reaction. The word "cytotoxic" is derived from the Greek word "cyto," which means cell, and is pronounced *sigh' toe*. The word "toxic" refers to damage by poison; thus, the word "cytotoxic" means cell poison.

The part of your body first damaged in a cytotoxic reaction is your white blood cells. When your white blood cells are killed, their powerful digestive enzymes are released into your blood. These digestive enzymes are then pumped throughout your body, breaking down and irritating any area of your body and causing many different symptoms.

The cytotoxic reaction was first observed by Arthur Black, MD. He was looking for a better way to test for delayed food allergies and did the first developmental work on a white blood cell test he named the "cytotoxic test." In 1956, his research was published in the medical journal *Pediatrics*.

The test was improved many times through the years. In 1988, a number of significant improvements came together. The new test significantly improved the accuracy of white blood cell testing. This improved test is called the Prime Test™ because it is the primary test to be used to discover delayed food allergies. The Prime Test uses white blood cells, known as leukocytes, and is in the general category called Leukocyte Antigen Sensitivity Test (LAST).

Discovering and avoiding delayed food and chemical allergies is a new approach to achieving health and is different from what is currently popular with most traditional doctors. They are trying to relieve symptoms with drugs, surgery, allergy injections or other techniques, rather than discovering the underlying causes of the symptoms and then removing the causes.

By testing to see if delayed allergic reactions to foods are the underlying reason for a health problem, doctors can promote healing without harming their patients. The Prime Test reveals a major cause of symptoms and makes possible a new approach for maximizing health and longevity without negative side effects.

If you know which foods are damaging your health, you have the opportunity to remove the major cause of your current and past symptoms. This awareness also empowers you to avoid new symptoms. To help accomplish this, read this book carefully and follow the recommendations of your specially trained doctor and counselor. If you just do enough to eliminate current symptoms, you are likely to experience problems in the future and be disappointed.

By being aware of your delayed food and chemical allergies, you have the information necessary to obtain your full health potential. You are responsible for your health.

Before taking the Prime Test you may have had some noticeable reactions caused by foods which are not compatible with your body. These may be the obvious or acute allergic reactions which are different from the hidden or delayed allergic reactions exposed by the Prime Test.

Professional help and expensive tests are not usually needed to discover acute reactions because your body will clearly warn you. When you are aware, you can avoid the damage caused by the acute allergy.

Food allergies are caused by more than one type of reaction. It is possible to have both acute and delayed reactions to the same food. Occasionally an allergy-causing food will show up on one type of test but not another. Some foods which cause acute or immediate reactions may not show up on the Prime Test.

With delayed allergies there may be no immediate symptoms when you eat an allergy-causing food. In fact, you may experience your old symptoms plus withdrawal symptoms when you first stop eating your allergy-causing foods. Fortunately, this only lasts for a few days and then all your symptoms usually go away. Delayed food and chemical allergies often become physical addictions.

A very strong desire for a food often indicates an addiction has developed to that food. This type of delayed food allergy reaction can be experienced during a meal containing the food or when the food is being avoided for a period of time. Food addictions involve the same inner body mechanisms which cause addictions to tobacco, alcohol, illegal drugs and prescription drugs.

Do not be surprised if you feel worse when you first discontinue the foods and chemicals you are allergic to. This withdrawal reaction is common and lasts about a week. Withdrawal will not cause lasting discomfort and differs for each person. When in withdrawal, your desire for offending foods may be severe, so plan ahead. It is helpful to remember that the withdrawal period often starts again each time you eat the food to which you are allergic and addicted.

*Let your food be your medicine
and your medicine be your food.*

Hippocrates
*Greek Physician, Father of Medicine, Author
Health Scientist and First Allergist — 460 to 377 BC*

The benefits from eating foods which are compatible with your body have to be experienced to be fully appreciated.

Healthy Ways of Eating

One approach for dealing with delayed food allergies involves avoiding the foods to which you are allergic and rotating your compatible foods. This is called a "Rotary Diversified Diet."

When you first become free of delayed food allergies, it is helpful to begin with a Rotary Diversified Diet to retest the foods your Prime Test indicated as not allergic.

One way to develop food allergies is to eat the same food every day. When you rotate your compatible foods, it is unlikely that you will start to react to them.

Rotary means to separate each individual food by at least three days and not eat it until the fourth day. As an example, if you have carrots at one meal on Monday, avoid them for at least three days and do not eat them again until Friday.

With some foods it is also helpful to rotate the food families so that a full day passes without eating any food from the same family. Carrots and celery are in the same family; therefore, carrots can be eaten at one meal on Monday, celery at one meal on Wednesday, and carrots at one meal on Friday.

Diversify your diet by adding several different foods from different food families. The foods are organized by families on the Prime Test panel to help you plan your meals.

Some foods are very closely related to others in their family and are sometimes identified by your white blood cells as the same food: for example, blackberry and strawberry are in the same closely related sub-family.

Close relationships within a food family are revealed on the Prime Test panel by the vertical line next to their number **1** boxes. See Panel A on page 37. When you react to a food, you need to avoid anything made with that food.

It is helpful to study the Example of Food Challenge Testing on page 143 before you make your own testing menu. Make copies of the blank Testing Menu form on page 141 so you will have a supply to work with. Fill in your compatible foods, properly rotated and diversified. Keep a record of any symptoms you have so you can identify reactive foods and chemicals. The Rotary Diversified Diet repeats so you can plan ahead and remember it without great difficulty.

After you have tested your foods twice over eight days and you are sure they are working fine, you may want to begin adding other foods which your Prime Test indicated as compatible.

In the beginning, it is best to eat only one or two foods at a meal to be sure those foods are compatible. Some foods are better digested when they are eaten alone.

The weights used for the foods on page 143 give a guide for choosing how much food to eat in a test meal. The weights are based on how the foods are usually purchased. When testing, eat enough to keep your energy levels up, but do not overeat.

To add more foods, try those which were not on your Prime Test but are in a family which tested largely compatible. You may find it helpful to make a copy of your menu to use as a shopping list and then place the original along with your Prime Test report on the inside of a kitchen cupboard door for easy reference. See chapter 5 for more information.

No allergy test is perfect and the Prime Test will occasionally indicate that a food is compatible when it is not. It is important to confirm the foods which the Prime Test indicates as being compatible with your body.

The first foods to test are those which you have not eaten frequently and have no other reason to suspect. Test by eating only one food at a meal, preferably at breakfast. If you did not react to carrots on your Prime Test, have a breakfast of carrots and keep track of how you feel. See the Example of Food Testing Log on page 145. It is helpful to make copies of the form titled Food Testing Log on page 144 and use them to keep track of how different foods affect you.

Buy the best quality foods available. Many foods are significantly contaminated with petrochemicals, pesticides and chemical fertilizers.

Additional allergy problems are caused from growth hormones, preservatives, food colorings and additives. Locate a reliable source of foods that are grown without pesticides or other chemicals. These foods are commonly referred to as "organically grown." It is important to avoid having a chemical-allergy reaction when eating a food and mistakenly believing it was a food-allergy reaction.

Almost all the foods used to make the Prime Test are organically grown so they will not cause a chemical-allergy reaction. Even if the food is not organically grown it is unlikely to cause a problem, because the amount of food used in the Prime Test is microscopic; thus, any residual chemical is so small it is unlikely to cause a reaction.

The Prime Test reports the damage to your blood cells on a scale of **1** through **4**. This scale does not necessarily indicate the degree of symptoms the offending foods may cause; therefore a number **1** reaction may cause symptoms as severe as a number **3** or **4** reaction. If you react to an item at any level, it is damaging to your body and needs to be avoided. It is important to avoid all foods for at least one month to which you have reacted.

After one month of avoiding a food, you may want to test to see if you have stopped reacting or "cleared" from your allergy to that food. If you have no adverse symptoms after eating a previously offending food two or three times, with seven days between exposures, you have probably cleared for that food. The best foods to test first are those with number **1** reactions because you are more likely to have developed a tolerance to them. Eat only one food at the test meal and eat a moderate amount, around 300 calories. If you eat other foods at the meal you may confuse the results of the test. Let at least three days go by before you test a second new food so you will not confuse a delayed reaction from the first new food as a reaction to the second new food.

There is a wide variation in how each person stops reacting, or "clears," from delayed food allergies. Most people will develop tolerance to many of their allergic foods and need to avoid a small number of continually damaging foods. If you have cleared regarding the tested food, you can occasionally return it to your menu. If you did not clear, you need to continue avoiding that food and test it once again in six months if the testing symptoms are not too severe.

There are a few foods which most people stay allergic to. These are often foods that their mother was allergic to, or foods which they ate before they were one year old, or foods which they have eaten repetitiously for most of their lives. These foods usually include coffee, yeast, wheat and dairy products.

For some people, reactions have spread to a large number of foods because of repetitious eating habits, combining reactive foods with compatible foods, overeating or an imbalance in their body. Other probable causes of delayed food allergies are eating large meals and eating excessive fat or protein.

By the time some people took their Prime Test, they were reacting to so many foods and chemicals they had trouble putting together a Four-Day Rotary Diversified Diet. In these cases, some compatible food may have to be used more often than once in four days.

There are additional approaches available that can be helpful for many people. They include pancreas supplements, neutralizing therapy, provocative testing and follow-up Prime Testing with counseling.

It is important to remember that virtually all drugs — over the counter, prescribed, and illegal — have damaging side effects on your body. Your white blood cells are particularly sensitive to drugs.

Top quality foods, those free from chemical sprays, are helpful for everyone, and are particularly important if you are allergic to chemicals.

New flavor preferences are developed by eating new foods several times. After you have eaten a compatible food several times, it is likely to become a favorite. When the new foods have provided a higher level of health, it is challenging not to overeat them.

Add new and different foods to your menu which your Prime Test indicates you are not allergic to. Be willing to experiment with a wide variety of foods. Buy most of your foods in the fresh produce department and avoid overeating packaged and canned foods.

It is important to eat three or four moderate size meals a day. Besides repetitive eating, overeating at one meal can create delayed food allergies.

Other Allergens

It is important to avoid other people's tobacco smoke because it can initiate an allergic reaction in your body. If you smoke, now is the best time to stop. Combine withdrawing from tobacco and food allergies and leave both of them behind you. When you are free from the damaging addictive reactions caused by foods, you will be better able to resist the residual temptation to smoke. Be careful to avoid inhaling other people's smoke. Feel free to ask smokers not to smoke in your area. Most people cooperate when they hear you are allergic to tobacco. There is no way to become fully well if you continue to smoke.

Remember, all alcoholic drinks contain yeast. If a single drink gives you mental or physical symptoms, you should strongly suspect an allergic reaction. See the alcohol ingredient chart on page 62.

Use the best water you can obtain. Many people react to the chlorine and other chemicals in tap water. Most glass-bottled spring or distilled water does not cause chemical allergy reactions and should be used for both drinking and cooking. Home water filters must combine a reverse osmosis filter with an activated charcoal filter to be effective. This type of unit often gives you better quality water than most bottled water and saves money in the long run.

It is essential to breathe clean air, as free as possible of chemicals such as smog, car exhaust, natural gas appliance fumes and formaldehyde.

The air also needs to be as free as possible of dust, dust mite fecal matter, mold, animal danders and pollens. In varying degrees, everyone's health is helped by clean air. Living and working in an area which has clean air and keeping a home clean is very important. Some people do not become well until they breath clean air and eat their compatible foods.

Clean air can be obtained by using a good air

filter — one which contains over four pounds of activated charcoal and a High Efficiency Particulate Air (HEPA) filter. The charcoal takes out most of the chemicals and the HEPA filter removes most particles. The flow rate should be over two hundred cubic feet of air a minute, through the filter, to be effective in an average size room. An activated-charcoal filter for cleaning the air in your car is also very important.

The Multifood Program™

Many people find it difficult to stay on a Rotary Diversified Diet. Fortunately, most are able to take advantage of an easier approach called "The Multifood Program" and continue rotating their compatible cereal grains.

Most people who have become free of their symptoms after following their personal Testing Menu are able to start combining their compatible foods. So long as you eat an equal amount of six or more compatible foods at each meal, it is unlikely you will start to react to any of them even though you no longer rotate your foods. However, this usually does not work with cereal grains. If you eat cereal grains, rotate them over four or more days. Eat no more than three ounces of fish or fowl a day. See your nutritional counselor for more information.

Small amounts of compatible fresh fruit may be all right for snacks; however, it is best to wait for an hour after meals before eating fruit. Fruit is high in simple sugars and should not make up an entire meal. For proper digestion, eat fruit by itself as a snack. Dried fruit and fruit juices have very high levels of simple sugars that are rapidly absorbed; thus they damage the body the same way refined carbohydrates do.

It is important to have meals high in complex carbohydrates and low in fat. The meals are physically larger because the foods have a high water content. You actually get to eat larger meals without consuming excess calories. Eating fewer calories has been shown in several animal studies to reduce disease and increase life span.

Have three compatible meals each day. The meals for adults should be between 300 and 800 calories depending on your body size and how active you are.

Notice how good you feel after you are on the program for a few weeks. If you later slip off the path, the memory of how good you felt will help you return.

You win two ways with The Quality Longevity Program. First, it is wonderful to be free of your health problems. Second, it is rewarding to help others become free of their health problems. Ask your doctor who specializes in food allergy for information that will help you share this health breakthrough with your friends.

Freedom from Degenerative Disease

Some foods are damaging to everyone and need to be avoided most of the time even if you are not allergic to them. It is important to remove foods from your regular diet which are not compatible with the human body. These foods are the ones which are dangerously high in fat, protein, refined sugar, cholesterol, or other harmful ingredients which cause heart disease, strokes, cancer, diabetes and other degenerative diseases.

The foods which are damaging to everyone are usually the most expensive. Many people find their food costs are significantly reduced by choosing foods with around 10 percent of total calories from fat and around 10 percent of total calories from protein. The remaining 80 percent are from complex carbohydrates. This is the 10–10–80 balance of macronutrients. Vitamins and minerals are micronutrients and are very important; however, they will not overcome a damaging balance of macronutrients.

The foods which cause degenerative diseases are identified on the Prime Test panel with a minus sign preceding the name. For example: -peanuts, -eggs, -coffee, -cows' milk, -beef.

Compare the foods you have eaten repetitiously with the ones to which you are allergic. There is often a correlation. The delayed allergic foods and chemicals which show up most often are those which are consumed most often. The twenty most common items causing delayed allergic symptoms are: -milk and all dairy products, -beef, wheat, -yeast, -eggs, -coffee, -tobacco, -pork, corn, -soy beans,

-sugar cane, oranges, potatoes, -chocolate, -peanuts, tomatoes, beets, apples, -food additives and -petrochemicals.

In countries where people consume rice or tea every day, these two items are in their top twenty most common allergy-causing items. If you eat carrots every day, you may develop a reaction to carrots. This also happens when people are regularly exposed to pollens, molds and other items in the air.

Some foods you have rarely or never eaten may cause allergic reactions. Your body may mistakenly identify a food to be the same as some other food which causes a reaction in your body.

It is interesting to note that of the top twenty reactors, thirteen have a minus sign in front of them because they have ingredients which cause degenerative diseases for everyone. It is important to avoid these damaging foods and chemicals even if you are not reactive to them. If you are allergic to them you have two good reasons to avoid them. It makes no sense to become free of chronic ailments by avoiding your delayed food allergies and then eat any significant quantity of foods which cause degenerative ailments such as heart disease, stroke and cancer.

Good circulation is essential to your health and longevity. A major cause of poor circulation is the clumping of red blood cells. This problem is called blood sludging and is created when red blood cells stick together. The two most frequent causes of blood sludging are allergic reactions and meals which have over 15 percent of total calories in fat.

It is important to digest what you eat. If you are eating meals with excessive fat, protein or simple carbohydrates, proper digestion will be impaired. This may be one of the underlying ways we develop delayed food allergies.

Specialized food combining has been heavily promoted in the last few years. When you are not eating foods and chemicals you are allergic to and are avoiding excess fat and protein, you do not have to worry about how you combine your foods. The exception is to eat fruits by themselves.

If you are overweight or think your weight is all right, you are likely to find your weight dropping rapidly during the first month you are free of reactions. This is mostly water loss and happens as allergic swelling goes down. Do not worry: this is desirable and is one indication your program is working. As the months go by you will also lose excess body fat. This is also desirable, and happens when you are no longer eating excess animal fat and vegetable oil.

The type of body weight you want to retain and build is lean muscle tissue. To be healthy and avoid being underweight, you need to exercise against resistance. Resistance exercise, also known as strength training, is usually done by raising and lowering your body or exercising with weights.

Your body's optimum weight for health and longevity is significantly below what the weight charts recommend and what you are used to seeing people weigh.

Continuous vigorous exercise (aerobics) is also essential for building and retaining health. Vigorous exercise includes uninterrupted long walks, jogging and swimming. Before starting, read *The New Aerobics,* by Kenneth H. Cooper, MD, MPH. When you have been eating foods compatible with your body, you have the energy and desire to exercise. You are also much less likely to have injuries.

Aerobic exercise will reduce the severity and length of food and chemical allergic reactions. This happens because your body becomes acidic from allergic reactions, while aerobic exercise helps your body become alkaline. Exercise also brings oxygen to your cells and takes toxins away. In addition, aerobic exercise frees the red blood cells which stick together after an allergic reaction. See the pictures at the back of the book.

Do not be surprised that many doctors do not believe in the importance of delayed food and chemical allergies, the 10–10–80 balance of macronutrients, or the Prime Test. Most food-allergy specialists have not had the opportunity to study and use the 10–10–80 balance of macronutrients. Most degenerative disease specialists have not had the opportunity to test the importance of delayed food allergies. Be sure to keep this in mind and be careful when reading health books. As often happens, well-informed individuals become aware of the overall picture before the specialists.

Discovering compatible foods by using an accurate white blood cell test for delayed food allergies is the first step toward removing the cause of a broad range of symptoms. Also, selecting foods low in fat, moderate in protein and high in complex carbohydrates will enable you to improve your health further and become free of additional symptoms. It is now possible to enjoy good health continually and fully live a much longer life.

A clean environment, in combination with aerobic and strength exercise, is necessary to regain and maintain health. Taking supplements to fulfill your unique vitamin and mineral requirements begins after your compatible foods are identified.

The Quality Longevity Program brings together, for the first time, the correct parts of the best health approaches. The combined effect of these breakthroughs enables you to become free of most allergic symptoms and degenerative ailments. You will be able to greatly exceed the average levels of health and longevity.

Summary

1. The Quality Longevity Program is designed to prevent damage to your body and mind, while removing symptoms. The Program helps you to stop reacting to foods currently causing damage. It also improves your circulation.

2. Frequent eating or overeating of currently compatible foods may cause you to become allergic to additional foods. When you eat foods out of rotation, eat very small amounts and chew thoroughly. It is important to rotate cereal grains.

3. Keep your Prime Test results with you for easy reviewing until they are clear in your memory.

4. Carefully follow your Testing Menu and record any symptoms. Do not rely on memory in the beginning.

5. For the first eight days, it is best to eat one or two foods at a meal to confirm their compatibly. Because of the accuracy of the Prime Test, it is usually not necessary to rotate the food families. However, it is best not to eat cereal grains daily.

6. Eat new and different foods which are compatible with your body. If you do not start to

feel better in two weeks, be suspicious of chemicals in your environment or in your food.

7. Very small amounts of an allergy causing food or chemical can cause severe reactions and prevent your symptoms from going away. If there is any amount in or on the food, the item must be carefully avoided. Know what is in an item before you put it into your body.

8. Be careful in the use of cosmetics, sprays, perfumes, colognes, deodorants, soaps, detergents, etc. Brush your teeth a little longer and use baking soda instead of toothpaste.

9. Be sure everything you ingest and have next to your body is compatible. Be continually aware of how you're feeling.

10. If you smoke, now is the best time to quit. If you do not smoke, do not breathe other people's smoke.

11. Reactions to drinks containing alcohol are common. They are caused by delayed allergic reactions to the yeast or to the foods from which the alcohol is made. Be suspicious if you drink alcoholic beverages often.

12. Be sure vitamins, minerals and other supplements you take are free of any items made from foods or chemicals to which you are allergic. Many contain cornstarch, yeast, milk or sugar.

13. Becoming free of acute and chronic ailments caused by allergic reactions is facilitated by improved circulation and digestion brought about by the 10–10–80 balance of macronutrients.

14. The type of weight you want to gain is lean muscle tissue. You want to be free of excess water from allergic swelling, and free of excessive body fat by eating around 10 percent of your total calories in fat and by avoiding most refined carbohydrates.

15. Clean food, water and air are important, as is regular aerobic and strength exercise.

16. Do not be impatient: it can take considerable time for your body to rebuild itself. Resist the temptation to try approaches which promise that you can eat whatever you want.

17. Some of the ways you can become allergic to foods are: overeating; not chewing thoroughly; eating compatible foods with the ones to which you are allergic; eating the same foods day after day; and eating excessive fat, protein or simple carbohydrates.

18. The Prime Test is designed to give results

11

similar to fasting and food-challenge testing. If you have significant symptoms, it is likely you will have several reactions on your test.

19. The Quality Longevity Program discovers the causes of current symptoms and prevents future symptoms from developing. To become healthy and then maintain great health, you need to have control over what goes into your body.

Whenever a breakthrough happens in health care, the establishment calls it controversial in order to slow down or stop the transition to the new approach. This is how traditional medical doctors cover themselves for having believed in obsolete thinking for so long. This enables them to maintain their credibility, and thus their power.

The allergy field is the best example of this problem. Traditional allergy approaches have been used extensively from 1980 to 1990. Yet the cases of asthma have nearly doubled, and asthma-caused deaths have gone up dramatically. People are weakened by traditional allergy drugs, and many become allergic to the drugs. This causes some people to become more allergic and develop asthma. Be careful to avoid most traditional allergy approaches.

Conclusion

The breakdown of the immune system is one of the fundamental causes of aging. By knowing and avoiding your delayed food and chemical allergies, you can eliminate the cause of symptoms and strengthen your immune system.

Each allergic reaction damages body cells. Most cells will repair but some amount of damage will be lasting. Your body will never be younger than it is today, nor better able to reverse the decline in health caused by allergic reactions. By starting now you are best able to become healthier as you grow older.

If you use only some of the parts of The Quality Longevity Program, you are likely to continue having discomfort and continue damaging your body. However, when you combine the important principles, the results exceed their sum. All other health programs lack this powerful synergistic effect.

It often takes months for your body to repair itself. Be careful not to credit some other approach you try after you have been eating your compatible

foods for a while. This often happens, and people credit the wrong factors or go back to eating their old foods, only to become sick again.

Search out health professionals who understand delayed food and chemical allergies, the Prime Test and the health building levels of macronutrients and supplements. Be cautious of advice from those who have not had the opportunity to study and test these fundamentals.

In the past, when breakthroughs have happened in medicine which are outside of regular approaches, such as using drugs or surgery, it has often taken about 50 years before the new idea has been widely accepted. If history repeats itself, the use of the awareness of delayed food allergies will not become a widely used, standard approach until the year 2000.

The better you understand and use The Quality Longevity Program, the better your health will be. Read and study as much information as you can find on delayed food and chemical allergies and the 10–10–80 balance of macronutrients, and carefully combine the two approaches. Tell your friends about The Quality Longevity Program. Life is more fun with healthy friends. With supporting friends, you are likely to be more successful.

Life is also more fun when we look better. The weight improvements are the most obvious; however, with improved circulation to our skin, a new radiance develops. With The Quality Longevity Program you have the energy and health to enjoy life more fully.

You have begun on a path which leads to higher levels of health than has been available before. It is not an easy path in the beginning. However, the continued rewards promote success. This approach is the essence of preventive care. Share your progress with your friends.

*You will observe with concern
how long a useful truth
may be known and exist,
before it is generally received
and practiced on.*

Benjamin Franklin
*Scientist, Author and A Founding Father
of the United States — 1706 to 1790*

Chapter 2
How Emotions Are Upset By Foods

When people eat foods or are exposed to chemicals which cause delayed allergic reactions, a damaging chain of events is started. First, the white blood cells are broken open and killed. This releases their chemicals, which in turn damages other cells, releasing more chemicals. These chemicals upset blood chemistry, which in turn upsets brain chemistry. This affects emotions by causing mild mood swings in some, fuzzy thinking in others, and full-blown mental illness in a few.

From minor emotional upsets to severe mental problems, upset brain chemistry causes almost as much suffering as all physical ailments combined. By knowing what actually causes severe emotional problems, people who have them can be helped effectively. Others who have lesser upsets can also become free of most of their discomfort.

Food-allergy specialists have demonstrated that most severe mental ailments are caused primarily by upset brain chemistry. Ironically, this is supported by the fact that prescription drugs for emotional problems work by changing brain chemistry. When they do change thinking and behavior, they are demonstrating that the ailment was not caused by something which happened in the past or by a wrong attitude. The drugs work by changing brain chemistry, not by changing past experiences. This helps explain why long-term psychoanalysis does not work well: it has little effect on brain chemistry.

Unfortunately, most psychiatrists have not fully grasped the significance of mind-altering drugs. Because some drugs temporarily stop some mental problems, the principal cause of these problems is not traumas from childhood, but upset brain chemistry.

If Freud were alive he would not be disappointed: shortly before he died he wrote that psychoanalysis was not practical except for doing research, and that the actual cause of madness was probably upset brain chemistry. His followers did not understand his final thinking on mental illness, and a huge industry continues today based on the long-term counseling known as psychoanalysis.

If Freud were a professor in medical school today, he probably would be teaching that upset brain chemistry is the main cause of abnormal behavior. Unfortunately, his followers are still treating mental problems by trying talk therapy and drugs instead of removing the primary cause: delayed food and chemical allergies which upset brain chemistry.

Some allergies involve the brain in such a way that exposure to the particular substance results in peculiarities of behavior.

Linus Pauling
Dual Nobel Laureate, Author and Founder of
Orthomolecular Medicine — 1901 to 1994

Upset brain chemistry contributes to the full range of emotional problems. The labels used for mental ailments go on and on, as does the number of drugs tried: Valium, Ritalin, Xanax, Zoloft, Prozac, Paxil, Lithium, Mellaril, Thorazine, etc. None of these drugs has been found to be free of serious side effects — including death, often by suicide.

Most mental patients feel so poorly when they are on mind-altering drugs they refuse to keep taking them, and many end up in trouble with the law and wandering the streets. Others become physically addicted to their prescription drugs and develop worse behavior while taking them. Even the mineral lithium, when given in medicinal doses, makes many people feel terrible, and in time it permanently damages the kidneys.

Doctors should not prescribe a mind-altering drug until they take it themselves and see how sick it makes them feel. This self-test technique would expose other damaging side effects, thereby reducing the use of drugs and dramatically increasing the use of delayed-allergy testing and counseling for emotional problems.

Some psychiatrists use large doses of vitamins to try to cure emotional problems. In some cases this is a real help for people. This is because delayed allergic reactions consume the body's reserves of vitamin C and some of the B vitamins. However, the benefits of this treatment, called the "orthomolecular" approach, usually do not last. Like most of traditional medicine, this approach is only treating symptoms without removing the cause.

When delayed food and chemical allergies are discovered and avoided, and specialized vitamins and minerals are taken, the benefits are often dramatic and lasting. Short-term counseling can be helpful for improving awareness and changing habits.

One type of emotional problem not helped much by being free from food and chemical allergies is neurosis. This type of disorder is largely caused by internalizing fear and pain from past experiences. It is best resolved by using emotion-release therapies which enable one to become free of the fear and pain. When brain chemistry is in balance, the chance of developing neurosis may be reduced.

The Search for the Cause of Madness

For thousands of years, mankind has been trying to discover what actually causes a few people to go crazy. The first record of this search started with Hippocrates about 400 BC. He wrote that some people became emotionally upset after they ate cheese.

He also noticed some people were tolerant of eating a small amount of a food, but a larger amount would make them ill. He wrote that serious diseases began "when they have merely taken twice a day the same food which they have been in the custom of taking once." This was later understood to be part of the addiction process. Also, some people have a genetic disposition for an ailment, and when they eat the wrong foods, they develop symptoms.

After Hippocrates, medicine, for the most part, entered the dark ages. The establishment believed "crazy people" were possessed by evil spirits. Today, many traditional doctors believe most emotional problems exist because parents mistreated their children, or because the person suffered from stress.

In 1905, Francis Hare, MD, wrote *The Food Factor in Disease* which reported health improvements when people stopped eating cereal grains. He mistakenly concluded the benefits came from eating more meat and thus more protein.

A landmark book was published in 1931 in the United States by Albert Rowe, MD, titled *Food Allergy: Its Manifestations, Diagnosis and Treatment*. With the 1951 book by Rinkel, Randolph and Zeller, titled *Food Allergy*, the foundation was laid for changing the way physical and mental illnesses are treated. Since then, traditional medicine often has been moving ahead at glacial speed or the movement has been in the wrong direction. Examples are the reliance on drugs, surgery, allergy injections and talk therapy.

Fortunately, with the advent of modern science, the function of the brain has begun to be understood. There are very fragile connective areas between brain cells which must have the correct balance of chemicals for the brain to work properly.

Theron Randolph, MD, though board certified in traditional allergy, became aware by 1944 that traditional skin tests and weekly allergy injections did not work for most allergy problems, and that most other medical approaches did not work well for common health problems. After developing an improved approach for treating illness by testing and counseling for delayed food allergies, he saw his patients, who also had emotional problems, become free of most of their physical *and* emotional problems at the same time.

Dr. Randolph began demonstrating his approach to psychiatrists, and by 1960, six traditional psychiatrists had changed the way they treated their psychiatric patients. A new day was dawning for people with mental diseases. Professionals are now beginning to learn that delayed allergic reactions to foods upset the chemical balance in the brain and thus cause many different types of mental problems.

This breakthrough is not widely known. People who have severe emotional breakdowns are still taken to traditional psychiatrists and are told to examine their childhoods, their parents, their relationships and the stress in their lives to find the cause of their problems. Most doctors will not admit that they do not know what causes severe emotional problems or even mood swings.

The exact contrary of what is generally believed is often the truth.

Jean de la Bruyere
French Philosopher — 1645 to 1696

It is now possible for a person to turn most emotional problems on and off. The relationship between delayed food and chemical allergies is as clear as the relationship between the light and the light switch. The switch is not the typical type of allergic reaction which allergists work with (known as an IgE reaction) but instead an IgG reaction, or immune complex reaction, or other mechanisms not yet fully understood. However, the following studies show that these delayed allergic reactions upset brain chemistry.

Dr. Randolph discovered the cause of madness in

some of his patients by fasting them on clean water in a clean environment. During the first four or five days, their symptoms often became worse because of withdrawal, and then their schizophrenia, manic-depressive bipolar behavior, chronic depression, hyperactivity and other symptoms usually went away.

When reintroduced to the foods they were allergic to, their problems came back. After avoiding the offending foods and chemicals again, their symptoms went away once more. (See how symptoms evolve and grow on pages 142 and 143.)

It may be helpful to understand your childhood and your parents. Forgiving all the people in your life who have been unkind to you helps you to enjoy life more fully. However, awareness of previous traumas does not correct brain chemistry or keep brain chemistry from becoming upset. Rough lives are not a significant cause of emotional breakdowns; if they were, we would have many more schizophrenics, manic depressives, etc. Traumatic events can trigger emotional breakdowns in people who have a predisposition to upsets and are eating foods and chemicals which upset their brain chemistries.

Two medical doctors who were not satisfied with traditional approaches for treating diseases studied the approach developed by Dr. Randolph. These doctors, Marshall Mandell, MD, a pediatric allergist, and William Philpott, MD, a psychiatrist, were working at Fuller Memorial Sanitarium. Many of the patients were in locked wards; some had been given surgical lobotomies and many were being given powerful drugs which caused chemical lobotomies.

Starting in 1971, Mandell and Philpott worked with more than 100 patients. Fasting them on clean water caused most to clear from their mental symptoms. The doctors were then able to bring the symptoms back by refeeding these patients foods to which they had delayed allergic reactions.

The traditional allergists and state regulators claimed that allergy testing should not be done in a mental hospital and blocked further progress. The doctors left the hospital and used their new knowledge in private practice, where they helped people who would otherwise have remained emotionally disturbed and damaged by traditional approaches.

Mandell and Philpott have published several papers outlining their successes, and have given numerous presentations to doctors from around the world. However, few medical doctors understand this breakthrough because it conflicts with their education and how they currently make money.

Double-Blind Studies

Double-blind studies are used to confirm the validity of some medical approaches. Neither doctor nor patient knows what the patient is eating, so expectations are not able to affect the outcome of the study. Thus, the placebo effect is eliminated.

One double-blind study was done with 150 men at the Veterans Administration Hospital in Pennsylvania. The men had been diagnosed as schizophrenics and had such severe symptoms they had to be kept in the locked ward. Half of the men were left on the Standard American Diet. Without the advantage of white blood cell testing, the doctors eliminated only wheat gluten and dairy products from the diets of the remaining patients. Some of these patients were secretly fed wheat gluten in their muffins as a double-blind control.

This study clearly showed that those who were free of wheat gluten and dairy products were discharged from the locked ward in half the time of those who made no changes in their diet or ate wheat gluten unknowingly in the double-blind part of the study. (Dohan DC, Grassberger JC: "Relapsed schizophrenics' earlier discharge from the hospital after cereal-free, milk-free diet" *Am J Psychiatry* 130;6 1973)

A similar double-blind study was done at the Bronx Psychiatric Center. When patients were free of wheat gluten and dairy products, they clearly improved, and when wheat gluten was reintroduced they regressed. (Singh M, Kay SR: "Wheat gluten as a pathogenic factor in schizophrenia" *Science* Jan 30, 1976)

Since these studies were done, it has been shown that patients do better when they avoid wheat entirely instead of just the gluten part. When patients avoid wheat, dairy products, and foods shown to be damaging on their Prime Test, their progress is dramatically improved. For people with no mental symptoms, there is often an improvement in mood and mental acuity when avoiding delayed allergies.

Emanuel Cheraskin, MD, did a study of 60 patients with one or more of the following symptoms: depression, anger, tension, sensitivity, anxiety and inadequacy. The patients were given a white blood cell test to find their compatible foods. After two months of avoiding their reactive foods, 76 percent of the patients experienced significant improvement in their emotional health. (Cheraskin E, Allen J, Zavik J: "The psychotherapeutic implications of cytotoxic testing." J Orthomolecular Psychiatry 1985; 14:128-135)

Additional studies of delayed allergies have been completed by other medical doctors and show similar success. One is by D. S. King, titled "Can Allergic Exposure Provoke Psychological Symptoms? A Double-blind Test," published in *Biological Psychiatry*, 6:3-19, in 1981. Another was done by R. Finn and T. M. Battcock, titled "A Critical Study of Clinical Ecology," published in *The Practitioner*, 229: 883-885 in 1985. Another was done by J. W. Crayton, S. Schilling and N. McGrath, titled "The Behavioral Effects of Milk, Wheat and Chocolate in Food-sensitive, Psychiatric Patients and Controls." This important paper was ready for publication in 1985; however, no traditional medical journal will print it.

There are numerous other studies which show that foods affect mind function because of delayed food and chemical allergies. The information is often buried in studies of other health problems. An example is an article in *The Lancet* titled "Is Migraine Food Allergy?" This double-blind study revealed that 41 of 88 children with migraine headaches also had behavioral disorders. Of these 41 with behavioral disorders prior to being tested for delayed food allergies, only five had behavior disorders after eating their compatible foods. This is one of the highest success rates ever achieved for helping people with behavioral problems.

A few double-blind studies of mental problems caused by delayed allergies have been recorded on video. This helps people see for themselves that foods and chemicals are the major cause of numerous mental and physical ailments.

Two Success Stories

When Kate Davies was 49, she had a severe skin rash which had started when she was an infant after she had been given cows' milk. Traditional allergists had been treating her for years, but their allergy injections and cortisone treatments helped her for only a short while, and then made her worse. The itchy rash spread all over her body, and she had to take an extra blouse to work because the first one had blood showing through it by noon.

She had her white blood cells tested for delayed food and chemical allergies, and started on The Quality Longevity Program. Her test discovered several foods and chemicals for her to avoid. It took a month before there was any change. Then, in a week, her rash was gone. Her rash reappeared when she eat the foods which showed up on her test.

Her daughter saw the improvements and decided to try the new life-style for herself. She had been fine until she was 14 years old. At that time she had an emotional breakdown and was diagnosed by some psychiatrists as a schizophrenic, and by other psychiatrists as a manic depressive. They kept her locked up, on and off, during the next 12 years and gave her drugs and talk therapy without success.

Her psychiatrists blamed everything from her childhood experiences to mistakes her parents had made in raising her. They had no idea the underlying cause of her mental symptoms was upset brain chemistry caused by delayed-type allergies.

After having her white blood cells tested and changing her foods, her brain chemistry normalized and her thinking cleared for the first time in years. She was able to go back to school, and received good grades. She was able to enjoy life again.

Later, she was assured by someone who did not understand delayed food allergies that she could eat whatever she wanted. She went back to eating wheat, dairy products, and a few other foods she was allergic to. In time she started hearing voices, became angry, hyperactive and then depressed. She had to be locked up in the hospital.

Her new psychiatrist prescribed the Prime Test. She went back to eating her compatible foods and her mind cleared again. So long as she avoids the food and chemicals to which she has allergic reactions, and does aerobic exercise, she is fine.

It is difficult to counsel people who have emotional symptoms. People with physical symptoms can easily understand the importance of food and chemical reactions because they can see their symptoms go away. And when they eat their damaging foods, their symptoms come back. However, people who have emotional symptoms have difficulty evaluating their behavior accurately because their brains do the evaluating, and their brains are not working properly.

These people need supporting friends in their lives who can help them control their behavior. Follow-up counseling is often helpful. Otherwise, they often do not make it through the first few weeks of withdrawal and end up angry. These people often try to control everyone around them as part of their attempt to control themselves. They often accept any other approach to their mental and physical problems rather than removing the cause.

Traditional doctors do not want to spend the money to test for the actual cause of emotional problems. However, families (or insurance companies, and, thereby, all of us) are often charged over eight thousand dollars *a week* for full-time psychiatric care, plus the cost of brain chemistry-altering drugs. The cost to test and counsel a person for delayed allergies is less than a thousand dollars.

One must be taught to suspect,
for if one does not suspect, one does not test,
and if one does not test, one does not know.

Herbert J. Rinkel, MD
Pioneer in field of food allergy and co-author with
Theron Randolph, MD, of the 1951 landmark
textbook Food Allergy — *1896 to 1963*

Getting the Word Out

The television network which has best informed the public about delayed food and chemical allergies is NBC. It had four segments in its award-winning *Today Show*. The first segment featured Dr. Randolph and how delayed food allergies cause arthritis. The second featured pediatric allergist Doris Rapp, MD, and how delayed food allergies cause hyperactivity (Attention Deficit-Hyperactive Disorder, or ADHD) in children. The third featured psychiatrist Bernard Raxlen, MD, and how delayed food allergies cause mental breakdowns. The fourth interviewed me and explained how delayed food allergies were tested for by using a person's white blood cells.

Dr. Raxlen commented on the value of using white blood cell testing for helping emotionally disturbed people, and stated that this approach to health care gave doctors a powerful new tool.

The head of the association of traditional allergists tried to keep NBC from airing these features. The vice president of NBC refused to be pressured, and the advantages of white blood cell testing were explained nationwide, as was the discovery that delayed allergies can cause sever mental disease.

Spokesmen for the traditional medical establishment brag that Americans have the best health care in the world. However, we are 17th from the best in infant mortality and 19th in longevity. In almost every category we are far from the top — except one. We pay more money per person for health care than any other country. If we had the best health care we would have one of the best levels of health and longevity. Instead, for developed nations, we have one of the worst.

The reason some foreigners come here to be treated is that we have spent most of our medical research money developing expensive procedures for people who are unaware or unwilling to use the breakthroughs in nutrition.

Much of our health-care crisis is caused by relying on obsolete, ineffective and costly drugs, surgeries and allergy injections. There is currently an all-encompassing monopoly strangling health care, a monopoly so vast that most people are not aware they are being controlled and kept unaware of the best preventive care.

Today, a small group of traditional medical doctors has control over how health-care dollars are spent. By influencing elected officials, the bureaucrats they appoint and insurance companies, this group dictates the type of therapies used by medical doctors, chiropractors and other health-care professionals. This group also controls where research money is spent, what studies are published and which approaches are taught in medical schools.

The suffering and expense caused by this archaic approach is most prevalent in the treatment of mental problems and chronic physical ailments caused by delayed food and chemical allergies.

Many physical ailments have increased in frequency and severity over the last 20 years; some have more than doubled. The increase in emotional problems has grown even faster as diets have become more repetitious and contaminated with chemicals. No traditional medical theory explains these increases; however, the science of delayed food allergies does.

In many areas of the country, 10 percent of children are on mind-altering drugs — by prescription. The drug is Ritalin and the problem is hyperactivity. Follow-up studies have shown that when these children grow up and are taken off Ritalin, they still have emotional problems and become involved in crime at a much higher rate than their contemporaries. With the crime rate accelerating out of control, can we afford not to use the knowledge that delayed food and chemical allergies upset brain chemistry and then behavior? Using this understanding of mental problems will dramatically reduce the crime rate.

All drugs that alter the mind to try and treat mental symptoms, only help in the short-term, at best, and cause *irreversible* symptoms in the long-term, even in very low doses. Peter R. Breggin, MD, a former teaching fellow from Harvard Medical School, has written a powerful book that explains how damaging these drugs are that his fellow psychiatrists are using. Read his book, *Toxic Psychiatry* before taking any drug for emotional problems.

When people are eating their compatible foods, several seemingly unrelated problems are substantially reduced because the total load on the body is reduced. Two common examples are depression and premenstrual syndrome (PMS).

When eating meals free from the foods and chemicals you are allergic to, you should feel good before and after meals. If, after a meal, you feel stimulated, irritable, depressed, sleepy, etc., be suspicious of one or more of the items in your meal.

When we look at what people are eating today, we see that fast foods are often made with wheat and dairy products. Even the health-food industry often uses the most reactive form of wheat — whole wheat. These two items, wheat and dairy products, cause more physical and mental health problems than any other foods. However, it is necessary to find most of the foods and chemicals which are causing the problem in order to achieve full reversal of symptoms.

Insurance companies and government programs must start reimbursing for what actually works, not for what has failed in the past. The current monopoly which controls health care is fighting to suppress the awareness of delayed allergies, and this damages our health and finances. Many of our companies are unable to compete in world markets because their health-care costs are double what they could be.

*Every age and generation must be as free
to act for itself, in all cases,
as the ages and generations which preceded it...
It is the living, and not the dead,
that are to be accommodated.*

Thomas Paine
A Founding Father of the United States, inspiration for the Declaration of Independence and Author — 1737 to 1809

While people are having severe emotional problems, much of their mental development is blocked. If an emotional breakdown happens when people are young, they often do not mature properly. This arrested development also happens while a person is taking mind-altering drugs — illegal or prescription. With their proper foods and avoidance of allergy-causing chemicals, their thinking and behavior are dramatically improved, but they are often immature. Counseling can help solve this problem when done by a specially trained person who understands upset brain chemistry caused by delayed allergies.

Counseling people is much more effective when they are not allergically reacting to a food or chemical. Have you ever tried to advise someone who is intoxicated by alcohol?

Delayed allergic reactions are a major cause of mood swings. When you stop eating your allergy-causing foods, you may experience withdrawal symptoms. Being aware of this will help you deal with this problem. Once you are free of delayed allergic reactions for a few weeks, you are likely to enjoy life more and have trouble remembering how often you were upset before. All you have to do is eat your old foods for a while to rediscover how life was before. These changes are often subtle, so observe closely and obtain feedback from your close friends. Romantic relationships are often improved by The Quality Longevity Program.

The most important factors which determine how much we enjoy life are our health and our emotions. By avoiding delayed food and chemical allergies and enjoying regular aerobic exercise, you will dramatically improve your physical and emotional health.

Eating the foods that keep your brain chemistry balanced is part of the foundation for enjoying life. Eating right facilitates everyone to: "Live in love," "Love your neighbor as you love yourself," "Love yourself — everything else will follow." Being in love does wonders for your immune system. You will instantly be healthier and better able to be good to yourself and everyone around you — the benefits escalate.

The time to be happy is now, the place to be happy is here and the way to be happy is to do the best you can for yourself and others.

*Come now and let us reason together,
let us hear all sides,
let us divest ourselves of prejudice
and the effects of early education.
Let us prove all things and hold fast
to that which is good.*

D. M. Bennett
Philosopher, Publisher and Author — 1818 to 1882

Chapter 3
Prevent and Reverse Chronic and Degenerative Diseases

When our white blood cells are killed by delayed allergic reactions, their powerful digestive enzymes are released. The enzymes are then free to flow throughout our bodies causing inflammation and damage. All diseases caused by this type of reaction are greatly relieved or eliminated by avoiding delayed allergies. In addition, diseases started by other causes are healed more rapidly because repair is facilitated by the absence of allergic reactions and destructive enzymes.

The terms "chronic" and "degenerative" are sometimes misused and often misunderstood. "Chronic" means constant or recurring, and chronic diseases can happen at any age. "Degenerative" means slowly deteriorating, and the damage from degenerative diseases accumulates with time. The word "disease" comes from the phrase "without ease" and means ailment.

The types of problems caused by killing white blood cells, and other reactions related to delayed food and chemical allergies, are in the category of chronic diseases and are those which cause symptoms for infants, children, adolescents and adults at any time during their lives. A chronic symptom may stay with us in varying degrees or it may go away and later return, or a new problem may develop.

Degenerative diseases are different. They start slowly, beginning in early childhood and build up throughout our lives, giving few recognizable warnings until blood cholesterol levels rise above 150. Later, there is some loss of hearing, eyesight or other vital functions, with most people ending up with a heart attack or stroke. Degenerative diseases are caused almost entirely by eating the wrong levels of macronutrients: more than 10 percent of calories from fat; more than 15 percent from protein; more than 80 milligrams of cholesterol a day; and by eating excessive amounts of sugar and other refined carbohydrates.

Most diseases are caused by improper eating, abusive life-style, a contaminated environment, infections, accidents and lack of exercise.

When we eat something not compatible with our bodies, we develop unpleasant symptoms.

The medical community has spent years defining those symptoms and labeling them as a particular ailment or disease. The goal of preventive care is to discover the *causes* of symptoms so that we can remove them from our lives, rather than hoping someone else or some drug will make our symptoms go away.

It is possible to believe you are free of symptoms because what you are feeling has always been with you. When people are not aware of their symptoms, they conclude what they are doing is fine. However, it often happens that a person is under the influence of a food or chemical and is not aware of the damage being done until a symptom becomes obvious.

By avoiding food reactions and improving the quality of the air and water consumed, most people can better tolerate their airborne allergies. Those who react to dust, molds, animals, pollens and other airborne allergens often find delayed food allergies to be the major cause of their symptoms.

Traditional doctors often complain that if delayed food and chemical allergies caused a broad range of chronic diseases, there would be supporting studies in the medical journals. The studies have been done and published. Most traditional doctors have not done their homework or have resisted acknowledging the significance of the studies.

Doris Rapp, MD, did an extensive review in 1989 of the medical literature and compiled the key studies done on how delayed food and chemical allergies cause some of the major chronic diseases. Most of the studies were in peer-review journals and some were double-blind (neither the doctor nor the patient knew what was being tested until the test was over). Her report revealed that for arthritis there were six studies; asthma, three; autism, three; chemical sensitivities, twelve; colitis, two; Crohn's disease, one; delinquency, four; eczema, two; epilepsy, four; fatigue, two; gynecologic problems, two; hyperactivity, twenty one; immune dysfunction, sixteen; irritable bowel, three; migraine headache, six; nephrosis, six; otitis, six; psychological dysfunction, two; Tourette's syndrome, one; and for vascular disease, fourteen.

She also located general studies on how delayed

food and chemical allergies cause symptoms. These include 26 positive double-blind studies, seven single-blind studies and ten non-blind studies which confirm that delayed food allergies cause a broad range of diseases.

CHRONIC DISEASES

The following chronic diseases are some of those commonly caused by delayed food and chemical allergies. These symptoms are often eliminated by avoiding the offending items, and can return by re-exposing yourself.

There are some other causes for the following symptoms; however, white blood cell reactions and related delayed food and chemical allergies are the most common cause and should be the first approach examined. It is possible to have delayed food allergies and not have recognizable symptoms.

This list comes from medical articles and books written by doctors with a successful history of treating these diseases. There are many other diseases which have been relieved which are not on this list.

If you have had or are having one or more of the following symptoms, it may get worse during the first week on The Quality Longevity Program as you go through withdrawal. Some symptoms leave slowly, some fluctuate, some leave rapidly.

Examples of Chronic Physical Symptoms

Head
Headache • Sinus headache • Migraine headache • Faintness • Dizziness • Feeling of fullness in the head • Hair loss • etc.

Eyes, Ears, Nose and Throat
Dark circles under the eyes • Swelling around eyes Pain in eyes • Watery eyes • Red bloodshot eyes Dilated pupils • Blurring of vision • Runny nose Stuffy nose • Bloody nose • Excessive mucus formation • Hay fever • Sneezing • Ringing in the ears • Ear ache • Fullness in the ears • Fluid in the middle ear • Hearing loss • Recurrent ear infections. Itching ear • Ear drainage • Sore throats Swollen tonsils • Changes in voice • Loss of voice Frequent "colds" • Chronic cough • Gagging Canker sores • Itching on the roof of the mouth Recurrent sinusitis • etc.

Heart and Lungs
Palpitations • Decreased heart rate • Low and high blood pressure • Rapid heart rate (tachycardia) • Irregular heart rate • Asthma • Chest congestion • Yawning • Hoarseness • etc.

Blood
Damaged or killed white blood cells • Low white blood cell count • Damaged or destroyed red blood cells • Blood sludging (rouleau formation) • Low red blood cell count • Enlarged red blood cells • Platelet clumping • Low percentage of segmented neutrophils (one type of white blood cell) • Increased eosinophils and basophils (types of white blood cells) • Low blood sugar (hypoglycemia) • High blood sugar (diabetes) • Increased blood enzyme levels such as LDH • AST (SGOT) • and ALT (SGPT) • High acid level in the blood (causing loss of bone calcium and mineral loss from organs and tissues) • etc.

Glands
Low thyroid levels • High thyroid levels • Low testosterone levels • Depressed pancreatic activity (thus low alkaline production and low digestive enzyme production) • Depressed or excessive sexual drive • Depressed adrenal function • etc.

Mouth
Bleeding gums • Sore tongue • Coated tongue • Bad breath • Cracked lips • Swollen lips • Ulcerations Loose teeth • Tooth loss • etc.

Gastrointestinal
Stomach ache • Nonulcer dyspepsia • Acid indigestion • Continually swollen stomach • Cramps Ulcers • Nausea • Vomiting • Bloating after meals Heartburn • Belching • Spastic colitis Ulcerative colitis • Celiac disease • Flatulence (passing gas) • Feeling of fullness in the stomach long after finishing a meal • Diarrhea Constipation • Rectal mucous • Abdominal pains or cramps • Appendicitis • Malabsorption • etc.

Skin
Hives • Rashes • Dandruff • Hair loss • Eczema Psoriasis • Dermatitis • Pallor • Pimples • Acne Dark circles under eyes • Bags under eyes Drooping eye lids • Swelling • etc.

Other Symptoms

Autoimmune diseases [Rheumatoid arthritis Juvenile-onset (type one) diabetes · Graves' disease Lupus · Multiple Sclerosis · Myasthenia Gravis] Adult-onset (type two) diabetes · Chronic fatigue Chronic fatigue syndrome · Chronic muscle fatigue Crohn's disease · Sleepy after meals · Insomnia Snoring · Sleep Apnea · Overweight · Malabsorption Underweight · Weakness · Muscle aches and pains Muscle spasms · Twitching · Stiffness · Joint aches and pains · Arthritis · Swelling of the hands, feet, or ankles · Phlebitis · Cold hands and feet · Restless leg syndrome (frequent movement) · Urinary tract symptoms (Pain, Frequency, Night urination, Bed wetting) · Impotency · Kidney Problems (Nephritis) Rectal itching · Sea sickness · Motion sickness Altitude Sickness · Chills · Sweats · Thyroid irregularities · Thirsty after meals · Back pain Premenstrual syndrome (PMS) · Yeast infections Vaginal inflammation · Sudden infant death syndrome (SIDS) · etc.

Examples of Chronic Mental Symptoms

Anxiety · Excessive talking · Fear · Depression Crying · Aggressive behavior · Delusions · Panic attacks · Hallucinations · Schizophrenia · Manic depressive · Irritability · Mental dullness · Poor concentration · Poor self control · Poor memory Mental lethargy · Confusion · Excessive daydreaming · Juvenile and adult hyperactivity Attention Deficit Disorder (ADD) · Juvenile and adult delinquency · Seizures · Epilepsy Restlessness · Learning disabilities · Poor work habits · Slurred speech · Stuttering · Inability to concentrate · Indifference · Poor coordination Compulsive behavior · Obsessions · Fear of eating Anorexia nervosa · Binge eating disorder (BED) Bulimia · Continuing desire for tobacco or alcohol Drug addiction · Being highly stressed · Sluggish in the morning · Suicide and attempted Suicide · etc.

Where to Find Foods that Can Cause Chronic Symptoms

The following lists are helpful in finding those foods that cause delayed food allergies. It is important to check labels; however, be aware that some labels are incomplete. Avoid items with food colorings and preservatives and try to locate a good source of foods which are grown free of pesticides and chemical fertilizers.

Items Often Containing Corn

Adhesives · Ales · Alcoholic beverages · Aspirin and other tablets · Baby foods · Bacon · Baking mixes (biscuits, pie crusts, doughnuts, pancake mixes) · Baking powders · Batters for frying · Beer Beverages (carbonated) · Bleached wheat flour Body and foot powders · Bourbon and other whiskies · Breads and pastries · Cakes · Candies Hard Candies · Canned peas · Cheeses · Chili Chocolate · Chop Suey · Coffee (instant) Cookies · Corn Flakes · Cosmetics · Cough syrups Cream pies · Dates · Confection · Deep-fat frying mixtures · Envelope adhesives · French dressing Fritos · Frostings · Fructose · Fruits (canned & frozen) · Fruit juices · Frying fats · Gelatin dessert (capsules) · Glucose products (this includes intravenous sugar solutions) · Graham crackers Grape juice · Gravies · Grits · Gum (chewing) Hams (cured/tenderized) · Ice creams · Inhalants Bath and Body Powders · Jams · Jellies · Catsup Meats (bologna · sausage · etc.) · Milk in paper cartons · Monosodium glutamate (MSG) Margarine · Peanut butters · Popcorn · Powdered sugar Prescription and over the counter drugs Preserves · Puddings (custards) · Rice (coated) Salad dressings · Sandwich spreads · Sauces for meats · Sherbets · Similac · Starch · String beans (canned and frozen) · Sorbet · Sorbitol · Soups (creamed and vegetable) · Soy bean milks Syrups · Karo · Sweetose · Talcum · Tapes · Teas (instant) · Toothpaste · Tortillas · Vegetables (canned, creamed and frozen) · Vanilla · Vinegar Vitamins (tablets, lozenges, suppositories, capsules) Wines (some American wines are corn-free) · Zest · etc.

Items Often Containing Egg

Baby foods · Baking powders · Batters for french frying · Boiled dressings · Bouillons · Breaded foods · Breads · Cake flours · Cakes · French toast Fritters · Frostings · Glazed foods · Griddle cakes Hamburgers · Hollandaise sauce · Ice cream · Ice milks · Icings · Livitin · Macaroni · Macaroons Marshmallows · Meat binders · Meat jellies · Meat loaf · Malted Cocoa drinks (Ovaltine and Ovomalt) Noodles · Ovomucoid · Pancake flours · Pastes Pretzels · Puddings · Salad dressings · Sauces Sausages · Sherbets · Souffles · Soups · Spaghetti Spanish creams · Tartar Sauce · Timbales · Vitelline Waffles · Wines clarified with egg whites · etc.

Items Often Containing Milk

Baby foods•Bread•Baking powder•Bavarian cream Biscuits • Bisques • Butter • Natural butter flavor Butter Buds•Butterscotch•Cakes•Candies•Casein Cheeses • Chocolate • Chowders • Chicken (butter injected) • Cocoa drinks • Cocaine (often cut with powdered milk)•Cooked sausages•Cookies•Cream Creamed foods • Cream sauces • Curds • Custards Doughnuts • Egg dishes • Flour mixtures • Foods prepared in factories or kitchens that also work with dairy products•Foods fried in butter•Foods prepared Au Gratin • Fritters • Ghee (clarified butter) • Gravies Hamburgers • Hard sauces • Hash • Herb tablets (lactose)•Hotcakes•Hydrolyzed lactalbumin•Ice creams Luncheon meats • Malted milk • Mashed potatoes Meat loaf • Milk chocolate • Margarines • Omelets Ovaltine • Ovomalt • Pie crusts • Prepared flour mixtures (biscuits, cake, cookies, doughnuts, muffins, pancakes, pie crusts, waffles) • Rarebits Salad dressings•Salad dressings at salad bars located near dressings with dairy products in them (spillage) Sherbets • Soda crackers • Sodium caseinate Souffles • Soups Turkeys (butter injected) • Wines clarified with milk • Whey • Zwieback • etc.

Items Often Containing Soybeans

Baby foods • bakery goods (breads, rolls, cakes, many pastries, biscuits, several crisp crackers) Candies (hard candies, nut candies, caramel) Cereals (Sunlets and Cellu Soy Flakes) • Crisco Spry and other shortenings • Dry lemonade mix Ready-to-eat cereals • Ice cream • Lecithin • Meats (pork link sausage and lunch meats) • Milk substitutes • Margarine and butter substitutes • Salad dressings•Sauces (La Choy Sauce, Lea and Perrins sauce, Heinz Worcestershire sauce) • Soy bean noodles • Tofu • Vegetable oils • Vitamin E • etc.

Items Often Containing Wheat

Alcoholic beverages (except Brandy and Wine) Baby foods • Bran • Breads (corn, gluten, graham, pumpernickel, rye, soy, wheat)•Cereals (bran, bran flakes, corn flakes, Crackels, cream of wheat, Farina, Grapenuts, Krumbles, Malted milk, Muffets, Ovaltine, Postum, puffed wheat, Ralstons wheat cereal, shredded wheat, Triscuits, Wheatena, Wheaties) • Flours (buckwheat flour, corn flour, durum flour, gluten flour, graham flour, lima bean flour, patent flour, rye flour, white flour, whole flour) Pastries and desserts (biscuits, cakes, candy bars, chocolate candy, cookies, crackers, doughnuts, frozen pies, muffins, pies, popovers, pretzels, puddings, rolls) • Wheat products (dumplings, macaroni, noodles, rusk, spaghetti, vermicelli, zwiebacks) Mustard • Miscellaneous (bouillon cubes, cooked meat dishes, foods fried in fats that have previously had wheat fried in them, gravies, ice cream, ice cream cones, matzos, mayonnaise, meat rolled in flour) • Sausages • Wieners • Bologna • Liverwurst•Lunch ham•Hamburger•Pancake mixtures Sauces • Soup thickeners (rue) • Some yeast products Tamari sauce (soy sauce)•Synthetic pepper•Waffles Wheat cakes • Wheat germ • Wheat grass juice Other types of wheat such as spelt and kamut • etc.

Items Often Containing Yeast

Alcoholic beverages (all) • Antibiotics • Barbecue sauce • Breads • Buttermilk • Catsup • Cheeses (all) Chili peppers • Citric acid • Condiments • Cookies Crackers • Dried fruit • Flour (enriched with vitamins from yeast) • French dressings • Frozen or canned fruit juices • Fermented products • Gerbers oat meal • Hamburger and hot dog buns • Horseradish • Malted products (including cereals, candy and malted milk drinks)•Mayonnaise•Meat (fried in cracker crumbs) • Milk (fortified with vitamins from yeast) • Mince pie • Monosodium glutamate (MSG) • Mushrooms • Olives • Pastries • Pickles Predigested protein products•Pretzels•Rolls•Root Beer • Salad dressings • Sauerkraut • Tamari sauce (soy sauce)•Tomato sauce•Truffles•Vinegars (all) Vitamin pills • Vitamin shots • etc.

Allergic and Toxic Reactions to Herbs

All foods and beverages are capable of causing delayed allergic reactions, especially if you consume them frequently or in large amounts. Herbal teas are no different. In addition, most have been discovered to have small amounts of damaging chemicals in them. Rose Hips and Linden Flower tea are the least toxic and if you are not allergic to them, you can drink them in rotation.

Most of the diseases herbs are supposed to cure are caused by delayed allergic reactions to foods and chemicals, or the wrong balance of macronutrients; therefore, they cannot work. However, there are some herbs and extracts from plants which can help your body to rebuild after you are on your optimum diet.

DEGENERATIVE DISEASES

The 10–10–80 balance of macronutrients is the part of The Quality Longevity Program which will prevent most degenerative diseases when it is begun around three years of age. Prior to that, infants need only mother's milk for one year and then a combination of foods which includes mother's milk and non-allergic foods for up to three years.

The Quality Longevity Program will begin reversing degenerative diseases as soon as it is begun. The sooner a person starts, the more effective it is. Most people experience dramatic improvements because symptom reversal is possible with a small increase in circulation. Many very ill people, some near death, started the 10–10–80 balance of macronutrients in their eighties and are now enjoying life again.

Degenerative diseases are almost entirely caused by eating outside the 10–10–80 balance. The calorie balance of the American diet in 1994 was approximately 36 percent fat, 12 percent protein, 27 percent complex carbohydrate and 25 percent refined carbohydrate. This 36–12–52 balance has over three times the fat we can tolerate and one third the complex carbohydrates we need. This unhealthy balance of nutrients is the major cause of death in America.

A 150-pound person can utilize no more than 46 grams of plant and animal protein a day; more is harmful. The average American eats around 100 grams. The excess typically comes from eating too much animal protein. Animal products are the only dietary source of cholesterol. We can tolerate eating about 80 milligrams of cholesterol a day — the average American eats around 500 milligrams. We can tolerate the amount of simple sugars found in a small amount of fresh whole fruit. However, most Americans eat over 20 percent of their calories from refined carbohydrates. An active person needs a total of 1200 to 2800 calories a day depending on body size, and yet the average American eats 3300 calories.

The recommendations of the American Heart Association, the federal government and similar organizations are damaging and have been shown in their own studies to create clogged arteries. They recommend up to 30 percent of one's calories from fat, over 15 percent from protein, only 55 percent carbohydrates and up to 300 milligrams of cholesterol.

Our government is under the influence of the traditional doctors. The medical establishment does not want to admit it has been so wrong for so long and that its entire orientation has been treating symptoms rather than discovering and removing the causes of disease. This is the essence of preventive care. Some of those in power feel the public could not handle the truth.

Excesses of fat, protein, refined carbohydrates, cholesterol and calories guarantee degenerative diseases and contribute to chronic diseases.

Examples of Degenerative Symptoms

Eyes, Ears, Nose and Throat

Cataracts • Glaucoma • Inability to focus eyes on nearby objects • Hearing loss • Loss of sense of smell and taste • Macular Degeneration (loss of vision) • etc.

Heart and Lungs

Angina • Emphysema • Heart attack • Hardening of arteries (arteriosclerosis) • Irregular heart rate Plaques in arteries, (atherosclerosis) • etc.

Blood

High cholesterol levels (above 150) • High triglyceride levels (above 100) • High fasting glucose levels (above 85) • High uric acid levels (gout) • Blood sludging (rouleau formation) • etc.

Mouth

Coated tongue • Bad breath • Loose teeth • Tooth loss • Cavities • etc.

Gastrointestinal

Appendicitis • Belching • Colitis • Constipation Diverticulosis • Gastritis • Hemorrhoids • Hiatus hernia • Indigestion • Liver diseases • Malabsorption • Polyps • Ulcers • etc.

Cancers

Breast • Bronchus • Colon • Intestine • Kidney Lung • Pancreas • Prostate • Rectum • Skin Stomach • Testicle • Trachea • Uterus • etc.

Other Degenerative Symptoms

Allergy (from mineral loss) • Aneurysm • Arthritis Claudication • Calcified organs • Adult-onset

(type 2) diabetes • Fatigue • Gallstones • Gangrene
Gout • High blood pressure • Hormone imbalances
Impotency • Kidney failure • Kidney stones • Loss
of skin tone • Mineral loss from bones • Multiple
sclerosis • Overweight • Poor circulation • Prostatitis
Reduced lung function • Reduced mental acuity
Senility • Stroke • Varicose veins • etc.

Foods which Cause Degenerative Diseases

Foods which cause degenerative diseases
are those which are high in fat, protein,
cholesterol and refined carbohydrates, or have
other ingredients which are damaging when
consumed in more than minute amounts.

Those foods causing the most damage are
pork (bacon, ham, sausages, etc.), beef (steak,
hamburger, etc.), cows' milk (butter, cheeses,
yogurt, etc.), lamb, vegetable oils (olive, safflower,
corn, peanut, coconut, soy, etc.), margarine, nuts
(all except chestnut), seeds (all), sugars (cane,
beet, corn, honey, maple, etc.), coffee (all forms),
tea, chicken eggs and legs, turkey legs, shellfish,
sardines, salmon, alcoholic drinks, dried fruit,
avocado, peanuts and soybeans.

Cancer

Whenever our cells are deprived of oxygen
they mutate to try to stay alive. Any additional
damage accelerates the process. These mutated
cells are cancer cells. In this mutated form
the cells are unable to stop reproducing and
overwhelm our body.

Eating over 10 percent of calories from
vegetable oils and animal fats deprives our
cells of oxygen. Allergic reactions impair
circulation. Toxic chemicals from smoking or
the environment accelerate the process. Recurring
tissue damage from the sun or continuing
irritation adds to the problem. Our bodies'
defenses can not keep up and cancer takes over.

Our white blood cells are constantly working
to keep our bodies free of cancer cells. They
search out mutated cancer cells and eat them.
When we avoid foods and chemicals which
damage our white blood cells and avoid vegetable
oils and animal fats, we have cancer prevention
working for us. This is much better than any
medical treatment for cancer after it has started.
See pictures of white blood cells, inside back
cover, and cancer charts on pages 58 and 59.

Stress

When we eat foods which damage our
bodies, high levels of stress are created. When
we are free from foods which are killing our
white blood cells, we have removed a major
cause of stress and are then better able to handle
the normal stress of living. Delayed food allergies
cause stress, and high levels of stress make people
more reactive. The regular problems of daily
life are not a major cause of excess stress.

When we eat meals high in vegetable oil,
animal fat, protein, cholesterol or refined
carbohydrates, we block our arteries with fat
and cholesterol and harden our arteries with
calcium. After eating incorrectly for years,
we get degenerative diseases. Stress is not a
significant factor in heart attacks, strokes or
cancer. However, excessive stress contributes
to chronic problems (see page 26).

Brief History

Effective treatment of diseases got off to
a good start with the brilliant work of
Hippocrates around 400 B.C. He became aware
that chronic diseases would occur when people
ate certain foods. Although he was confident
that eating properly was the foundation of
health, he was unaware that foods eaten every
day could cause intermittent symptoms.

Hippocrates' understanding about the
importance of eating compatible foods was lost
until the first part of the twentieth century,
when many chronic diseases were shown to
be caused by delayed food allergies. These
discoveries were made by Francis Hare, MD,
Arthur Coca, MD, Albert Rowe, MD, Herbert
Rinkel, MD, Theron Randolph, MD, and others.
Dr. Randolph has made major contributions
to the understanding of food and chemical
reactions and has shared these insights
continually over the last 50 years.

By 1980 there were approximately 800
scientists and doctors with the understanding
that food and chemical allergies are the
underlying cause of most chronic diseases. By
1993 there were probably over 8000 scientific
and health professionals with this new
awareness of food and chemical reactions. The
number of people going to traditional allergists
has been dropping steadily for the last ten years.

Unfortunately, most traditional allergists still use scratch tests on the skin and have their patients come back for injections every week for years. This lucrative approach has given traditional allergists the power to control what insurance companies will cover and to manipulate state and federal governments to force competitors out of business. In addition, they have suppressed information from the public and other health professionals. Supporting scientific references on how the hidden and delayed type of food and chemical allergies cause chronic diseases are in chapter 11, page 93.

A different group of scientists and doctors discovered that foods high in fat and protein are the cause of degenerative diseases.

The awareness that eating excessive fat and cholesterol causes degenerative diseases and deaths was missed until the first part of the twentieth century. In the early thirties, I. M. Rabinowitch, MD, successfully treated diabetics by lowering fat intake and increasing carbohydrate intake. His 1935 report demonstrated significant improvements for diabetics with the unexpected finding that patients had a 20 percent reduction in blood cholesterol levels and a corresponding reduction in atherosclerosis.

The second major clue came during the Second World War. When the Nazis overran a country and took the expensive "rich" foods, the local people ate less fat and cholesterol. Even though the local people lived under greatly increased stress, carefully kept records show that cardiovascular deaths declined sharply. After the war was over, the old foods were eaten again and the heart disease rate went back up, even though stress went down to normal levels.

The third major clue came from Ancel Keys, MD. In 1958 and in 1970, he revealed that wherever people around the world ate low-fat, low-cholesterol diets, they had low blood cholesterol levels and low levels of heart disease. It has since been shown, without exception, that all groups around the world which eat high-fat, high-cholesterol diets have severe artery damage, and the resulting degenerative diseases.

These discoveries and others led Nathan Pritikin to test the 10–10–80 balance of macronutrients. He published the first medical study in 1975 which demonstrated that a diet with 10 percent fat and under 20 milligrams of cholesterol a day would reduce blockages in the arteries. The blockages were shown to be reduced by a 5700 percent increase in the ability of patients to walk and by x-rays. (Pritikin N, Pritikin R, Kern J, Kaye SM: Diet and exercise as a total therapeutic regime for the rehabilitation of patients with severe peripheral vascular disease. Archives of Phys Med Rehab 1975; 56:558.)

This breakthrough has helped thousands of people reverse their degenerative diseases and avoid dangerous drugs and surgery. By 1980 there were nearly a thousand scientists and doctors recommending the 10–10–80 balance of macronutrients. By 1993 there were thousands of scientists and doctors who knew the 10–10–80 balance works for people over three years old. However, so much money is being made selling drugs and then performing surgery that some traditional doctors have misled most people into believing 15 to 30 percent of our calories from fat is fine and 300 milligrams of cholesterol a day will not hurt them.

It is now hard for world-renowned heart specialists to admit they have been mistreating their patients by giving them drugs or coronary bypass or other types of surgery.

There are a few doctors who understand the causes of both chronic and degenerative diseases. They are testing their patients for delayed food reactions and recommending the 10–10–80 balance of macronutrients.

The opposition to new, effective approaches often lasts until those in power retire or die. Most of the doctors who are resisting the awareness of delayed food and chemical allergies and white blood cell testing are elderly. The use of these scientific discoveries is growing rapidly.

Every new theory encounters opposition
and rejection at first. The adherents to the old,
accepted doctrine object to the new theory,
refuse it recognition and declare it to be mistaken.
Years, even decades, must pass before it
succeeds in supplanting the old one.
A new generation must grow up
before its victory is decisive.

Ludwig von Mises
Philosopher and Economist — 1881 to 1973

Where Stress Comes From and The Total Load Concept

Painful Symptoms Begin

Components That Make Up Our Total Stress Load

Typical Person

| Regular Upsets in Life and Relationships |
| Chronic Infections |
| Miscellaneous Allergies |
| Airborne Allergies |
| Chemical Allergies |
| Food Allergies |

Example A

| A New Problem in Life or Relationships |
| Regular Upsets in Life and Relationships |
| Chronic Infections |
| Miscellaneous Allergies |
| Airborne Allergies |
| Chemical Allergies |
| Food Allergies |

Example B

| Regular Upsets in Life and Relationships |
| Chronic Infections |
| Miscellaneous Allergies |
| Airborne Allergies |
| Chemical Allergies |
| Food Allergies |

Example C

| Regular Upsets in Life and Relationships |
| Chronic Infections |
| Miscellaneous Allergies |
| Airborne Allergies |
| Chemical Allergies |
| Food Allergies |

This chart explains how delayed allergies cause stress and symptoms. Many people live with high levels of stress caused by delayed allergic reactions without realizing it. See example at the left side of chart.

In Example A, a new problem pushes the person up to the level where symptoms begin. In Example B, the person eats the wrong foods, creating added stress, and symptoms. If people are not aware of how delayed food and chemical allergies cause stress, they often blame someone or something else in their life.

In Example C, you see the low levels of stress you can achieve when you are free of your delayed food and chemical allergies.

When you live life free of most stress, you are able to enjoy each day more. When a problem does come along, you can handle it without having physical or emotional symptoms and becoming sick.

Chapter 4
Improved Allergy Testing for Foods and Chemicals

Doctors who are aware of the importance of delayed food and chemical allergies significantly improve the health of over 90 percent of their patients. Often, these patients have been to several different types of doctors without receiving lasting benefit. Unfortunately, traditional allergists and their trade organizations claim food allergies are rare, occurring in only three percent of adults. Also, most of these traditional allergists mistakenly believe children outgrow their allergies and that chemical allergies do not exist. However, there are now several published double-blind studies done in the United States and Europe which clearly demonstrate that traditional allergists do not understand the nature or importance of delayed food and chemical allergies.

Most traditional allergists miss this most common type of allergic reaction because their test, known as the skin test or prick test, does not detect any allergic reactions other than the acute, rapid-acting, IgE antibody type. Because traditional allergists rely on this insensitive and often inaccurate skin test, they agreed to change the word "allergy" to mean *only* IgE reactions. This artificial definition limits awareness and makes traditional allergists hostile toward doctors who help people with delayed food allergies.

Delayed allergies are not the same as acute IgE allergies, and are caused by different mechanisms, including antibodies IgA, IgD, IgG, IgM and immune complexes. Traditional skin tests do not detect delayed food or chemical allergies.

It is rare for people to have acute type IgE allergies to foods. Less than three percent of the population has this type. Usually, people know if they have the acute type of reaction without being skin tested. Skin tests inherently cause some harm to people and can cause severe reactions and even death. In contrast, blood tests for delayed food and chemical allergies do not harm people.

It would be difficult for traditional allergists to change their thinking and practices, because their economic base and political power would be lost to preventive care doctors. They would also have to admit they are ineffective and have been mistreating their patients for years.

It is not necessary for doctors to refer their patients to traditional allergists — those who certify themselves to be "board certified allergists." Now all doctors can help their patients by performing allergy tests in their offices by using the improved type of white blood cell test called the Prime Test.™

One fundamental advantage of the Prime Test over other types of tests for allergies is that it shows the actual damage to the white blood cells and other blood components. Other blood tests are indirect and measure only the levels of IgE or IgG antibodies which may cause damage to the white blood cells. In addition, they do not demonstrate whether the antibodies are actually causing reactions, and they do not reveal reactions if other mechanisms are involved. The Prime Test is superior because it shows the result of several different types of allergic reactions.

The Prime Test also demonstrates reactions which cause damage to white blood cells but do not kill them. Changes in platelets and red blood cells are observed. White blood cell counting tests miss these three types of reactions and thus miss many delayed food allergies.

You can measure the accuracy of any test for food and chemical allergies by testing symptom-free, very athletic young people who have no apparent health problems and then testing people with different levels of health. By doing this, it was discovered that very healthy people usually have around 15 damaging reactions out of 100 foods and chemicals. People with significant health problems often have over 25 reactive items and very sick people sometimes have 60 reactive items. Forty compatible foods to start with are enough to turn a person's health around.

By removing the reacting items, there will be a marked improvement in most peoples' health. When the foods or chemicals are again consumed, the symptoms often return. The above ratios are true for the Prime Test and for fasting and food-challenge testing. Any test which does not match these parameters is not accurate or sensitive enough for delayed food and chemical allergy testing. Other testing methods often reveal few or no reactions for people with severe delayed food and chemical allergies.

The Prime Test is helpful for improving the health of most people. It gives them an awareness that delayed food and chemical allergies are a major health problem. In addition, it does not harm their health and costs much less than other types of tests.

Preventive Care and the Prime Test

Doctors who use the Prime Test are interested in finding the underlying causes of ailments and removing them. This differs from the traditional approach of coming up with a name for the symptom, called a diagnosis, and then trying approaches to suppress the symptom by using drugs, surgeries and allergy injections. Any approach which only suppresses symptoms is dangerous to your health.

Most traditional medical approaches work well for accidental injury and almost as well for infections. However, they do not work well for most other types of health problems.

Accidents and infections cause about 20 percent of health problems in the industrialized world. In the long run, the remaining 80 percent are usually made worse by relying on traditional approaches such as drugs, surgeries and allergy injections. The large majority of health problems are caused by mistakes in life-style, and most of these can be avoided or reversed by avoiding damaging foods and chemicals.

Many ear, nose and throat (ENT) specialists have been using white blood cell testing for years. They use the first procedure developed, which is called the cytotoxic test.

They already knew drugs and surgeries were of little help and led to larger problems later. After trying the traditional allergist's drugs, skin tests and twice-weekly allergy injections which go on for years, ENT specialists could clearly see their patients did not improve and were often being made worse. Besides unnecessary suffering, their patients were spending large sums of money, and insurance companies began raising their rates. Soon doctors began losing their patients. Most ENT specialists who are aware of delayed food and chemical allergies stopped using traditional skin tests and ineffective, though lucrative, allergy injections.

Many allergy specialists who have a comprehensive knowledge of delayed food and chemical allergies belong to the American Academy of Environmental Medicine. They include some of the first doctors who helped their patients by using the original cytotoxic test.

Many doctors who practice preventive care have specialized in delayed food and chemical allergies and have helped their patients by using the original cytotoxic test. Their approach is designed to find the causes of patients' health problems and then help patients eliminate the cause, which is often reactive foods and chemicals.

When it is not possible to remain free of a particular item, doctors are sometimes able to neutralize the reaction. Instead of using trial and error to find the items, the Prime Test enables the doctor to discover rapidly which foods and chemicals need neutralizing therapy.

Theron Randolph, MD, the father of Environmental Medicine, has stated that over 60 percent of the people who came to his office had first learned of the cause of their health problems by taking the original cytotoxic test.

Doctors in the United States and Europe are now using the Prime Test to help people attain excellent health as rapidly as possible. This is accomplished at less expense than traditional allergy approaches and without causing harm to the person.

Insurance companies are being informed about the cost savings and health benefits of the Prime Test so that more people will be reimbursed without delay.

Advantages of the Prime Test

The Prime Test visually exposes actual white blood cell damage and death, rather than counting the cells before and after exposure to a food or measuring the levels of antibodies. The following outline explains several areas where the Prime Test has advantages over other blood tests and skin tests for allergies.

1.0 Advantages of the Prime Test Slide

1.1 The liquid antigen (food or chemical) is

instead of from the top. This creates an even deposition of antigens on both surfaces. When antigens are dried from the top, the antigen coatings are too thin in some areas and too thick in others. As much as 40 percent of the slide is not covered at all. The Prime Test slide also creates an even coating of antigens on the slide and on the underside of the permanently attached cover slip; thus, there is no area of high concentration of antigen on the slide surface. The top and bottom surfaces end up with half the thickness of antigen coating; the original cytotoxic test has all of its coating on one surface. See diagrams on page 31.

1.2 The antigen chamber is designed so it cannot trap air; thus, the coating is uniform. The coating is so thin it is hard to see.

1.3 The space between the slide cover and slide surface is a uniform .006 of an inch. Thus, the white blood cells are always within .003 of an inch from an antigen-coated surface. This significantly improves the reproducibility of the test. The distance from the white blood cells to the antigen in the cytotoxic test varied from .010 to over .050 of an inch.

1.4 Because the Prime Test antigen chamber volume is tightly controlled, the ratio of white blood cells to antigens is constant. This increases reproducibility.

1.5 This chamber is less than half the size used with the cytotoxic test. Thus, less blood is needed to perform the Prime Test.

1.6 The Prime Test antigen chambers do not leak as Vaseline rings occasionally do, nor can they overflow and cross-react as can other types of plastic chambers.

1.7 Saline solution need not be added to the serum because the new slide gives improved cell mobility without drying problems.

1.8 The special slides make it easier for the laboratory technician to see the different reactions; thus, people can learn to read the test with less training.

2.0 Advantages of Prime Test Antigens

2.1 The antigens are prepared using a significantly improved technique. There are several important changes from the original cytotoxic test. The antigens are carefully formulated to give test results which parallel the reactions actually taking place in the person's body. This work was never done for the original cytotoxic test. After working with numerous patients, we have been able to correlate the reactions seen on the Prime Test with the food or chemical which is causing symptoms.

2.2 In order to break down natural toxins, and to convert the active ingredients of the antigens into solution, the appropriate antigens have been heated.

2.3 Because so little antigen is needed for the Prime Test, the antigen pH is unimportant.

2.4 The antigens are usually made from pesticide-free and chemical-free materials. The amount of food is so small that any pesticide left is too small to cause a reaction.

2.5 Selected antigen solutions are run through micropore filters to remove particles.

2.6 The antigens have been processed using methods which prevent contamination.

3.0 Advantages of Prime Test Report Form

3.1 Many foods, chemicals, vitamin supplements, medications and other items are available for testing. This enables the counselor to prescribe the best health program without having to guess which items are compatible.

3.2 The foods are listed by food families, thus facilitating nutritional counseling and patient understanding.

3.3 Foods and chemicals which cause non-allergic health problems are identified by a small minus sign in front of the item.

3.4 Closely related foods are identified by one vertical line in front of their boxes.

3.5 Reactions are separated into four levels. The number **1** level designates platelet aggregation. This important type of reaction is missed with other tests. Numbers **2**, **3** and **4** designate increasing levels of damage to white blood cells and reactions involving red blood cells.

3.6 The test form gives valuable information which helps people understand their results.

4.0 Cost Advantages of the Prime Test

4.1 The Prime Test slides have improved optics, so reading time is reduced.

4.2 There are ten antigen chambers per slide, which means less loading and unloading of the microscope compared with three-chamber slides.

4.3 Glass slides, cover slips, antigens and supplies no longer must be purchased.

4.4 Glass slides no longer must be carefully cleaned and specially coated.

4.5 Antigens no longer must be formulated and specially preserved.

4.6 Vaseline rings no longer must be made.

4.7 Cover slips no longer must be placed over the chambers after the blood cells have been added.

4.8 Additional, specially trained personnel are not needed to manufacture test kits.

Other testing methods cost over twice as much as the Prime Test, require expensive equipment, and have fewer foods and chemicals available for testing. Also, other types of tests miss many of a person's allergy causing foods and chemicals. The soon-to-be-patented Prime Test is a trademark of Advanced Health Center.

Conclusion

The Prime Test is the primary and optimum test for delayed food and chemical allergies. It is more accurate and less expensive than other tests and can be done in the doctor's office.

*Give the people the light
and they will find their own way.*

Thomas Jefferson
A Founding Father of the United States, Author of the Declaration of Independence, Inventor, Architect, Author and Third President of the United States — 1743 to 1826

Shared Experiences

In 1978 I was looking for the answer to my health problems and discovered they were caused by a type of food allergy which does not show up on traditional allergy tests. Fortunately, I was able to find an improved type of white blood cell test and became free of my symptoms.

I was able to become well because I was free to choose the approach which worked for me. If the medical establishment and government had blocked me from finding out about delayed food allergies and the Prime Test, I would have suffered unnecessarily for years.

The Quality Longevity Program helped me take the correct action to improve my health. The change was so dramatic I decided to study the research behind the program. The information was so valuable I decided to change my career in 1980 and started counseling people so they could also take advantage of this improved approach to health.

One of my life's greatest joys is the pleasure of passing this awareness to others and watching their many health improvements.

Mark Matulis, Health Consultant
Monarch Beach, California

The shared experiences are from correspondence on file.

Mark has been able to sort out the facts from all the information available. He is doing a good job of helping a lot of people become informed.

William H. Philpott, MD, Psychiatrist,
Author of the books, *Brain Allergies* and
Victory Over Diabetes

The white blood cell test identified some delayed food allergies that were causing my chronic joint pain and contributing to bronchial and sinus disorders. An unexpected benefit has been a new sense of mental clarity.

Elizabeth Freeman, Registered Nurse

Twenty years ago I was looking for the solution to my health problem. After seeing many doctors and engaging in a week of medical tests at a world-famous medical clinic in the Midwest, I was unable to find answers of any value.

Ultimately I found a physician who understood food allergies and with his advice I was able to regain my health. Through the years since then, with the aid of white blood cell testing, I have been able to remain in excellent health.

Stephen White, Newport Beach, California

Prime Test™

Side View of Prime Test Slide
Not To Scale

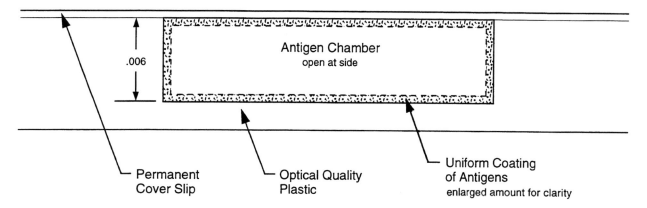

.006

Antigen Chamber
open at side

Permanent
Cover Slip

Optical Quality
Plastic

Uniform Coating
of Antigens
enlarged amount for clarity

Uniform coating of the antigens is now possible because the antigen solution dries from the side. This controlled drying prevents the antigen coating from being too thin in one area and too thick in another. This is one of several improvements which make it possible to obtain accurate, reproducible results.

Another improvement made possible by the new design is that the antigen coating is on both the slide and the underside of the cover slip. The chamber height is uniform and only .006 of an inch, and thus the white blood cells are always within .003 of an inch from an antigen-coated surface. Damaging reactions can be clearly seen with a microscope.

Doctors interested in performing the Prime Test in their office can contact Advanced Health Center, 34146 Selva Road, Suite 200, Monarch Beach, California, 92629. Phone (714) 661- 4001.

Side View of Cytotoxic Test Slide
Not To Scale

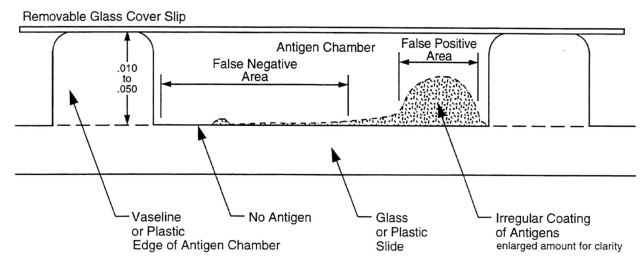

Removable Glass Cover Slip

.010
to
.050

Antigen Chamber

False Negative
Area

False Positive
Area

Vaseline
or Plastic
Edge of Antigen Chamber

No Antigen

Glass
or Plastic
Slide

Irregular Coating
of Antigens
enlarged amount for clarity

The diagram above is representative of different types of cytotoxic tests. When liquid antigens dry on a flat surface they deposit their ingredients irregularly.

Therefore, with the cytotoxic test it is possible for the laboratory technician to get false negatives and false positives depending on the areas studied.

Shared Experiences

Thank you for your invaluable help concerning my health problems. Your test is great and very informative. Everyday I feel better.

Mike Cramer, La Habra, California

My family doctor diagnosed my "chronic" hives, swelling of my eyes, lips, and hands as nerves. He treated me with cortisone and benadryl. After approximately two months, I still needed help.

I decided to try your white blood cell test and in a week began The Quality Longevity Program. My hives cleared up, and I was surprised that other symptoms I had been suffering from for years went away, including headaches and being moody. My compatible foods helped me to lose 16 pounds. My skin is softer and smoother than it has ever been. My whole attitude changed when I changed my foods.

I tested myself by eating the wrong foods. In two days my eyes would swell and the headaches would start. My whole attitude would change. I felt miserable.

I can't say enough for the program; it has helped me in many ways. I have learned so much about nutrition. I am much happier and healthier than I have ever been.

Gayle Nejman, Anaheim, California

I am very grateful for the healing which resulted, and still continues. I hesitated at first because The Quality Longevity Program seemed so expensive, and when I did start, it was very rough going. It was such a change of life for me, but it has been well worth all of it. I am very thankful for what it has done for me. The benefits are multiple.

My hope was that I might be able to overcome the irritating rashes that constantly plagued me for years. Medical doctors had no satisfying answers, stating the rashes were caused by allergies. Under your nutritional counsel, the irritations were not immediately brought under control, but began to diminish. I learned a new way of diet and more than one and a half years later they rarely flare up. When they do, I know how to handle them and I live in comfort.

The other things that happened to my health are even more spectacular. I lost considerable weight (28 pounds), although I still have trouble keeping it down. My borderline high blood pressure is down — I am off medication which a doctor had said I would have to use for life. My painful arthritis, which I was medicating very heavily, rarely pains me, and I do not take the medication any more. My general health and stamina are so much improved that I am now able to live a much fuller life, even at age 68. Thank you so much.

Reverend Herman T. Petersen
San Diego, California

I must admit I was initially a bit skeptical about how white blood cell testing and nutritional counseling could help solve the health problems I have had to tolerate for so many years. My doubts vanished, however, when a six year old, who attended the school I direct, went through The Quality Longevity Program.

The child's learning ability increased dramatically. He no longer needed an afternoon nap or to be calmed down from hyperactivity. The puffiness in his face disappeared, and overall he became a happier, more productive child — all in a matter of weeks!

I immediately started the program myself and within three weeks my headaches ended, I lost the 15 pounds that even consistent, vigorous exercise never affected, and the excessive mucous in my sinuses and throat cleared; no more itchy eyes. I am less moody, I have abundant energy and am more clear and focused. My skin looks so good that people are remarking about it! My teaching staff even claims I am more enjoyable to work with!

I hope all the parents of my students will be as wise as the parent of that six year old. At the height of the running nose season, you'll often hear me say to a parent, "Ever had your child checked for delayed food allergies?" Why allow children, or anyone at any age, to go through life tied to medications for this or that ailment when all they would be doing is treating the symptoms of a delayed food allergy?

I will continue to recommend your program highly to the many people I have in my life.

Shelly De Groot, Directress
Crown Hill Montessori School, Seattle, Washington

Chapter 5

How to Use Your Prime Test Results

Experience how enjoyable life can be when you are not going up and down on the addiction roller coaster. The difference between being addicted to cocaine, heroin, alcohol, tobacco, corn, coffee, wheat or dairy products is a matter of degree. Your health and life will deteriorate if you are consuming anything you are addicted to. Enjoy life fully by being free of drug addiction and food addiction.

It is important to avoid foods to which you are allergic and eat the correct balance of macronutrients. However, most health professionals and the majority of the public do not realize how common delayed food allergies are and they do not understand the importance of eating the foods that make up the 10–10–80 balance of macronutrients.

Repetitiously eating a food may cause you to become allergic to it; however, stuffing yourself or eating when you are not hungry increases your chances of developing delayed food allergies. By eating small or moderate meals of around 600 calories, and by rotating your compatible foods, you can avoid becoming allergic to them.

Young people's digestive systems are often powerful enough that they can make mistakes and not feel the damage. The problems start showing up as we become older.

It is not possible to be overweight and be healthy. The excess fat and cholesterol that is eaten travels along the arteries, building blockages before being deposited in the vital organs and fat cells.

There is an added need for taking vitamin C if you are eating cereal grains or dried beans because these foods have no vitamin C. Other vitamins may be needed if there is a deficiency discovered by testing, or if a special therapy is being used.

Mineral supplementation is helpful to reverse the mineral loss caused by a high protein diet or allergic reactions. Be sure to select vitamins and minerals which are free of sugar, yeast, milk or food binders. A very small amount of an allergy causing food can cause serious problems and prevent you from breaking the addiction to that food.

Several thousand people have been tested for delayed food allergies in the United States over the last 40 years; however, the information on the 10–10–80 balance of macronutrients was not available to them.

Since 1976, several million people have started on the 10–10–80 balance of macronutrients. Most of them have not heard about the need to test for delayed food allergies. Many people have developed delayed food allergies and related health problems by eating the same food every day. Others find their chronic symptoms become worse when they eat larger quantities of foods to which they are already allergic.

As more people combine the advantages of eating non-allergic foods with the 10–10–80 balance of macronutrients and engage in regular exercise, the full benefits of The Quality Longevity Program will become better known.

This program eliminates the cause of most chronic diseases. It also stops the progression of, and begins to reverse, degenerative diseases. It strengthens our immune system and helps us avoid and fight infection. Removing excess fat from your diet is the healthy way to reduce the high calorie content of the Standard American Diet. This dramatically increases your chances of living more than 100 years.

When we avoid chronic diseases, we accelerate the reversal of degenerative diseases. When we avoid degenerative diseases, we facilitate becoming free of chronic diseases.

The life of man is formed from the things he eats. Prepare simple meals, chew well, and sup lightly.

Leonardo da Vinci
Father of Anatomy, Engineer, Botanist,
Artist and Inventor — 1452 to 1519

There are no known negative side effects of The Quality Longevity Program. One unforeseen advantage is the reduced need for anesthetic drugs if one must have surgery. If you are going to have surgery, tell your doctor that you are on a 10 percent fat diet and will need less anesthetic.

How to Use Your Prime Test Form

On the test forms on pages 37 through 39, the space between the number and the name of the food is provided so you will have a record of how often you have been eating the food or item in the past. If you usually have bread for breakfast and a roll or other bread product for dinner, that would be two exposures to baker's yeast a day; thus you would write the number 14 in the space to indicate the approximate number of times you are having baker's yeast each week. If you have mushrooms once a month or less, put the letter "R" for rarely.

For any allergy test to be fully helpful, it must include enough foods to reveal the offenders as well as reveal those foods which are compatible so a health program can be put together without guessing at what the compatible foods are. Test Panel G tests for 220 items, which includes a broad range of foods, seasonings, vitamins, chemicals and other allergens. See pages 37 and 38.

Panel D tests for 110 items, which is the minimum number of foods and other items needed so an accurate health program can be put together for those with moderate problems. See page 39.

The Rotary Diversified Diet

The foods are arranged in their families on the test panels to help you rotate them more easily. Identify which families work best for you so that you can test additional foods in those families which are not included in your Prime Test. If you have a large number of reactions, you may not be able to rotate all of your compatible foods by families. However, be careful to rotate the individual foods to reduce the chances of becoming allergic to them.

By planning ahead and taking food with you when traveling, you can eliminate the times you are stuck eating foods which do not support your health and longevity. Complex carbohydrates are digested more efficiently, and when they are used up your body will let you know it is time to eat again. It is important to have good foods available and ready, so you won't be tempted to eat something damaging.

By using a Rotary Diversified Diet in the beginning, you will learn how different foods affect your body and mind. You will be able to tell which foods work best, which foods have to be carefully rotated, and which foods need to be completely avoided.

The terms "delayed food allergy," "hidden food allergy," "food sensitivity" and "food intolerance," when used properly, mean the same thing — an abnormal and damaging reaction to the body's cells.

Mistaken Criticisms of White Blood Cell Testing

The type of testing performed by traditional allergists around the country misses many of a person's reactive foods and therefore has little value. This has been well documented by food allergy specialists who isolate food allergies by having their patients fast for five or more days until their symptoms go away, and then test them with one food per meal for several weeks.

In 1977, I began working with people who had fasted and food-tested to discover which foods were causing their symptoms. We made major improvements in the cytotoxic test so people were able to get results similar to testing by fasting on water for five days and then food-challenge testing. For the first time, people were able to find out which foods were good for them and which were causing symptoms without having to undergo lengthy, frustrating, health damaging and painful testing.

In 1988, a breakthrough in allergy testing began with the introduction of the Prime Test.™ This white blood cell test has significant improvements over the cytotoxic test and other tests for delayed chemical allergies. However, most doctors are not yet aware that delayed food allergies are a major cause of diseases and thus are negative about any test which reveals this reality.

As of 1994, this medical breakthrough is not taught in any medical school. Do not be surprised if the doctors you talk with do not understand delayed food and chemical allergies.

Another criticism of white blood cell testing is that different laboratories give different results. This is true, because most laboratories are not using the latest techniques.

A common misunderstanding about white blood cell testing is that it does not test for what the body is actually exposed to. Some people feel the body is only exposed to a food after it has been broken down by digestive enzymes. This is not true. The body actually assimilates whole food molecules through the tissue under the tongue and reacts to the food without it being swallowed. This has been clearly demonstrated by the sublingual method of food allergy testing. One drop of an allergy causing food can be placed under the tongue of a fasting patient and cause obviously damaging and painful reactions. The white blood cells circulating inside the body are damaged by a food reaction the same way they are damaged outside the body during the Prime Test.

After taking the Prime Test and utilizing the results properly for two months, people agree that delayed food allergies are a fundamental cause of health problems. In time, people often modify their dietary programs to try to remain symptom-free with less effort. Our bodies change with time and follow-up testing is often helpful.

The evidence is overwhelming that delayed food and chemical allergies are a major cause of numerous health problems and that the Prime Test for this type of allergy is the optimum first test.

Avoid being discouraged by those who say food allergies are not the cause of your symptoms. Most of the press and most doctors are under the influence of traditional allergists. The sad fact is that traditional allergists do not understand allergy.

In order to become a medical doctor, one has to take dozens of courses, many of which are incomplete or obsolete. If the students do not agree with the approach being taught, they have to go along or they do not graduate. After this, the person is subjected to an exhausting internship which often exhausts the desire to be open and compassionate. Many traditional doctors end up with the wrong information and no longer care about the health of the people who come to them.

How You Can Test a Food

The Prime Test will occasionally miss a reactive food so it is helpful to confirm your results by eating only one food at a time. If you have completely avoided a food for several weeks, it is possible to have a meal of only that food to see if it is now compatible for you.

It is a good indication the food is compatible when you feel fine from the time you start eating the food until after the next meal. An additional indicator is your pulse. If your pulse rises or declines more than 12 beats per minute, it is likely that the food is a reactor. Compare your pulse rate at the start of the meal with your pulse rate at 20, 40, and 60 minutes after you have eaten. The pulse test works only when your heart is one of the organs being affected. Most people find that less than 25 percent of their reactive foods effect their heart rate. See the Example of Food Testing Log on page 145 and make yourself copies of the Food Testing Log on page 144.

If you have avoided a food for two weeks or more, it may not cause symptoms the first time you eat it. Therefore, the test results you obtained from eating a food cannot be relied upon until you have confirmed the results by eating the food once a week for several weeks.

Avoid adding salt to test meals or regular meals. Unprocessed foods provide the proper amount of salt for your body. Added salt causes swelling, weight gain, inflammation, and sometimes contributes to high blood pressure.

Summary

All of the fat, protein, carbohydrate, fiber, vitamins and minerals we need are supplied by eating compatible plant foods as grown, with occasional small amounts of fish or fowl. There is no food we need to eat every day, or even once a week, to achieve and maintain great health.

The Quality Longevity Program works for adults and children. Infants need to get a good start by consuming only mother's milk for the first year of life, and then begin adding foods which are compatible with their bodies.

One problem with The Quality Longevity Program is that you will soon feel so good you will think that you can eat anything. Fortunately, our bodies give us symptoms to help us be good to ourselves. Be an honest observer of your body and mind.

Leave your drugs in the chemist's pot if you can heal the patient with food.

Hippocrates
Greek Physician, Father of Medicine,
Health Scientist and First Allergist — 460 to 377 BC

Quality Longivity

Prime Test™

Designed to facilitate accurate nutritional
counseling. Not for diagnosis of disease.

Panel G
Side 1

Name (print) _____ Home Phone (_____) _____
　　　　　　　Last　　　　　　　　　　First　　　　　　Initial　　　　　　　　　　　　area code

Address _____ Work Phone (_____) _____
　　　　　　Street　　　　　　　　　　　　　　　　Apt. #　　　　　　　　　　　area code

City _____ Sex M ☐ F ☐
　　　　　　　　　　　　　　　　　　　State　　　Zip

Test Date _____ Birth Date _____ Age _____ Time blood sample drawn _____ Time of last meal _____

☐ Complete Blood Count and Blood Chemistry, _____

Referred by _____ Parent or Guardian _____

IMPORTANT INFORMATION ABOUT YOUR TEST

The Prime Test exposes foods, chemicals and other items which are damaging to you. This is accomplished by combining your living white blood cells, platelets, red blood cells and plasma with a microscopic amount of the item to be tested. Then a laboratory technician studies your cells using a high-powered microscope. If no damage is seen, the item is not reactive and no mark is placed on the test form. However, if damage is seen and your cells react and become damaged or killed, you need to avoid that item. A black mark is placed in the appropriate box to indicate the amount and type of reaction. The Prime Test is the primary and optimum first screening test for discovering delayed reactions. It exposes hidden or delayed reactions often missed by other types of tests.

There are four levels of reactions; however, a low level **Number 1** reaction may cause severe symptoms in your body like a more damaging higher level reaction. If you react at any level, you need to avoid the item.
Number 1 indicates the item is a reactor due to platelet aggregation.
Number 2 indicates the item has caused damage to approximately 25% of the white blood cells.
Number 3 indicates the item has caused damage to approximately 50% of the white blood cells.
Number 4 indicates the item has caused damage to more than 90% of the white blood cells and some damage to the red cells.

(a) Avoid all forms of a food when you react to any product made with that food. These items are identified by a double line next to their number 1 boxes. See the example 131 through 135. **(b)** The foods on your test are listed in their families. Reactive foods often show up in groups by families and sub-families. The sub-families are identified by a vertical line next to their number 1 boxes. Be cautious of families and sub-families where you have reactions. See the example of a sub-family, number 36 through 40. **(c)** On side two, item 149 is a combination of petroleum by-products. If you reacted to this item, you need to minimize your exposure to car exhausts, gas appliances, sprays, smog, etc. * Item 139: this and most vitamin C is made from corn. Item 145 is from the Konsyl Company; item 146 is "Vitamin & Mineral Insurance Formula," and 147 is "Super B," both from Bronson Pharmaceuticals; and item 150 is the food colors FD and C Yellow #5, Red #40, Blue #1, and Red #3, from McCormick.

The Prime Test is calibrated to parallel the results of fasting and individual food-challenge testing. Occasionally, the test will miss a food you are sensitive to. The test does not detect acute IgE type reactions. Do not eat any foods that you already know cause problems. If you have avoided a reactive food for more than one week prior to taking your test, it may not react on the Prime Test. Skin tests are not usually able to detect delayed food and chemical reactions and the Prime Test is not usually able to detect dust, mold, pollens and other airborne reactions. It is desirable to confirm the results of your test by eating meals of a single food which tested compatible to be sure you do not have a reaction the test missed.

HOW TO PREPARE FOR YOUR TEST

There is often a correlation between repetitiously eaten foods and delayed food reactions. Put the average number of times you have eaten a food per week on the line before the food. If you have eaten the food less than once a week, put the letter **L** on the line. If you have eaten the food rarely, put the letter **R**, and if never, put the letter **N**.

On the day before the test, eat no foods after dinner, drink only spring or distilled water, and do not brush your teeth or eat until after the test the next morning. With the help of your doctor, avoid any drugs containing steroids and hydrocortisone for 48 hours before the test; this includes skin creams. Avoid smoking, or other people's smoke, and any other exposure which may cause a reaction, from dinner until the time you give your blood sample. Reschedule your test if you develop a cold, flu or other infectious disease prior to your appointment.

List any additional items you are taking more often than once a week such as vitamins, medicines, herbs, spices, etc. — _____

_____

_____

List your current and past health problems — _____

_____

Remarks — _____

Prime Test™

Designed to facilitate accurate nutritional
counseling. Not for diagnosis of disease.

Name _____

Control Number _____

Date _____ **Panel G**

Total Reactions _____ Side 2

Controls	1 2 3 4	
1 ___ negative control ª .... ▢▢▢▢ 1	A
2 ___ positive control .... ▢▢▢▢ 2	
Fungus	
3 ___ mushrooms .... ▢▢▢▢ 3	
4 ___ -yeast – baker's .... ᵇ ▢▢▢▢ 4	
5 ___ -yeast – brewer's .... ▢▢▢▢ 5	
Cereal Grains (Grasses)	
6 ___ barley .... ▢▢▢▢ 6	
7 ___ wheat .... ▢▢▢▢ 7	
8 ___ rye .... ▢▢▢▢ 8	
9 ___ wild rice .... ▢▢▢▢ 9	
10 ___ oats .... ▢▢▢▢ 10	
11 ___ rice .... ▢▢▢▢ 1	B
12 ___ millet .... ▢▢▢▢ 2	
13 ___ -sugar cane .... ▢▢▢▢ 3	
14 ___ corn (maize) .... ▢▢▢▢ 4	
Cyperaceae	
15 ___ water chestnut .... ▢▢▢▢ 5	
Palm	
16 ___ -coconut .... ▢▢▢▢ 6	
17 ___ -date .... ▢▢▢▢ 7	
Farinosa	
18 ___ pineapple .... ▢▢▢▢ 8	
Lily	
19 ___ asparagus .... ▢▢▢▢ 9	
20 ___ onion .... ▢▢▢▢ 10	
21 ___ garlic .... ▢▢▢▢ 1	C
Banana	
22 ___ banana .... ▢▢▢▢ 2	
Ginger	
23 ___ ginger .... ▢▢▢▢ 3	
Orchid	
24 ___ vanilla .... ▢▢▢▢ 4	
Pepper	
25 ___ -black pepper .... ▢▢▢▢ 5	
Walnut	
26 ___ -walnut .... ▢▢▢▢ 6	
27 ___ -pecan .... ▢▢▢▢ 7	
Beech	
28 ___ chestnuts .... ▢▢▢▢ 8	
Mulberry	
29 ___ fig .... ▢▢▢▢ 9	
Buckwheat	
30 ___ buckwheat .... ▢▢▢▢ 10	
Pink	
31 ___ beet .... ▢▢▢▢ 1	D
32 ___ Swiss chard .... ▢▢▢▢ 2	
33 ___ spinach .... ▢▢▢▢ 3	
Myristiceae	
34 ___ nutmeg (mace) .... ▢▢▢▢ 4	

Laurel	1 2 3 4	
35 ___ -avocado .... ▢▢▢▢ 5	
36 ___ cinnamon .... ▢▢▢▢ 6	
Brassica	
37 ___ kale .... ▢▢▢▢ 7	
38 ___ cabbage .... ▢▢▢▢ 8	
39 ___ Brussels sprouts .... ▢▢▢▢ 9	
40 ___ broccoli .... ▢▢▢▢ 10	
41 ___ cauliflower .... ▢▢▢▢ 1	E
42 ___ radish .... ▢▢▢▢ 2	
43 ___ mustard .... ▢▢▢▢ 3	
44 ___ turnip .... ▢▢▢▢ 4	
45 ___ rutabaga .... ▢▢▢▢ 5	
46 ___ bokchoy .... ▢▢▢▢ 6	
47 ___ horseradish .... ▢▢▢▢ 7	
48 ___ watercress .... ▢▢▢▢ 8	
Rose	
49 ___ blackberry .... ▢▢▢▢ 9	
50 ___ raspberry .... ▢▢▢▢ 10	
51 ___ strawberry .... ▢▢▢▢ 1	F
52 ___ apple .... ▢▢▢▢ 2	
53 ___ pear .... ▢▢▢▢ 3	
54 ___ plum (prune) .... ▢▢▢▢ 4	
55 ___ -almond .... ▢▢▢▢ 5	
56 ___ peach .... ▢▢▢▢ 6	
57 ___ apricot .... ▢▢▢▢ 7	
58 ___ nectarine .... ▢▢▢▢ 8	
59 ___ cherry .... ▢▢▢▢ 9	
60 ___ rosehips tea .... ▢▢▢▢ 10	
Legume	
61 ___ alfalfa sprouts .... ▢▢▢▢ 1	G
62 ___ licorice .... ▢▢▢▢ 2	
63 ___ azuki bean .... ▢▢▢▢ 3	
64 ___ carob .... ▢▢▢▢ 4	
65 ___ lentil .... ▢▢▢▢ 5	
66 ___ split pea .... ▢▢▢▢ 6	
67 ___ -peanut .... ▢▢▢▢ 7	
68 ___ kidney bean .... ▢▢▢▢ 8	
69 ___ string bean .... ▢▢▢▢ 9	
70 ___ pinto bean .... ▢▢▢▢ 10	
71 ___ black bean .... ▢▢▢▢ 1	H
72 ___ navy bean .... ▢▢▢▢ 2	
73 ___ mung bean .... ▢▢▢▢ 3	
74 ___ lima bean .... ▢▢▢▢ 4	
75 ___ fava bean .... ▢▢▢▢ 5	
76 ___ pea .... ▢▢▢▢ 6	
77 ___ chick pea (garbanzo) ... ▢▢▢▢ 7	
78 ___ blackeyed pea .... ▢▢▢▢ 8	
79 ___ -soybean .... ▢▢▢▢ 9	
80 ___ jicama .... ▢▢▢▢ 10	

Rue	1 2 3 4	
81 ___ lemon .... ▢▢▢▢ 1	I
82 ___ orange .... ▢▢▢▢ 2	
83 ___ tangerine .... ▢▢▢▢ 3	
84 ___ grapefruit .... ▢▢▢▢ 4	
85 ___ lime .... ▢▢▢▢ 5	
Spurge	
86 ___ curry .... ▢▢▢▢ 6	
87 ___ tapioca (cassava) ...... ▢▢▢▢ 7	
Cashew	
88 ___ -cashew .... ▢▢▢▢ 8	
89 ___ -pistachio .... ▢▢▢▢ 9	
90 ___ mango .... ▢▢▢▢ 10	
Maple	
91 ___ -maple sugar .... ▢▢▢▢ 1	J
Buckthorn	
92 ___ grape .... ▢▢▢▢ 2	
Mallow	
93 ___ okra .... ▢▢▢▢ 3	
94 ___ -cotton seed oil .... ▢▢▢▢ 4	
Sterculia	
95 ___ -chocolate (cocoa) ..... ▢▢▢▢ 5	
Theaceae	
96 ___ -tea (green or black) ... ▢▢▢▢ 6	
Caricaceae	
97 ___ papaya .... ▢▢▢▢ 7	
Myrtle	
98 ___ clove .... ▢▢▢▢ 8	
Carrot	
99 ___ carrot .... ▢▢▢▢ 9	
100 ___ celery .... ▢▢▢▢ 10	
101 ___ parsnip .... ▢▢▢▢ 1	K
102 ___ caraway .... ▢▢▢▢ 2	
103 ___ dill .... ▢▢▢▢ 3	
104 ___ parsley .... ▢▢▢▢ 4	
Heath	
105 ___ blueberry .... ▢▢▢▢ 5	
106 ___ cranberry .... ▢▢▢▢ 6	
Oleaceae	
107 ___ -olive .... ▢▢▢▢ 7	
Flaxseed	
108 ___ -flaxseed oil .... ▢▢▢▢ 8	
Canola	
109 ___ -canola oil .... ▢▢▢▢ 9	
Algae	
110 ___ kelp .... ▢▢▢▢ 10	

ª, ᵇ See Side 1 for explanation of footnotes.

Prime Test is a trademark of Advanced
Health Center, 34146 Selva Road, #200,
Monarch Beach, California 92629, USA
Phone (714) 661-4001 ©1988 Rev. 1/95

Prime Test™

Designed to facilitate accurate nutritional counseling. Not for diagnosis of disease.

Name _____

Control Number _____

Date _____ **Panel G**

Side 3

Nightshade   1 2 3 4
- 111 ___ potato .... ☐☐☐☐ 1 ⌐L
- 112 ___ eggplant .... ☐☐☐☐ 2
- 113 ___ tomato .... ☐☐☐☐ 3
- 114 ___ -tobacco .... ☐☐☐☐ 4
- 115 ___ chili pepper .... ☐☐☐☐ 5
- 116 ___ paprika .... ☐☐☐☐ 6
- 117 ___ bell pepper .... ☐☐☐☐ 7

Nightshade — Mint
- 118 ___ peppermint .... ☐☐☐☐ 8
- 119 ___ sage .... ☐☐☐☐ 9
- 120 ___ basil .... ☐☐☐☐ 10
- 121 ___ rosemary .... ☐☐☐☐ 1 ⌐M
- 122 ___ marjoram .... ☐☐☐☐ 2
- 123 ___ sage .... ☐☐☐☐ 3
- 124 ___ oregano .... ☐☐☐☐ 4
- 125 ___ thyme .... ☐☐☐☐ 5

Nightshade — Morning Glory
- 126 ___ yellow sweet potato .... ☐☐☐☐ 6
- 127 ___ "yam" (maroon sweet potato) .... ☐☐☐☐ 7

Nightshade — Pedaliaceae
- 128 ___ -sesame .... ☐☐☐☐ 8

Madder
- 129 ___ -coffee .... ☐☐☐☐ 9
- 130 ___ -decaffeinated coffee ... ☐☐☐☐ 10

Gourd
- 131 ___ cucumber .... ☐☐☐☐ 1 ⌐N
- 132 ___ zucchini squash .... ☐☐☐☐ 2
- 133 ___ yellow neck squash .... ☐☐☐☐ 3
- 134 ___ scallop squash .... ☐☐☐☐ 4
- 135 ___ butter nut squash ..... ☐☐☐☐ 5
- 136 ___ banana squash .... ☐☐☐☐ 6
- 137 ___ acorn squash .... ☐☐☐☐ 7
- 138 ___ pumpkin .... ☐☐☐☐ 8
- 139 ___ cantaloupe .... ☐☐☐☐ 9
- 140 ___ watermelon .... ☐☐☐☐ 10

Bellflower
- 141 ___ iceberg lettuce .... ☐☐☐☐ 1 ⌐O
- 142 ___ romaine lettuce .... ☐☐☐☐ 2
- 143 ___ artichoke .... ☐☐☐☐ 3
- 144 ___ chamomile tea .... ☐☐☐☐ 4
- 145 ___ sunflower seed .... ☐☐☐☐ 5

Birch
- 146 ___ -filbert .... ☐☐☐☐ 6

Sapucaya
- 147 ___ -Brazil nut .... ☐☐☐☐ 7

Protea
- 148 ___ -macadamia nut .... ☐☐☐☐ 8

Linden
- 149 ___ linden flower tea .... ☐☐☐☐ 9

Dillenia   1 2 3 4
- 150 ___ kiwi fruit .... ☐☐☐☐ 10

Ginger
- 151 ___ turmeric .... ☐☐☐☐ 1 ⌐P

Myrtle
- 152 ___ allspice .... ☐☐☐☐ 2
- 153 ___ clove .... ☐☐☐☐ 3

Araliaceae
- 154 ___ -ginseng .... ☐☐☐☐ 4

Mollusks
- 155 ___ -scallop .... ☐☐☐☐ 5
- 156 ___ -oyster .... ☐☐☐☐ 6
- 157 ___ -clam .... ☐☐☐☐ 7

Crustaceans
- 158 ___ -shrimp .... ☐☐☐☐ 8
- 159 ___ -lobster .... ☐☐☐☐ 9
- 160 ___ -crab .... ☐☐☐☐ 10

Cartilaginous Fish
- 161 ___ -shark .... ☐☐☐☐ 1 ⌐Q

Bony Fish
- 162 ___ -sardine .... ☐☐☐☐ 2
- 163 ___ -salmon .... ☐☐☐☐ 3
- 164 ___ trout .... ☐☐☐☐ 4
- 165 ___ catfish .... ☐☐☐☐ 5
- 166 ___ cod .... ☐☐☐☐ 6
- 167 ___ bass .... ☐☐☐☐ 7
- 168 ___ -tuna .... ☐☐☐☐ 8
- 169 ___ -butter fish .... ☐☐☐☐ 9
- 170 ___ -swordfish .... ☐☐☐☐ 10
- 171 ___ halibut .... ☐☐☐☐ 1 ⌐R
- 172 ___ sole .... ☐☐☐☐ 2
- 173 ___ perch .... ☐☐☐☐ 3
- 174 ___ mahi mahi .... ☐☐☐☐ 4

Poultry
- 175 ___ chicken .... ☐☐☐☐ 5
- 176 ___ -chicken egg .... ☐☐☐☐ 6
- 177 ___ turkey .... ☐☐☐☐ 7
- 178 ___ -duck .... ☐☐☐☐ 8

Mammals
- 179 ___ -pork .... ☐☐☐☐ 9
- 180 ___ -beef .... ☐☐☐☐ 10
- 181 ___ -cows' milk .... c ☐☐☐☐ 1 ⌐S
- 182 ___ -butter .... ☐☐☐☐ 2
- 183 ___ -cheese mix .... ☐☐☐☐ 3
- 184 ___ -yogurt .... ☐☐☐☐ 4
- 185 ___ -lamb .... ☐☐☐☐ 5
- 186 ___ rabbit .... ☐☐☐☐ 6
- 187 ___ -goats' milk .... ☐☐☐☐ 7

Other   1 2 3 4
- 188 ___ -honey .... ☐☐☐☐ 8
- 189 ___ bee pollen .... ☐☐☐☐ 9
- 190 ___ -spirulina .... ☐☐☐☐ 10
- 191 ___ aloe vera .... ☐☐☐☐ 1 ⌐T
- 192 ___ pau d'arco tea .... ☐☐☐☐ 2
- 193 ___ psyllium seed .... ☐☐☐☐ 3
- 194 ___ tap water .... ☐☐☐☐ 4
- 195 ___ amaranth .... ☐☐☐☐ 5
- 196 ___ quinoa .... ☐☐☐☐ 6

Cleaning Agents
- 197 ___ Ivory soap .... ☐☐☐☐ 7
- 198 ___ Dial Gold soap .... ☐☐☐☐ 8
- 199 ___ Neutrogena soap .... ☐☐☐☐ 9
- 200 ___ Shaklee Basic H .... ☐☐☐☐ 10
- 201 ___ Amway LOC .... ☐☐☐☐ 1 ⌐U

Chemicals
- 202 ___ -BHT .... ☐☐☐☐ 2
- 203 ___ -sodium bisulfide .... ☐☐☐☐ 3
- 204 ___ -formaldehyde .... ☐☐☐☐ 4
- 205 ___ -aspirin .... ☐☐☐☐ 5
- 206 ___ -Tylenol .... ☐☐☐☐ 6
- 207 ___ -Ibuprofen .... ☐☐☐☐ 7
- 208 ___ -saccharin .... ☐☐☐☐ 8
- 209 ___ -Equal (aspartame) ..... ☐☐☐☐ 9
- 210 ___ -MSG .... ☐☐☐☐ 10
- 211 ___ -food coloring .... ☐☐☐☐ 1 ⌐V
- 212 ___ -phenol .... ☐☐☐☐ 2
- 213 ___ -natural gas extract ... ☐☐☐☐ 3
- 214 ___ -petroleum by-products .... ☐☐☐☐ 4

Airborne Allergens
- 215 ___ dust .... ☐☐☐☐ 5
- 216 ___ grass pollen mix .... ☐☐☐☐ 6
- 217 ___ tree pollen mix .... ☐☐☐☐ 7
- 218 ___ mold .... ☐☐☐☐ 8
- 219 ___ cat danders .... ☐☐☐☐ 9
- 220 ___ dog danders .... ☐☐☐☐ 10

c See Side 1 for explanation of footnotes.

The Prime Test does not disclose IgE type allergies. IgE allergies are a common cause of airborne allergies and an uncommon cause of food or chemical allergies.

Prime Test is a trademark of Advanced Health Center, 34146 Selva Road, #200, Monarch Beach, California 92629, USA Phone (714) 661-4001 ©1988 Rev. 1/95

Prime Test™

Designed to facilitate accurate nutritional
counseling. Not for diagnose of disease.

Name _____

Control Number _____

Date _____   **Panel D**

Total Reactions _____   Side 2

Controls

	1 2 3 4	
1 ___ negative control .... ▢▢▢▢ 1	A
2 ___ positive control .... ▢▢▢▢ 2	

Fungus

| 3 ___ -yeast mix .... ▢▢▢▢ 3 |

Cereal Grains (Grasses)

| 4 ___ barley .... ▢▢▢▢ 4 |
| 5 ___ wheat .... ▢▢▢▢ 5 |
| 6 ___ rye .... ▢▢▢▢ 6 |
| 7 ___ oats .... ▢▢▢▢ 7 |
| 8 ___ rice .... ▢▢▢▢ 8 |
| 9 ___ millet .... ▢▢▢▢ 9 |
| 10 ___ -sugar cane .... ▢▢▢▢ 10 |
| 11 ___ corn (maize) .... ▢▢▢▢ 1 | B |

Palm

| 12 ___ -coconut .... ▢▢▢▢ 2 |

Farinosa

| 13 ___ pineapple .... ▢▢▢▢ 3 |

Lily

| 14 ___ asparagus .... ▢▢▢▢ 4 |
| 15 ___ onion .... ▢▢▢▢ 5 |
| 16 ___ garlic .... ▢▢▢▢ 6 |

Banana

| 17 ___ banana .... ▢▢▢▢ 7 |

Orchid

| 18 ___ vanilla .... ▢▢▢▢ 8 |

Pepper

| 19 ___ -black pepper .... ▢▢▢▢ 9 |

Buckwheat

| 20 ___ buckwheat .... ▢▢▢▢ 10 |

Pink

| 21 ___ beet .... ▢▢▢▢ 1 | C |
| 22 ___ spinach .... ▢▢▢▢ 2 |

Laurel

| 23 ___ -avocado .... ▢▢▢▢ 3 |

Brassica

| 24 ___ cabbage .... ▢▢▢▢ 4 |
| 25 ___ Brussels sprouts .... ▢▢▢▢ 5 |
| 26 ___ broccoli .... ▢▢▢▢ 6 |
| 27 ___ cauliflower .... ▢▢▢▢ 7 |
| 28 ___ mustard .... ▢▢▢▢ 8 |

Rose

| 29 ___ strawberry .... ▢▢▢▢ 9 |
| 30 ___ apple .... ▢▢▢▢ 10 |
| 31 ___ pear .... ▢▢▢▢ 1 | D |
| 32 ___ plum (prune) .... ▢▢▢▢ 2 |
| 33 ___ -almond .... ▢▢▢▢ 3 |
| 34 ___ peach .... ▢▢▢▢ 4 |
| 35 ___ apricot .... ▢▢▢▢ 5 |
| 36 ___ nectarine .... ▢▢▢▢ 6 |

Legume

	1 2 3 4	
37 ___ carob .... ▢▢▢▢ 7
38 ___ lentil .... ▢▢▢▢ 8
39 ___ split pea .... ▢▢▢▢ 9
40 ___ -peanut .... ▢▢▢▢ 10
41 ___ kidney bean .... ▢▢▢▢ 1	E
42 ___ pinto bean .... ▢▢▢▢ 2
43 ___ string bean .... ▢▢▢▢ 3
44 ___ navy bean .... ▢▢▢▢ 4
45 ___ lima bean .... ▢▢▢▢ 5
46 ___ mung bean .... ▢▢▢▢ 6
47 ___ pea .... ▢▢▢▢ 7
48 ___ chick pea (garbanzo) ... ▢▢▢▢ 8
49 ___ blackeyed pea .... ▢▢▢▢ 9
50 ___ -soybean .... ▢▢▢▢ 10
51 ___ alfalfa sprouts .... ▢▢▢▢ 1	F

Rue

| 52 ___ lemon .... ▢▢▢▢ 2 |
| 53 ___ orange .... ▢▢▢▢ 3 |
| 54 ___ grapefruit .... ▢▢▢▢ 4 |

Buckthorn

| 55 ___ grape .... ▢▢▢▢ 5 |

Sterculia

| 56 ___ -chocolate (cocoa) ..... ▢▢▢▢ 6 |

Theaceae

| 57 ___ -tea .... ▢▢▢▢ 7 |

Caricaceae

| 58 ___ papaya .... ▢▢▢▢ 8 |

Carrot

| 59 ___ carrot .... ▢▢▢▢ 9 |
| 60 ___ celery .... ▢▢▢▢ 10 |

Heath

| 61 ___ blueberry .... ▢▢▢▢ 1 | G |
| 62 ___ cranberry .... ▢▢▢▢ 2 |

Oleaceae

| 63 ___ -olive .... ▢▢▢▢ 3 |

Nightshade

| 64 ___ potato .... ▢▢▢▢ 4 |
| 65 ___ tomato .... ▢▢▢▢ 5 |
| 66 ___ -tobacco .... ▢▢▢▢ 6 |
| 67 ___ chili pepper .... ▢▢▢▢ 7 |
| 68 ___ bell pepper .... ▢▢▢▢ 8 |

Nightshade — Morning Glory

| 69 ___ yellow sweet potato ... ▢▢▢▢ 9 |
| 70 ___ "yam" (maroon sweet potato) ... ▢▢▢▢ 10 |

Nightshade — Pedaliaceae

| 71 ___ -sesame .... ▢▢▢▢ 1 | H |

Madder

	1 2 3 4	
72 ___ -coffee .... ▢▢▢▢ 2

Gourd

| 73 ___ cucumber .... ▢▢▢▢ 3 |
| 74 ___ winter squash .... ▢▢▢▢ 4 |
| 75 ___ summer squash .... ▢▢▢▢ 5 |
| 76 ___ cantaloupe .... ▢▢▢▢ 6 |
| 77 ___ watermelon .... ▢▢▢▢ 7 |

Bellflower

| 78 ___ lettuce .... ▢▢▢▢ 8 |
| 79 ___ -safflower oil .... ▢▢▢▢ 9 |

Crustaceans

| 80 ___ -shrimp .... ▢▢▢▢ 10 |
| 81 ___ -lobster .... ▢▢▢▢ 1 | I |
| 82 ___ -crab .... ▢▢▢▢ 2 |

Bony Fish

| 83 ___ -salmon .... ▢▢▢▢ 3 |
| 84 ___ cod .... ▢▢▢▢ 4 |
| 85 ___ bass .... ▢▢▢▢ 5 |
| 86 ___ -tuna .... ▢▢▢▢ 6 |
| 87 ___ halibut .... ▢▢▢▢ 7 |
| 88 ___ sole .... ▢▢▢▢ 8 |

Poultry

| 89 ___ chicken .... ▢▢▢▢ 9 |
| 90 ___ -chicken egg .... ▢▢▢▢ 10 |
| 91 ___ turkey .... ▢▢▢▢ 1 | J |

Mammals

| 92 ___ -pork .... ▢▢▢▢ 2 |
| 93 ___ -beef .... ▢▢▢▢ 3 |
| 94 ___ -cows' milk .... ▢▢▢▢ 4 |
| 95 ___ -lamb .... ▢▢▢▢ 5 |

Other

| 96 ___ -honey .... ▢▢▢▢ 6 |

Vitamins

| 97 ___ B-complex .... ▢▢▢▢ 7 |

Chemicals

| 98 ___ -BHT .... ▢▢▢▢ 8 |
| 99 ___ -sodium bisulfide .... ▢▢▢▢ 9 |
| 100 ___ -formaldehyde .... ▢▢▢▢ 10 |
| 101 ___ -aspirin .... ▢▢▢▢ 1 | K |
| 102 ___ Ivory soap .... ▢▢▢▢ 2 |
| 103 ___ -saccharin .... ▢▢▢▢ 3 |
| 104 ___ -Equal (aspartame) ..... ▢▢▢▢ 4 |
| 105 ___ -MSG .... ▢▢▢▢ 5 |
| 106 ___ -food coloring .... ▢▢▢▢ 6 |
| 107 ___ -petroleum by-products ... ▢▢▢▢ 7 |

Airborne Allergens

| 108 ___ dust .... ▢▢▢▢ 8 |
| 109 ___ mold .... ▢▢▢▢ 9 |
| 110 ___ pollen mix .... ▢▢▢▢ 10 |

Shared Experiences

I feel The Quality Longevity Program is of unquestionable benefit to me. The money was well spent. This program has brought relief where drugs could not. I believe in what you are doing and have recommended you to others.

Carrie Lynch, Irvine, California

It has been several months now since my white blood cell test, and I am so pleased and relieved. I want to thank you for the time you spent with me and for having the test available.

The most important result of the program for me is the absence of the headaches that have plagued me most of my life. One of the unexpected benefits is that my weight has returned to normal for the first time in twenty-five years. Before, I had fallen short of achieving my normal weight even when strictly dieting.

I now have the energy and desire to exercise. My husband says he can't keep up with me. This is all like a miracle to me because I have spent many years and dollars trying to gain better health.

Everywhere I go, people tell me how good I look. I know it because I feel so good.

Willa Blomgren, Friday Harbor, Washington

I wish to put in writing that the white blood cell testing was very beneficial to my allergy conditions.

During the spring I lived on pills to keep from sneezing and itching to death. After the testing I lived through spring without any pills. I didn't believe I could ever do that. I also needed less sleep and felt an increased motivation for physical exercise.

I've been to many doctors and have had skin tests and injections. Believe me, none of these helped half as much as the information I gained through white blood cell testing. You may send any government agency to me for further documentation. I was totally thrilled with this new insight to living!

Diane Hardison, Teacher, Newport Beach, CA

My first encounter with psoriasis was in 1960. In 1970 it had spread over 80% of my body. I saw many doctors and tried many remedies but nothing achieved any long-lasting positive results.

Last year my oncologist, after checking out The Quality Longevity Program, gave me the go-ahead to try white blood cell testing and the nutritional counseling program. Being a professional home economist, I thought I already ate well, but I went ahead and approached this new system of eating with a positive attitude. Within six weeks my skin had cleared by 90%! Amazing! A wonderful side benefit was the loss of 25 pounds. My doctor was as delighted as I was and totally approved of the food plan, no matter what the ailment.

Because my food plan omitted dairy products, I was concerned about my body's calcium level. My doctor furnished me with the following encouraging blood test results. Before the program: Calcium 9.3, Triglycerides 152, Glucose 93, Cholesterol 195. After being on the program: Calcium 9.5, Triglycerides 119, Glucose 79, Cholesterol 169.

It has been 12 months since I changed my eating patterns, and I plan to stick with it. Even though 10% of the time I make "moderate exceptions," I have kept my weight down, stayed healthy and feel good. My psoriasis is 95% clear, which is the longest and best clearing I've had in 10 years.

I advise anyone with psoriasis to try the program. You have nothing to lose (except a lot of scales, aggravation and excess weight) and everything to gain — good health!

Arlene Harrison, Bellevue, Washington

Thank you for helping me and my family to improve our standard of health.

Before we arrived in California, we suffered for years from various health problems including continual colds, flus, overweight and fatigue. I never realized our frequent infections and illnesses were directly related to our eating habits and resulting weakened immune systems.

I learned a great deal from working with you and saw how much I was helping other people. The specialized nutritional counseling together with the testing is definitely a most useful and beneficial health aid. My conventional learning in nutrition was constructively and logically rebuilt. In doing this, I regained my good health.

Linda Rubin, Laboratory Supervisor
Tustin, California

Chapter 6

Understanding Your Complete Blood Count and Blood Chemistry Levels

The test called Complete Blood Count (CBC) reveals your total number of white blood cells. You have several different types of white blood cells, also called leukocytes. Your report gives you their individual names and what percent of the total white blood cells the different types are.

The report also reveals your total number of red blood cells, also called erythrocytes, and their condition.

The "normal ranges" listed on your test reports are not averages from healthy people but are averages of all the people who have taken these tests in the past several years. Many of those people were not healthy; thus, the normal, or Average Ranges, often do not reflect good health.

For some tests, calling the ranges "normal" inaccurately implies that the level indicates health. No large-scale tests have been run on fully healthy people — those free from infections and delayed allergic reactions and a lifetime of eating the improper balance of macronutrients (fats, proteins, carbohydrates) and cholesterol. Different laboratories often have different ranges.

The Optimum Ranges that follow are the best estimates available to help you maximize your health. If any of your results are out of the Optimum Ranges, it is important to correct nutritional errors, obtain follow-up tests and listen carefully to knowledgeable professional advice. Be careful of the numbers used by most traditional doctors and the media — they do not reflect the latest scientific research.

To help you compare your levels and measure your progress, transfer the numbers from your past, present and future tests into the boxes to the right of the Optimum Range numbers. Record the dates of your tests in the boxes below. Using the correct principles for eating, combined with regular aerobic exercise, should rapidly move your blood levels into the Optimum Ranges and keep them there.

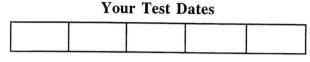

Your Test Dates

YOUR WHITE BLOOD CELLS

1. **WBC** is the abbreviation for White Blood Cells.

You have approximately one white blood cell for every 800 red blood cells. Your white blood cells have the ability to identify problems in your body and to correct them. They search out, attack and kill bacteria and viruses. They identify your body's damaged or sick cells and remove them. Every day they are searching out pre-cancerous cells and eating them so they do not multiply.

When your white blood cells are healthy, they are your main defense against infection and cancer.

Problems that cause a very low white blood cell count are: typhoid, chronic infections, mononucleosis, some cancers, various drugs, and delayed allergic reactions to foods and chemicals which kill white blood cells.

When foods or chemicals damage and kill the white blood cells, it is called a cytotoxic reaction. Avoiding hidden food allergies and performing regular aerobic exercise will help strengthen your white blood cells. When you are eating your compatible foods, your white blood cell count may be low because there is less need for them to work on allergic reactions.

A high white blood cell count often indicates a battle is going on in your body between your white blood cells and some type of bacteria. White blood cell counts often go up shortly after a food allergy reaction and slowly drop to below "normal" levels. However, if you have been running a low white blood count and get an infection, it may increase your levels to the mid-range. See items 9 through 15 for further information on the different types of white blood cells.

The range is measured in thousands per cubic millimeter.
Average Range
4.8 through 10.8

Optimum Range — estimated

3.7 through 10.8					

YOUR RED BLOOD CELLS

2. **RBC** is the abbreviation for Red Blood Cells.

Low red blood cell counts are referred to as anemia. Low counts are caused by several different problems, including: impaired red blood cell production, internal bleeding, poor iron assimilation, lack of aerobic exercise and damage caused by food and chemical allergy reactions.

Production may also be depressed by allergic reactions. Removing allergic exposures and enjoying regular aerobic exercise helps to bring up a low red blood cell count.

Delayed food and chemical allergies and eating over 10 percent of total calories in fat will cause the red blood cells to stick together, creating blood sludging and poor circulation. Avoiding allergic reactions and excess fat and adding aerobic exercise improves circulation.

The range is measured in millions per cubic millimeter, for male (M) and female (F).
Average Range
M 4.6 through 6.2
F 4.2 through 5.4

Optimum Range — estimated

M 5.0 through 6.4					
F 4.8 through 5.8					

3. **HgB** and **HB** are abbreviations for Hemoglobin.

HgB relates to the oxygen-carrying capacity of the blood. The ability of your hemoglobin to carry oxygen is chemically destroyed by carbon monoxide from cigarette smoke, vehicle exhausts, natural gas appliance fumes, etc. Low levels indicate a reduced oxygen-carrying capacity and high levels cause blood sludging

and increased stroke risk. The function and level are improved by breathing clean air free of any cigarette smoke and other chemical pollution, avoiding delayed allergic reactions and by doing aerobic exercise every day.

The range is measured in grams per deciliter which is abbreviated as Gm/dl.
Average Range
M 14 through 18
F 12 through 16

Optimum Range — estimated

M 14 through 14.9					
F 12 through 13.9					

4. **HcT** is the abbreviation for Hematocrit.

HcT is that percent of your blood which is made up of red blood cells. Most of the remainder is serum. In addition, there are small amounts of life-saving white blood cells and platelets.
Average Range
M 42 through 52%
F 37 through 47%

Optimum Range — estimated

M 42 through 52%					
F 37 through 47%					

5. **MCV** is the abbreviation for Mean Corpuscular Volume.

MCV relates to the size of the red blood cell. The red blood cells may become enlarged when allergic reactions are occurring and may then have difficulty circulating through the small capillaries.

The range is measured in cubic microns.
Average Range
M 80 through 94
F 79 through 97

Optimum Range — estimated

M 80 through 94					
F 79 through 97					

6. **MCH** is the abbreviation for Mean Corpuscular Hemoglobin.

MCH indicates the weight of hemoglobin in

each red cell and is often low when the hemoglobin is low. See preceding item 3.

The range is measured in picograms.
Average Range
27 through 35

Optimum Range — estimated

27 through 35					

7. **MCHC** is the abbreviation for Mean Corpuscular Hemoglobin Concentration. MCHC is the Mean Corpuscular Hemoglobin expressed in percentage.
Average Range
30% through 36%

Optimum Range — estimated

30% through 36%					

8. **PLATELETS**

The platelets help stop bleeding and are decreased by many drugs, including aspirin. A very high level may indicate cancer. Platelets often stick together during delayed allergy reactions and this can create serious circulation problems and cause the release of the chemical serotonin; thus, upsetting blood and brain chemistry. Platelets are measured in thousands.
Average range
150 to 450

Optimum range — estimated

150 to 450					

TYPES AND PERCENTAGES OF YOUR WHITE BLOOD CELLS

9. **LYMPHOCYTE**

This type of white blood cell should be a lower percentage than neutrophils (item 11). It is damaged in delayed allergy reactions and its quantity should increase by avoiding foods and chemicals which are not compatible with your body and by doing aerobic exercise.
Average Range
30% through 38%

Optimum Range — estimated

30% through 38%					

10. **MONOCYTE**

This type of white blood cell is damaged by delayed allergic reactions. Its quantity and condition should be improved by avoiding delayed allergic reactions and by doing aerobic exercise.
Average Range
0% through 6%

Optimum Range — estimated

0% through 6%					

11. **NEUTROPHILS** are also segmented neutrophils or polys.

Neutrophils are the type of white blood cells which suffers the most damage during delayed allergy reactions. Their quantity, vitality and percentage often increases when avoiding delayed food and chemical allergies and by doing aerobic exercise.
Average Range
50% through 62%

Optimum Range — estimated

50% through 62%					

12. **EOSINOPHILS**

This type of white blood cell is sometimes increased when allergic acute reactions are prevalent.
Average Range
0% through 5%

Optimum Range — estimated

0% through 3%					

13. **BASOPHIL**

It is a type of white blood cell which is sometimes increased with delayed allergic reactions and with pregnancy. Avoiding delayed allergic reactions, or having the baby, should decrease a high percentage.
Average Range
0% through 2%

Optimum Range — estimated

0% through 1%					

14. **STAB** is one name for Band Neutrophil.

The stab is a young, immature, segmented neutrophil.
Average Range
0% through 5%

Optimum Range — estimated

0% through 5%					

15. **OTHER** is short for Other Immature White Blood Cells.
Average Range
0% through 3%

Optimum Range — estimated

0% through 3%					

16. **CELL MORPHOLOGY** relates to a visual examination of the blood cells and comments are made regarding variations. Examples are: (a) Normal (b) Anisocytosis refers to a variation in the size and hemoglobin content of your red blood cells, (c) Poikilocytosis refers to abnormalities in the shape of your red blood cells, (d) Schisocytes refers to fragments of red blood cells.

Cell condition					

BLOOD CHEMISTRY

Your blood has four major components: white blood cells, red blood cells, platelets and plasma. The plasma is a clear liquid that contains chemicals and enzymes. It also carries your blood cells throughout your body. After your blood is centrifuged, the clotting factors are removed from your plasma and the remainder is called serum.

The serum is the transparent liquid that remains after the white blood cells, the red blood cells and the platelets have been removed. The blood chemistry test is done on the serum part of your blood and reveals the chemical balances and metabolic processes of your body and can discover several diseases.

This test is also called SMAC because it is often run on a SMAC computer, or a Chem 24 because it gives 24 different reports on your blood chemistry.

The average American range is often called "normals," but is often different from the healthy Optimum Range, due to years of improper diet. The "normals" or "Average Ranges" can be a clear danger signal.

Remote groups of people who eat differently and have blood tests in the Optimum Ranges throughout their lives are free from the ailments that are the major killers of Americans and Europeans. The Optimum Ranges can be obtained when you are free of food and chemical allergies and are balancing the macronutrients calories at 5 to 10 percent fat, 10 to 15 percent protein and 80 percent complex carbohydrates. Enzyme levels in the blood should decrease when allergic reacting foods and chemicals are discovered and removed. See the explanation after item 4, below.

1. **GLUCOSE**
This level measures blood sugar in the serum. This is the primary test for diabetes, and may also indicate liver or kidney problems. Fasting blood sugar levels above 110 indicates diabetes. By avoiding delayed allergic reactions and other harmful foods your blood sugar levels should not become elevated or depressed. In addition, your insulin works more efficiently when you are avoiding damaging vegetable oils and animal fats. Therefore, your fasting blood sugar level stays in the Optimum Range.

The range is measured in milligrams per 100 milliliters and is abbreviated mg/100 ml. This is sometimes reported in milligrams per deciliter, which is abbreviated as mg/dl.
Average Range
65 through 100

Optimum Range — estimated

65 through 85					

2. **BUN** is the abbreviation for BLOOD UREA NITROGEN and is a normal metabolic waste.

This is a measure of the kidney's ability to rid the body of the waste products from protein metabolism. Slight elevations indicate excessive protein intake. Marked elevations indicate kidney disease. When protein is 10 to 15 percent of total calories, there is a desirable decrease in your blood urea nitrogen.

The range is measured in mg/dl.

Average Range
10 through 25

Optimum Range — estimated

10 through 15					

3. CREATININE is a normal metabolic waste.

This is a much more sensitive measure of kidney function, which is independent of protein ingestion. Elevations indicate kidney disease. The range is not affected by diet.

It is measured in mg/dl.
Average Range
0.7 through 1.3

Optimum Range — estimated

0.7 through 1.3					

4. BUN / CREATININE RATIO

The ratio of BUN to creatinine is an index of kidney function. This ratio will become smaller as the BUN decreases with decreased protein intake.
Average Range
10 through 35

Optimum Range — estimated

10 through 25					

ENZYME LEVELS IN YOUR BLOOD

The next four tests, AST (SGOT), ALT (SGPT), LDH and alkaline phosphatase are measures of enzyme levels in the blood serum. When there is a rise in an enzyme level, it reflects tissue damage. When cells are killed their enzymes are released into the blood serum. If any one of the first three, AST (SGOT), ALT (SGPT) or LDH is elevated or there is any history of allergic symptoms, taking the Prime Test is indicated because destruction of white blood cells releases enzymes into the serum.

The Optimum Range for enzymes has to be estimated because no studies have been done on groups of people free from delayed food and chemical allergies.

Not all allergic reactions cause the type of damage which releases enzymes; however, if the enzymes are elevated, it is probable that allergic reactions are taking place.

5. AST (SGOT)

AST is an enzyme contained in all your body cells, including your white blood cells and red blood cells. Very high levels indicate a recent heart attack, liver disease or muscle failure. If you are at the high end of this range, the Prime Test is indicated. AST is also elevated following ingestion of aspirin, codeine, or cortisone. A gradual decrease will occur when foods and chemicals that are damaging to your body are avoided.

The range is measured in international units per liter at 37° C. and is abbreviated to U/L.
Average Range
0 through 41

Optimum Range — estimated

0 through 25					

6. ALT (SGPT)

ALT is an enzyme which is not contained in white blood cells but is contained in red blood cells. Very high levels indicate a recent heart attack, liver disease or muscle failure. Red blood cells are affected to a lesser degree than white blood cells by allergic reactions. However, if you are in the upper end of this range, the Prime Test is indicated. A gradual decrease will occur when foods and chemicals that are damaging your body are avoided.

The range is measured in U/L at 37° C.
Average Range
0 through 45

Optimum Range — estimated

0 through 25					

7. LDH

White blood cells contain the LDH enzyme. When they are destroyed in a white blood cell reaction, your LDH level goes up and the white blood cell count goes down. Greatly elevated levels indicate heart or lung damage or muscle failure. If you are at the high end of this range, the Prime Test is indicated for delayed food and chemical allergies. A gradual decrease will often occur when the foods and chemicals damaging to your body are avoided for several weeks.

The range is measured in U/L at 37° C.

Average Range
60 through 175

Optimum Range — estimated

40 through 100					

8. G. G. T.

G. G. T. is the abbreviation for Gamma Glutamyl Transforase. It is sometimes abbreviated to G. G. T. P.

This enzyme goes up when there is damage to the liver. The alcohol in one beer will cause this level to go up. This test is often used to screen for alcohol abuse.

The range is measured in U/L at 37° C.
Average Range
0 through 65

Optimum Range — estimated

0 through 30					

9. TOTAL BILIRUBIN

This test measures liver function or the breakdown products of red blood cells. Elevated values indicate liver disease or hemolytic anemia. The range is not usually affected by diet.

The range is measured in milligrams per decaliter and is abbreviated as mg/dl.
Average Range
0.1 through 1.2

Optimum Range — estimated

0.1 through 1.2					

10. ALKALINE PHOSPHATASE

Elevation of this enzyme reflects liver, gall bladder or bone disease. Elevations also indicate increased bone metabolism while growing or during the healing of a fracture. The range is not affected by diet.

It is measured in U/L at 37° C.
Average Range (adult)
30 through 110

Optimum Range (adult) — estimated

50 through 110					

11. TOTAL PROTEIN

This level indicates the total protein content of the serum. A very high or very low level indicates numerous ailments. The Optimum Range is slightly reduced from the Average Range when eating properly.

The range is measured in grams per deciliter which is abbreviated as Gm/dl.
Average Range
6.8 through 8.5

Optimum Range — estimated

6.0 through 8.0					

12. ALBUMIN

Albumin is one of two major proteins in the serum. Marked elevations or depressions indicate numerous ailments. The Optimum Range is slightly reduced from the Average Range when eating properly.

The range is measured in Gm/dl.
Average Range
3.2 through 5.0

Optimum Range — estimated

3.0 through 4.7					

13. GLOBULIN

This is the other major protein measured in the serum; when added to the albumin you get the total protein. Elevations are seen in malignancies and infections. Not diet affected.

It is measured in Gm/dl.
Average Range
1.5 through 3.5

Optimum Range — estimated

1.5 through 3.5					

14. A / G RATIO

This is an abbreviation for the albumin to globulin ratio. Changes in this ratio reflect numerous diseases, particularly malignant diseases. The range is slightly affected by diet.
Average Range
1.1 through 2.5

Optimum Range — estimated

1.1 through 2.5					

15. URIC ACID

This level measures the by-products of protein metabolism. High levels may reflect anemia, leukemia or eating excessive animal protein. This can cause gout, which seriously damages your joints. By temporarily avoiding most animal products, high uric acid levels often drop rapidly.

The range is measured in mg/dl.

Average Range
M 4.0 through 8.0
F 2.0 through 6.5

Optimum Range — estimated

M 3.0 through 6.0					
F 2.0 through 5.0					

16. TOTAL CALCIUM

This level is very sensitive to hormonal and metabolic changes. It is maintained by your body very rigidly between the levels of 9 and 10.5. Abnormal levels may indicate parathyroid disorder or bone disease. The blood calcium level is not usually changed by calcium in the diet; however, bone calcium levels are improved by a low protein diet and by avoiding delayed food and chemical allergies.

The range is measured in mg/dl.

Average Range
9 through 10.5

Optimum Range — estimated

9 through 10.5					

17. PHOSPHORUS — SERUM

Phosphorus and calcium are in dynamic equilibrium and therefore complement each other. As the phosphorus goes up, the calcium level comes down and vice-versa. The blood phosphorus range is not usually changed by diet.

The range is measured in mg/dl.

Average Range
2.5 through 4.5

Optimum Range — estimated

2.5 through 4.5					

18. SODIUM

Sodium is an electrolyte and the level is maintained by your body within the boundaries of 135 to 148. Changes reflect metabolic and hormonal disturbances. Your blood levels of sodium are not changed much by eating salt. The damage of a high salt and high sodium diet is not reflected in the serum sodium.

The range for electrolytes is measured in milliequivalent per liter and is abbreviated mEq/L.

Average Range
135 through 148

Optimum Range — estimated

135 through 148					

19. POTASSIUM — SERUM

Like sodium, potassium is an electrolyte and the level is maintained by your body within very specific levels of 3.3 through 5.8. Your blood levels of potassium are not changed much by eating it, but reflects kidney function and other metabolic processes.

The range is measured in mEq/L.

Average Range
3.3 through 5.8

Optimum Range — estimated

3.3 through 5.8					

20. CHLORIDE

Like sodium, chloride is an electrolyte and is maintained by your body within very specific limits. It is governed primarily by the metabolism of your body and elevations outside of the normal levels reflect some form of metabolic disturbance. Your blood levels of chloride are not changed much by eating salt (sodium chloride).

The range is measured in mEq/L.

Average Range
95 through 110

Optimum Range — estimated

95 through 110					

21. CARBON DIOXIDE

The carbon dioxide level is a by-product of metabolism and is the indicator of acidity of the blood. An increase in carbon dioxide indicates a decrease in acidity. The range is not affected by diet.

The range is measured in mEq/L.

Average Range
24 through 30

Optimum Range — estimated

24 through 30					

22. ANION GAP

This is a calculation between your positive and negative electrolytes. When out of the normal range, it is likely your sodium, potassium, chloride or carbon dioxide are out of their proper range.

Average Range
0 through 25

Optimum Range — estimated

0 through 25					

23. TRIGLYCERIDE

This blood fat is very sensitive to dietary intake. Elevated levels increase the risk of degenerative diseases such as atherosclerosis, heart disease and diabetes. Your triglyceride level can be used with your cholesterol level and age to predict accurately the amount of artery damage.

A high triglyceride level falls rapidly by avoiding all vegetable oils and animal fats above 10 percent of total calories. It is also important to avoid refined carbohydrates, sugars, honey, dried fruits, fruit juice and to eat only small amounts of fresh fruit. Triglyceride levels remain low with proper diet and regular aerobic exercise.

The range is measured in mg/dl.

Average Range
30 through 175

Optimum Range

30 through 100					

24. TOTAL CHOLESTEROL

This level reflects the sum of dietary cholesterol and cholesterol made by the body. Elevated levels put you at great risk from artery damage called atherosclerosis and the resulting

degenerative diseases. High cholesterol levels will drop rapidly when less than 1 ounce of fish or fowl is eaten a day while avoiding all dairy products, eggs and red meats. This amount represents about 20 milligrams of cholesterol a day. The western industrialized diet contains around 500 milligrams a day, derived from dairy products, eggs and red or white meat.

There are different types of cholesterol: high density lipoprotein, low density lipoprotein and very low density lipoprotein. These factors have a small secondary importance; however, the most important factor is having your blood cholesterol level below 150. Having your high density lipoprotein (HDL) above 30 percent of your total blood cholesterol level is of some help when your total level is over 150.

When your blood cholesterol is under 150 and stays there for a few years, your chance of having a heart attack falls to nearly zero. The American Heart Association claims your blood cholesterol level is fine if it is under 200. However, 20 percent of heart attacks happen between 150 and 200. This misinformation helps millions of people to have unnecessary heart attacks each year. People almost never have a heart attack if their blood cholesterol level is under 150. Healthy babies are born around 70.

Total cholesterol decrease is a good indicator of how well the 10-10-80 balance works. Dangerously high cholesterol levels — those above 150 — drop dramatically during the first month and continue to improve by eating under 20 milligrams of cholesterol per day. After your blood level is under 150 you can keep it there, in most cases, by not eating more than 80 milligrams — about four bites of fish or fowl — a day. It is helpful to read the information on pages 55 and 78 and the charts on 60 and 61.

The range is measured in mg/dl.

Average Range
150 through 330

Typical inaccurate recommendations:

Desirable: less than 200
Borderline: 200 — 239
High risk: 240 or more

Optimum Range

70 through 150					

25. IRON

A low level indicates an iron storage problem or anemia. A high level indicates excess iron in the diet, or a liver malfunction such as Hemochromatosis, or elevated red blood cell level such as Polycythemia.

The range is measured in micrograms per deciliter and is abbreviated mcg/dl.

Average Range
40 through 175

Optimum Range — estimated

40 through 175					

26. DIRECT BILIRUBIN

Bilirubin is left over from broken down red blood cells. This is a more specific test of liver function and the liver's capacity to handle bile pigments. Elevated levels indicate liver disease or gall bladder disease. The range can be effected by delayed food allergies.

The range is measured in mg/dl.

Average Range
0.0 through 0.5

Optimum Range — estimated

0.0 through 0.5					

27. INDIRECT BILIRUBIN

This is a measure of red blood cell breakdown as well as liver function. Elevations indicate hemolytic anemia, gall bladder disease, or liver disease. The range is not usually affected by diet but delayed food allergies can break down red blood cells. This test is often not run unless the total Bilirubin indicates a problem.

It is measured in mg/dl.

Average Range
0.1 through 1.2

Optimum Range — estimated

0.1 through 1.2					

Summary

There are several CBC and Blood Chemistry results that relate to the Prime Test, and it is desirable to have the three done at the same time so comparisons can be made and a baseline can be established.

The Average Ranges are from the Massachusetts General Hospital and the Medical Science Institute in Los Angeles, and are often mistakenly referred to as "normals."

If some of your diet-affected blood levels on the CBC and Blood Chemistry report are out of the Optimum Range, it is desirable to have them re-checked after you have corrected your diet for one month. If some of the values that are not related to diet are out of the Optimum Range, it is desirable to get re-tested sooner to see if it was a temporary body condition or a testing problem with your blood sample. If the variations repeat, it is important to discover the cause. Many problems contribute to delayed food and chemical allergies.

Helpful Reading

The first books to read are Dr. Randolph's *An Alternative Approach to Allergies* and *Dr. Mandell's 5 Day Allergy Relief System*. Avoid Randolph's and Mandell's recommendations to eat high fat and high cholesterol foods. Also avoid their suggestion to fast. There are often lasting problems caused by fasting. For fasting to bring about reliable food testing results, it must be done in a specially designed facility that is free of chemicals, pollens, molds, etc. During the fast, the only liquid consumed must be non-contaminated water. Serious withdrawal symptoms can come up during the fast which need specialized help. Damaging reactions may show up after people eat a food allergic to them, and they may need assistance to deal with the discomfort.

Other helpful books on delayed food and chemical allergies are: *The Food Sensitivity Diet* by Doug Kaufmann and Racquel Skolnik; *Dr. Berger's Immune Power Diet,* by Stuart Berger, MD; *Brain Allergies, The Psychonutrient Connection* by William Philpott, MD, and Dwight Kalita, PhD; *The Yeast Connection* and *Solving the Puzzle of Your Hard-to-raise Child* by William G. Crook, MD; *Food Allergy and Intolerance* by Jonathan Brostoff, MD, and Linda Gamlin; *Nutritional Medicine* by Stephen Davies, MD, and Alan Stewart, MD; *The E. I. Syndrome* by Sherry A. Rogers, MD, and *Allergies and the Hyperactive Child* and *Is This Your Child?* by Doris Rapp, MD. For more help read *The Allergy Self-help Book* and *The allergy Self-help Cookbook* by Sharon Faelten.

Read about delayed chemical allergies in,

Why Your House May Endanger Your Health by Alfred V. Zamm, MD. Also read, *Your Home, Your Health and Well Being* by David Rousseau, William J. Rea, MD, and Jean Enwright.

After you have a solid understanding of the importance of avoiding delayed food and chemical allergies, read the books which explain how to avoid and reverse degenerative diseases. These ailments and many of the benefits of the 10–10–80 balance are explained in the books, *Live Longer Now* by Jon Leonard, J. L. Hofer and Nathan Pritikin; *The Pritikin Program* and *The Pritikin Permanent Weight Loss Manual* by Nathan Pritikin; *The McDougall Plan for Super Health and Life-Long Weight Loss* by John McDougall, MD; *Reversing Heart Disease* and *Reversing Diabetes* by Julian Whitaker, MD, and *Dr. Dean Ornish's Program for Reversing Heart Disease* by Dean Ornish, MD. Avoid the recommendations of these degenerative disease specialists to eat a repetitious diet made up primarily of allergy-causing cereal grains.

Eating right does not work without exercise, both aerobic and strength. Read *The New Aerobics* by Kenneth Cooper, MD, and *Fit or Fat* by Covert Bailey. Find a good gym and trainer.

The animal studies done on longevity have shown that reducing the total number of calories significantly, as much as 40 percent, has reduced the incidence of disease and dramatically increased life span. Because this has worked with a broad range of animals, there is every reason to believe it will work with humans. If it turns out not to work for humans, there are no negative side effects, and you will be slender and have the extra money you would have spent on food. The best way to eat fewer calories is to eat less fat and protein. You do this naturally by taking advantage of the 10–10–80 part of The Quality Longevity Program. Two good books to read about the advantages of lowering your caloric intake are *Maximum Life Span* and *The 120 Year Diet* by Roy L. Walford, MD.

The importance of sunlight is well presented by Zane R. Kime, MD, in his book *Sunlight Could Save Your Life*. A good book to read about health problems caused by the different types of sugars is *Lick the Sugar Habit* by Nancy Appleton, PhD.

The best health magazines to read regularly are *Longevity* and *Lets Live*. Most of the other health magazines and health letters are promoting obsolete information or have been taken over by traditional medical doctors. One of the least competent magazines to evaluate health issues is *Consumer Reports*. It's traditional doctors did not understand the importance of the 10–10–80 balance of macronutrients when they reviewed Pritikin's work. Later, they were totally lost when they commented on delayed food allergies.

Most university health letters are written to support traditional medical approaches and keep their medical graduates employed.

After following The Quality Longevity Program for several weeks, your body should be greatly strengthened by your improved eating and exercise. You may be tempted by your improved health to eat carelessly. You may also be encouraged to go back to the old ways of eating by well-meaning but uninformed people who do not believe that delayed food allergies exist and are just in your mind.

Acknowledge the rewards of your efforts and avoid the mistake of crediting your successes to something else. Our bodies give us valuable information only when we understand how to read it. We then have the power to become healthy.

The first few times you reintroduce a food to which you are still allergic, you may get a stimulant reaction and wrongly believe the food is fine for you. If you are stimulated by a damaging food, you may not notice that your health is starting to decline.

This approach to health is difficult during the first few weeks as you learn how to prepare new foods and eat differently. Some new foods may not be your favorites; however, they often become enjoyable. By staying on The Quality Longevity Program, you continue to improve your health and add years to your life span.

The harder I work the more I live,
I rejoice in life for its own sake.
Life is no brief candle...
To me it is a sort of splendid torch
which I have got hold on for the moment...
I want to make it burn as brightly as possible
before handing it on to the future generations.

George Bernard Shaw
Dramatist, Essayist and Critic — 1856 to 1950

Chapter 7

The Helpful Science of Fats, Proteins, Carbohydrates, Cholesterol and Alcohol

Over the last 50 years, there has been a great deal of public awareness of how vitamins and minerals, the micronutrients, operate in our bodies. However, very little public awareness exists of how fats, proteins and carbohydrates work in our bodies. These are the macronutrients. They are the major components of our foods and have a great impact on our health. The wrong balance of these major components causes a broad range of ailments throughout the human body.

Information about all the health problems caused by dietary fats began to reach the public several years ago. However, some of this information was dangerously wrong. Fortunately, there are now comprehensive research studies available on how fats operate inside our bodies.

There are two basic categories of fats: saturated fat, which is solid at room temperature, and unsaturated fat, which is liquid at room temperature.

Saturated Fat

Saturated fat causes several health problems. It is concentrated in foods from animals such as red meat, fish, fowl, eggs and dairy products. Saturated fat also comes from a few vegetables, such as coconut oil and palm oil.

Saturated fat clogs up our circulation by staying in our blood for about six hours after we eat it. By that time, our bodies have either deposited the fat in our fat cells or in lumps along our artery walls. A small amount is converted into glucose for energy. When saturated fat comes from animals it contains cholesterol. It also contains toxins, because the animal's body concentrates and stores pesticides, chemicals, antibiotics and hormones in the fat cells. When we eat animal fat, we concentrate the animal's toxins throughout our bodies.

Saturated fat creates additional problems because it causes our liver to produce more cholesterol. Saturated fat thus accelerates the build-up of blockages in all of our arteries. It is a major cause of impaired circulation, degenerative diseases plus a major factor in obesity.

Vegetable Oil

Most people have been told that eating vegetable oil is good for your health and we can eat up to 30 percent of our total calories from fat, so long as the fat is primarily made up of vegetable oil. However, this belief has been shown to be false, and diets based on this belief have turned out to be deadly.

One missing piece of information is that all types of vegetable oil take nine hours to clear out of our blood. This type of fat stays in our circulation for *three hours longer* than saturated fat before our bodies can clean it out of the blood and store it in fatty tissue. During the time vegetable oil is in the blood, it coats our red blood cells, causing them to stick together and clog up our circulation. This deprives our bodies of the oxygen they desperately need. Because vegetable oil, which includes the monounsaturated and polyunsaturated types, stays in the blood longer, it clogs up circulation longer, and this accelerates a number of disease processes.

Vegetable oil is 100 percent fat and it helps to think of it as plant fat. As bad as saturated fats are, we are better able to clear them from our circulation.

In many cases, cancer gets started because the cells are deprived of oxygen. Vegetable oil increases your risk of coming down with cancer more than saturated fat. The advice to switch from saturated animal fat to polyunsaturated vegetable oil has turned out to be very dangerous: we need to avoid them both.

When you look at the fat and cancer charts on pages 58 and 59, you see that the Israelis and South Africans have much more cancer than would be expected for the amount of fat they eat. This is happening because the medical profession and government in Israel have been very successful at selling people on switching from animal fat to vegetable oil. In South Africa the cancer rate is higher than expected because peanuts grow easily, are cheap and are thus a large part of the diet. Peanuts are 70 percent fat when measured by calories. Notice that many Italians and Portuguese are also in trouble: olive oil is a big part of their diet.

When you look at the research on vegetable

oil, you can see why so many health professionals are confused. When people eat more vegetable oil and less animal fat, their blood cholesterol levels go down. This looked good, but they did not ask where the cholesterol was going. Researchers later found that the vegetable oil was coating the walls of the arteries and making them sticky. The cholesterol was going out of the blood, where it is an *indicator* of potential artery damage, and imbedding in the artery walls, where it *does* the damage.

Studies using animals have been done to try to find a vegetable oil that does not cause the build up of these blockages, called plaques, in the arteries. They tried combining each type of vegetable oil with a little cholesterol and then feeding it to test animals. They discovered that all types of oils, when combined with a little cholesterol, caused severe blockages to develop.

One oil was more damaging than the rest. Peanut oil caused the plaques to grow larger, faster. The researchers had no idea why. I suspect that peanuts, and thus peanut oil, were as highly allergic for the test animals as they are for humans. This may have caused inflammation in the walls of the arteries and thus promoted the rapid growth of blockages.

There are other serious problems caused by vegetable oils. Removing the oil from the vegetable turns about 15 percent of the oil into trans fats, and trans fat are the same cancer-causing type created when you turn vegetable oil into margarine.

We have no enzymes in our bodies to break down trans fats, and there is no way our bodies can use them in making healthy cells. Trans fats are mistakenly incorporated by our cells and become part of the wall of our cells. The trans fats do not fit correctly in the cell wall and this causes the cells to leak. It does not make any difference whether it's safflower oil, sunflower oil, olive oil, canola oil or any other oil. All of them develop trans fats when they are processed, sometimes as much as twenty percent of the total oil.

If unsaturated fats aren't good for us and saturated fats aren't good for us, what is good for us? Well, what is good for us is the level of fats we get when we eat primarily fresh vegetables and other complex carbohydrates. If you eat fresh vegetables and other complex carbohydrates, your diet turns out to be around 10 percent total calories in fat. This level of fat is what our bodies can handle without causing health problems.

In order to obtain this level of fat, there are a few animal products and vegetables to avoid. Red meats are around 60 percent fat by calories after you have trimmed off all the visible fat. Eggs are 65 percent fat and most dairy products are between 30 and 100 percent fat. Nuts and seeds are around 75 percent fat, peanuts and avocados are 70 percent fat and soy is 35 percent fat. It is the total percentage of fat that is important, not whether the fat is monounsaturated or polyunsaturated.

It is important to measure fat by percentage of total calories; otherwise, you can easily be mislead. When fat is measured as a percent of the total *weight* of a food, the numbers look low because most foods have much of their weight made up of the water that is in them. As an example, low-fat dairy products look low in fat because they claim 2 percent fat on the label. That is 2 percent fat by weight, but in reality it is 30 percent fat by calories. When an advertisement claims a product is 98 percent fat free, it may be 30 percent fat by calories and thus dangerously high in fat.

Some people worry that if they don't get enough fat in their diets they will get sick. There are no cases on record of people's having health problems because of a fat deficiency. Our bodies can make different types of fats, called fatty acids, from the carbohydrates we eat, except for one. It is called an essential fatty acid and its name is linoleic acid. This fatty acid must come from our diet.

How much linoleic acid we need from our diet was carefully researched when scientists studied how to put together a diet for astronauts who were going to travel through space. They needed to know this because they had not been able to invent a toilet that would work in space and thus had to put together a diet that would fulfill all nutritional requirements, without anything being left over, so the astronauts would not have any bowel movements.

Careful studies showed that when only *one* percent of a person's total calories was from fat and that fat was high in linoleic acid, all their fat requirements were fulfilled.

It is virtually impossible to have your dietary fat level below five percent, even if you eat all vegetables. However, special synthetic diets have been put together which have one percent fat. People have been put on these special ultra-low-fat diets for years without causing health problems.

The special diet powder was called Vivonex and it was going to be given to astronauts. However, someone invented a toilet that would work in zero gravity and the diet was never used in space. The diet powder was then used to help children who were unable to metabolize one of the amino acids. These children grew well and their health improved dramatically when eating ultra low-fat and low-protein Vivonex.

There are some special fats which do help the immune system. They are called omega three and omega six fatty acids. These are the kinds of special fats that are in mothers' milk. We received them from our mothers if we nursed. The omega three fatty acid is found in flaxseed oil. It is often helpful to take small amounts of the omega six fatty acid from evening primrose oil or borage oil. However, the supplementation needs to be at very low levels. These fatty acids can be utilized much more effectively when the rest of the diet is very low in fat. Therefore, the 10 percent fat diet, with some of these supplements, can help the immune system without damaging circulation.

Some think fish oil being is health building because of studies done on Eskimos; however, there are complications with fish oil. You would have to take such high amounts that the oil would cause health problems because it would add to total fat consumed. Also, fish oil is often contaminated with pesticides and toxins like PCB.

Heart disease problems experienced by Eskimos and everyone else can be prevented by eating a 10 percent fat diet with a maximum of 80 milligram a day of cholesterol. Adding fish oil to an inherently unhealthy diet causes problems.

We need a very small amount of the essential oil called linoleic acid for our bodies to function properly. We get over ten times the amount of linoleic acid we need on a diet that contains 10 percent of its total calories in fat.

One of the additional complications of fat is that it turns rancid very quickly. As an example, when peanuts are ground to make peanut butter, oxygen contacts the oil in the peanuts and the oil starts to become rancid. This is true of all vegetable oils and the fat from animals.

We can detect the rancid problem with fish oil, because when it is exposed to oxygen, the fish starts to rot and we can smell it. Unfortunately, when vegetable oil starts to become rancid, it is hard to smell it, so you don't have a good way of detecting it. However, it starts to become rancid immediately, and

within days of being processed there is a significant amount of rancidity in all oils.

Rancidity creates free radicals and these molecules contribute to cancer, heart disease and other health problems. The free radicals travel through our bodies like x-rays, damaging cells. Thus, rancid oils and fats create additional health problems throughout our bodies. Reduce free radicals by avoiding added fats.

Research done in 1991 by Darshan Kelley, PhD, has shown that as we eat less fat, our immune system becomes stronger. The improved immune function was measured by the increased performance of people's white blood cells.

Proteins

Proteins are used as building blocks by our bodies. However, if we take in too many of these building blocks, we create serious health problems. When our bodies cannot use the proteins, they have to be converted to either carbohydrates or fats. They cannot be stored as we store fat in fat cells. When our bodies process proteins, several toxic chemicals are created. Two of these chemicals are ammonia and ketone. These chemicals are very hard on the filtration system of our bodies — the liver and kidneys.

The damage caused to the kidneys by protein has been clearly demonstrated in studies with people who already have damaged kidneys. In the past, when people had kidney failure, they would either die, go on a kidney machine or have a kidney transplant. All three approaches have serious drawbacks. Now, people can eat no more than ten percent total calories from protein and prevent kidney failure. They stay in good health with their remaining kidney function.

There is now overwhelming evidence that every time you eat excess protein you are causing some damage to your kidneys. This damage will often not be apparent for most people until they are over fifty years old.

High-protein diets and even moderate-protein diets diminish our essential mineral levels. When we eat protein, an acid residue is left in the body. This acid residue has to be neutralized, otherwise, the acidity would break down our cells. The body does this by drawing calcium out of our bones and other minerals out of our tissues to offset the acid condition. After the acid has been neutralized, many of these minerals are lost with our urine. Thus, people on the typical Western European and American diet already have significant bone loss by the time they are in their thirties and forties. By the time they are in their fifties, sixties, or seventies, their bones are starting to break with normal activity. This is a very significant problem for women because they start out with less bone mass in the first place. However, too much protein damages everyone's bones and causes the loss of numerous vital minerals.

We need protein for building and repairing our bodies. But, do we need 70 to 140 grams of protein per day? That is the amount in the Standard American Diet.

When we go back to the study done by NASA for their astronauts, it was found that people were healthy on seven percent of total calories from protein or about 30 to 40 grams of protein a day. This is about half the amount of the Standard American Diet and enables people to grow well and be healthy without protein deficiency or protein toxicity.

The public has been heavily pressured into believing that more protein is better. Most people believe there is a world protein shortage. This is not true. There is a calorie shortage, and what people need are complex carbohydrates, not more proteins and fats. We do not want a worldwide campaign to catch and raise foods that are high in protein. People need to grow and eat foods high in complex carbohydrates. These foods are the natural energy-providing fuels for the body, and they have all the protein and fat in them needed for great health.

For years it was thought that different foods had to be eaten together so we would receive the proper balance of amino acids. We were told to combine beans and corn and to combine dairy products with other foods to make the amino acids complete. This has turned out to be untrue.

The food designed for rapid growth of human infants is mothers' milk. When you study the amino acid balance of mother's milk you discover it is very similar to the amino acid balance of fresh vegetables. Thus, a diet high in fresh vegetables gives people the ideal amino acid balance. You don't need to combine your beans and corn or add dairy products to your vegetables to get the best amino acid balance.

Carbohydrates

The remaining major component of our diet is carbohydrates. Carbohydrates come in two basic forms: simple and complex.

Simple carbohydrates are white sugar (cane or beet), brown sugar, honey, corn fructose, glucose, lactose and the sugars that are in fruit and vegetable juices. They are assimilated very quickly by the body so that when we eat simple carbohydrates, they overwhelm the body's sugar balance. Our bodies must turn these sugars into fat very rapidly, or they will damage our cells. The fat is then deposited all over our bodies.

What we do not need for energy is a flood of simple carbohydrates into our bodies. A sugar flood causes a rebound reaction that leaves us with low blood sugar. We need an even and constant flow of blood sugar from complex carbohydrates as they are slowly digested. When we eat fresh vegetables and other complex carbohydrates, they break down slowly as they go through the digestive tract over the next several hours. The energy keeps flowing into our blood stream over an extended period of time, giving us energy until the next meal.

An analogy is what happens when you pour fuel directly into your carburetor — you flood the engine and it dies. However, if you meter it in slowly from the gas tank and through the carburetor, the car runs fine.

The human body runs very much the same way. Pour the sugar in by eating sweetened foods or fruit juices and you will flood your body and damage your health. With complex carbohydrates, energy flows into your body slowly over an extended time, and you do not run into the problems of overloading your body with sugar. Your body runs smoothly, and you have continuous energy until it is time to eat again.

Dr. Sanchez did a study at Loma Linda University which discovered one of the ways sugar affects our immune system. After giving people complex carbohydrates, he measured how well people's white blood cells ate germs. The cells worked fine. When he gave people white sugar he noticed their white blood cells got sick and they could not eat the germs as fast as the germs would multiply.

He then tried brown sugar, fructose, glucose, honey and orange juice and found that all these simple carbohydrates made peoples' white blood cells get sick and slow down. What have we been giving children when they catch a cold virus? Orange juice! When you make juice out of oranges you cause their sugar to be rapidly absorbed by the body.

Many people have observed that they feel sick after eating sugar, and think they are allergic to the sugar. That happens; however, they may be suffering a more severe allergic reaction to the food they ate along with the sugar. This can happen because their white blood cells are made weaker by the sugar and thus, more die when they eat the delayed allergy-causing food.

When we eat meals high in complex carbohydrates, portions need to be larger because these foods have a high water content. Thus, we get to eat significantly larger portions and three meals a day including a couple of compatible snacks. This keeps energy flowing into our bodies throughout the day.

When we eat proteins and fats and they are metabolized by our bodies, numerous toxic by-products are formed. Our organs have to work hard to free us of these toxins.

Complex carbohydrates are metabolized easily and cleanly by our bodies. When they are broken down the energy they provide is utilized. There are two non-toxic by-products; one is carbon dioxide which we exhale away; the other is water which we sweat and urinate away.

Our bodies are designed to run on complex carbohydrates. They are the best source of energy, they give our muscles the fuel to move and our brain the energy to think clearly. We need a diet that has about 80 percent of total calories from complex carbohydrates.

Cholesterol

Another item in our diet surrounded with a great deal of misunderstanding is cholesterol. Cholesterol is referred to as a lipid; however, when you look at the scientific structure of cholesterol, you see that it is a crystal and not actually a fat. These crystals are like little pieces of very thin broken glass, square in shape and microscopic in size.

The cholesterol crystals in our blood have very sharp edges and pass through the inner wall of our arteries. It is like having a piece of broken glass under the skin of your finger.

The cholesterol crystals begin to cut and tear the delicate inner walls of our arteries. Our bodies build up fatty deposits around the sharp cholesterol crystal to protect itself. The fat and cholesterol become a lump or fatty deposit. These lumps grow in the walls of our arteries, cutting off our circulation and causing heart attacks and impaired circulation throughout our bodies.

In the United States alone, heart disease kills someone every 32 seconds. That equals a fully loaded 747 airplane crashing every three hours. If that many 747s were crashing, the plane would be grounded immediately and not used until it was changed. The Standard American Diet needs to be changed. The minor changes recommended by the American Heart Association have been proven by their own research studies to fail at lowering the fat and cholesterol intake enough to be of any real value. This has misled some to believe that changing diet is of little help.

Heart attacks are now so common they are considered a natural part of aging. In fact, it is entirely abnormal to have a heart attack — you have to eat excess fat and cholesterol for over thirty years before you can have one. By starting The Quality Longevity Program now, you can start cleaning out your arteries and dramatically reduce your chances of ever having a heart attack.

The amount of cholesterol we need is fully provided by our bodies' own production of cholesterol. There is no need to eat cholesterol.

One of the old arguments against a very low cholesterol diet is that we won't be able to build the hormones we need to have children. The Chinese are on a very low cholesterol diet, and there is no indication that they are having a problem reproducing. People are free of most degenerative diseases in the areas of the world where they eat virtually no cholesterol at all. Their glands work fine, and the people are prolific.

Can we eat cholesterol and be healthy? Yes we can. Our bodies are able to tolerate around 80 milligrams of cholesterol a day without our levels of blood cholesterol becoming dangerously high. If our blood levels are already high — above 150 — we need to eat less than 80 milligrams a day for a while to offset having over-eaten cholesterol in the past. In that case, we need to eat around 25 milligrams or less a day until we lower our blood levels under 150.

There is a great deal of misunderstanding about cholesterol. There are three different ways cholesterol is bound together in our blood: high density lipoproteins, low density lipoproteins, and very low density lipoproteins. The high density lipoproteins, known as HDL cholesterol, are thought to be the good cholesterol. Actually, cholesterol is cholesterol, and the HDL cholesterol is bound up in a way that does not cause damage to the arteries as does the low density lipoproteins (LDL) cholesterol.

LDL implants cholesterol rapidly into the walls of the arteries. Thus, people with a high level of LDL cholesterol have more heart disease than people who have high HDL cholesterol. However, research in Japan shows that high HDL levels deposit cholesterol in the skin. The correct goal is to have low HDL and very low LDL.

The emphasis needs to be on having your total blood cholesterol level under 150, not on your HDL and LDL cholesterol. When you are using the best approach for lowering your blood cholesterol, the 10–10–80 balance, you are doing what works best to bring about the optimum levels of HDL and LDL.

The most important steps are: eating a diet containing less than 25 milligrams of cholesterol a day until your blood cholesterol is under 150, and then eating under 80 milligrams; and avoiding saturated fats and vegetable oils by eating a diet with around 10 percent of its total calories derived from fat and performing regular aerobic exercise. These steps are necessary for lowering your blood cholesterol under 150, and they also support other areas of your health.

The cholesterol chart on page 61 is from the Framingham Study. It shows the blood cholesterol levels of people when they died. Notice that about 20 percent of the people who died of coronary artery disease had blood cholesterol levels between 150 and 200. There is a lower death rate when people are between 150 and 200; however, the death rate is still very high. Notice there are *no* deaths from coronary artery disease when the blood cholesterol levels are under 150.

The goal is to have your blood cholesterol

level under 150. How low can you go and still be healthy? When we look for remote groups of people that do not have heart disease, we find a few groups that have been carefully studied. One is the Tarahumara Indians in central Mexico. These people have a diet that is around ten percent fat, ten percent protein, eighty percent complex carbohydrate and very little dietary cholesterol.

The Tarahumara Indians have great endurance, regularly running a 50 mile foot race. When their blood cholesterol levels were measured, they averaged around 70 milligrams. All of the evidence shows that you can be fully healthy if your blood cholesterol level is between 70 and 150. Most people build blockages in their arteries at 160, and virtually everybody builds blockages at 170 and above.

There is one group of people who have very low levels of blood cholesterol and are very sick. People with advanced cancer often have low blood cholesterol levels because cancer cells lose the ability to make their own cholesterol and have to obtain their cholesterol from the blood. It may help to starve out cancer cells by having very low levels of blood cholesterol.

One reason why some health professionals are confused about blood cholesterol and diet is that when you are on the Standard American Diet, you can dramatically increase your dietary cholesterol, causing your blood cholesterol to go up a small amount or even go down a small amount. You can even cut your dietary cholesterol in half and see very little change. This happens because most people's digestive tracts become saturated starting at around 200 milligrams of dietary cholesterol a day. The Standard American Diet has around 500 milligrams a day. If you add a dozen eggs to your daily diet you are eating around 3000 milligrams a day; however, you are still *absorbing* only 200 milligrams a day because most people's digestive tracts can not absorb any more cholesterol.

If you cut the standard 500 milligrams of dietary cholesterol a day in half you are then eating 250 milligrams but you are still absorbing around 200 a day. To keep your blood cholesterol under 150 you need to eat no more than 80 milligrams a day. To get your blood cholesterol down to 150 you need to eat under 25 milligrams a day.

With all of the available evidence, why has the American Medical Association, the American Heart Association and the other associations of traditional doctors not given this information to you? One possible reason is that some of these people may not have done their homework. Another possible reason is that they figured the American public is simply not able to deal with the reality of how bad their diet is. Thus, they are trying to get the public to take a little step in the right direction.

People deserve the truth. Then, let them decide how many steps they want to take in the right direction. Let them know the scientific facts, instead of telling them they can eat 300 milligrams of cholesterol a day, and that a diet with 20 to 30 percent fat builds health.

There is no scientific evidence to support the high levels of cholesterol and fat currently recommended by the American Heart Association and the American Cancer Society. When most people know the truth, I believe a high percentage of them will take advantage of the health building 10–10–80 balance of nutrients. When a significant percentage of people become aware, most of the rest follow rapidly.

Another reason why the correct information about what makes a health building diet has not been given to the public is the influence of the industries which produce the damaging foods. When you look at the foods to be avoided, you see that the industries which produce those foods are some of the most powerful in the country. They are the dairy industry, the meat industry and the egg industry.

The dairy industry is one of the highest contributors to and manipulators of politicians, schools of nutrition, and the medical profession. The industry is trying to keep this health saving information from the public.

Once people learn what is truly optimum for their health, they see that dairy products, red meats, eggs and vegetable oils are obsolete. Industries which produce them are going to fall further into disrespect and financial hard times when people learn the truth and stop buying foods which damage their health.

Alcohol

The problems caused by drinking alcohol have filled books. Alcohol kills cells in the mouth, throat, stomach and small intestine. Then, by way of the circulatory system, cells throughout the body and brain are damaged and killed. Most cells are replaced, but some cannot be and are lost forever, such as brain cells. Do you have any brain cells you do not need?

When new chemicals are tested on animals to see if they are harmful, one important test is to see if any damage is done to fetuses. Any damage and the chemical is abandoned. In studies with humans, it was discovered that any alcohol consumed during pregnancy damages the fetus.

Deaths caused by drinking alcohol are more than 20 times greater than those caused by all illegal drugs combined.

The studies which suggest that one or two drinks a day help people avoid a heart attack and that drinkers are healthier than non-drinkers, are seriously flawed. They did not take into account that the people who did not drink were often sickly because they used to drink or had other health problems. One drink a day, or even one drink a week, often leads to severe alcohol addiction. Alcohol also contributes to delayed food and chemical allergies.

The chart on page 62 shows the wide range of allergy-producing foods and numerous chemicals which are in alcoholic beverages. Dr. Theron Randolph discovered in 1948 that alcohol addiction is a delayed allergy reaction. This breakthrough is just now being used to achieve a high success rate, for the first time, in helping alcoholics. Alcoholics Anonymous and other approaches which use group support and talk therapy, without the food addiction awareness, have less than a 20 percent success rate.

While you are working to improve your health, it is important to stay free of alcohol. All alcoholic beverages have traces of yeast left in them from the brewing process. When becoming free of alcohol, it helps to remember that alcohol is made by yeast eating a food and then excreting alcohol. Thus, alcohol is yeast urine.

Start taking correct steps toward great health. As you feel better you will want to take more steps. Preventive care helps you to feel great.

*Can you afford to live your life
as if there is nothing you do not know,
when knowing it would transform your life?*

Dietary Fat Is Shown To Be The Primary Cause Of Breast Cancer

There is the same direct cause and effect relationship for several other types of cancer and artery disease.

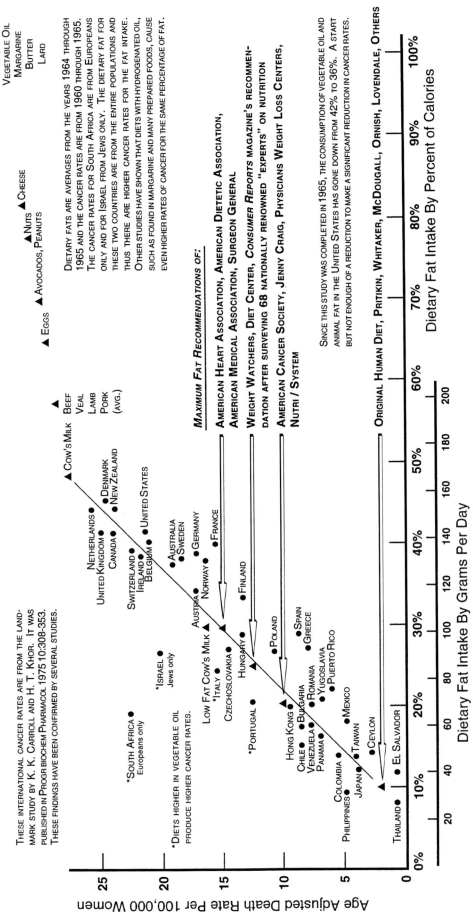

These international cancer rates are from the land-mark study by K. K. Carroll and H. T. Khor. It was published in Progr Biochem Pharmacol 1975 10:308-353. These findings have been confirmed by several studies.

Dietary fats are averages from the years 1964 through 1965 and the cancer rates are from 1960 through 1965. The cancer rates for South Africa are from Europeans only and for Israel from Jews only. The dietary fat for these two countries are from the entire populations and thus there are higher cancer rates for the fat intake. Other studies have shown that diets with hydrogenated oil, such as found in margarine and many prepared foods, cause even higher rates of cancer for the same percentage of fat.

Maximum Fat Recommendations of:

American Heart Association, American Dietetic Association, American Medical Association, Surgeon General

Weight Watchers, Diet Center, Consumer Reports magazine's recommendation after surveying 68 nationally renowned "experts" on nutrition

American Cancer Society, Jenny Craig, Physicians Weight Loss Centers, Nutri / System

Since this study was completed in 1965, the consumption of vegetable oil and animal fat in the United States has gone down from 42% to 36%. A start but not enough of a reduction to make a significant reduction in cancer rates.

Original Human Diet, Pritikin, Whitaker, McDougall, Ornish, Lovendale, Others

Age Adjusted Death Rate Per 100,000 Women

Dietary Fat Intake By Grams Per Day

Dietary Fat Intake By Percent of Calories

In Thailand, one woman out of one thousand develops breast cancer. In the United States, one woman out of *nine* develops breast cancer.

The above chart gives a clear picture of the importance of a very low-fat diet. When fat is 10 percent of total calories, breast cancer is almost nonexistent. At 20 percent fat, the chance of getting breast cancer goes up 300 percent. At 30 percent fat, there is an epidemic of breast cancer.

Notice the straight line relationship: women who eat more fat get more breast cancer.

During 1991 in the United States, 175,000 women discovered they had breast cancer; over 45,000 died. When used from infancy, a reduction of over 70 percent is possible by using only the low fat part of The Quality Longevity Program.

Breast feeding gives up to a 50 percent reduction. Genetics and avoiding pesticides are important, but dramatically lowering vegetable oil and animal fat intake and having healthy white blood cells are primary for preventing breast cancer. Stress and what we think are important, but they contribute little to what actually causes cancer.

Preventing cancer is more effective than trying to cure it. White blood cells continually attack pre-cancerous and cancerous cells. Cancer treatment should include testing for delayed food allergies.

Dietary Fat Is Shown To Be The Primary Cause Of Prostate Cancer

There is the same direct cause and effect relationship for several other types of cancer and artery disease.

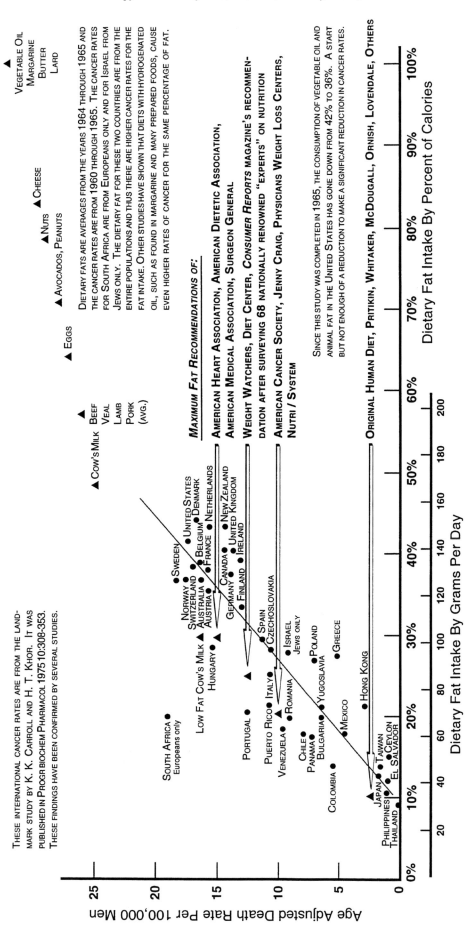

Prostate cancer is so common in men who eat the traditional American and European diet that 60 percent of the men who live to be 70 years old have it. The longer men stay on a "moderate" or high fat diet the greater their chance of developing prostate cancer. By the time these men reach 90, virtually 100 percent have this disease. More men would die of prostate cancer except for the fact it is slow growing and most men die first from heart disease or some other fat and cholesterol-caused disease.

In the United States in 1992, 165,000 men were diagnosed with prostate cancer and 35,000 died. All types of added vegetable oils contribute to prostate cancer and red meat and butter dramatically increase the chance of it being fatal. Elevated blood cholesterol levels, those above 150, add to the problem. The cholesterol crystals accumulate in the prostate and cut up the tissue.

Men need regular PSA blood tests, starting at age 50, for detecting this cancer. With accurate diet plus hormone treatments, most prostate cancer can be stopped and surgery can be avoided.

For men, women and children who want to avoid cancer and other degenerative diseases, 10 percent fat and less than 80 mg. of cholesterol a day are the only levels that work for each body size, shape and "type." Use preventive care and test.

Dietary Effect On Total Blood Cholesterol Levels

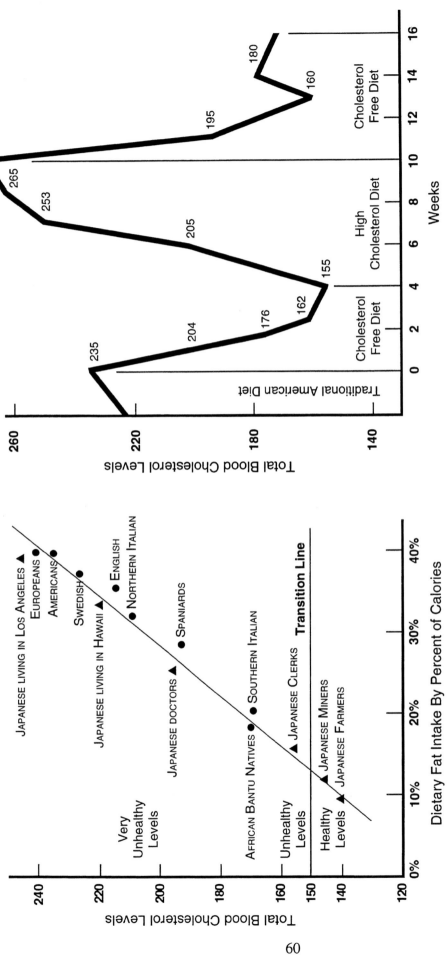

The chart on the left shows the effect of dietary fat on 1288 men, aged 40 to 49, from different countries. The amount of fat intake parallels the cholesterol intake, with those eating 10 percent fat also eating low cholesterol diets. Notice how blood cholesterol levels rise with increased fat intake, even for people from the same ethnic group (see Japanese and Italians). This study was done by Ancel Keys, MD, in 1958 and is titled "Lessons to be learned from serum cholesterol level."

There have been studies on 25 different cultures who's members eat around 10 percent fat and heart disease is virtually unknown. When some members of these groups started eating the Standard American Diet, they developed fatal heart disease and other degenerative diseases.

The chart on the right shows that when a study is designed properly, people can dramatically reduce their total blood cholesterol levels. Most studies reported in the popular press only reduce the daily intake from 500 milligrams of cholesterol to 200 or more. To achieve a change, the intake needs to be 30 milligrams or less. There are 10 studies which have confirmed these results.

A few people have low blood cholesterol levels even though they are eating high amounts of cholesterol and fat. This happens because they have impaired absorption, rapid transfer of the cholesterol from the blood to the arteries or a cancer that is eating their blood cholesterol.

Low Blood Cholesterol Levels Prevent Heart Disease

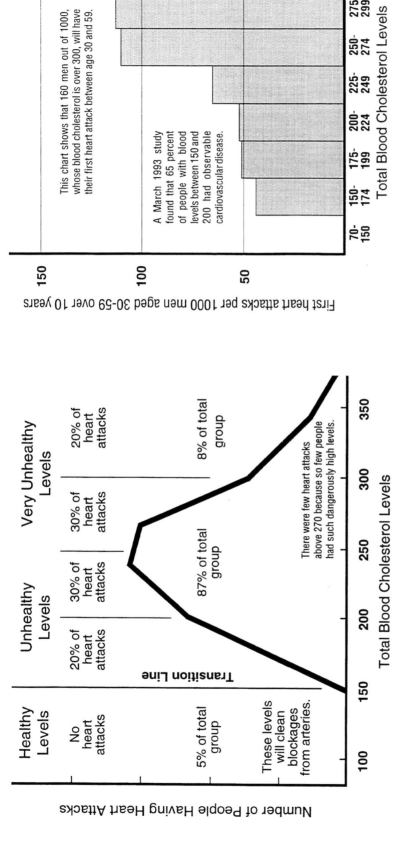

This chart shows that 160 men out of 1000, whose blood cholesterol is over 300, will have their first heart attack between age 30 and 59.

A March 1993 study found that 65 percent of people with blood levels between 150 and 200 had observable cardiovascular disease.

First heart attacks per 1000 men aged 30-59 over 10 years

Total Blood Cholesterol Levels

70-150 | 150-174 | 175-199 | 200-224 | 225-249 | 250-274 | 275-299 | Over 300

Healthy Levels — No heart attacks — 5% of total group — These levels will clean blockages from arteries.

Transition Line

Unhealthy Levels — 20% of heart attacks — 30% of heart attacks — 87% of total group

Very Unhealthy Levels — 30% of heart attacks — 20% of heart attacks — 8% of total group

There were few heart attacks above 270 because so few people had such dangerously high levels.

Number of People Having Heart Attacks

Total Blood Cholesterol Levels

The chart on the left is from the Framingham Study. It has been monitoring the health of all the people of Framingham, Massachusetts for more than 40 years to discover how to avoid heart attacks and the premature deaths they cause.

The research demonstrated there were no heart attacks when blood cholesterol levels were under 150. However, 20 percent had heart attacks between 150 and 200. The internationally renowned heart-disease specialist and director of the study, William Castelli, MD, stated that it is best to have your blood cholesterol under 150 if you want to avoid having a heart attack.

Many people under 150 had stressful lives, but none had heart attacks. Thousands die each month of heart attacks with their cholesterol in the "recommended" range of 150 to 200. Studies from around the world confirm these numbers.

The chart on the right combines the results of several major studies and confirms that the higher your blood cholesterol level is above 150, the greater your risk of heart attack. This is also true for several other degenerative diseases.

The above information has not been given to the American public by any medical association. Over half of the doctors treating degenerative diseases would be out of work if people ate properly. And health care costs would drop in half. Over 90 percent of the adults in America have cholesterol levels above 150 and most do not know they are in trouble.

In China the average cholesterol level is 127. Heart disease is almost unknown and stroke, cancer and other degenerative diseases are low.

Ignore the American Heart Association's unsupported recommendation that "You are fine if your blood cholesterol is under 200 and you can eat up to 300 milligrams of cholesterol a day and up to 30 percent of your calories in fat and be healthy."

Eating under 25 milligrams of cholesterol a day and around 10 percent of your calories from fat can lower your blood cholesterol to under 150. Then you will start to have healthy arteries. Later you can eat up to 80 milligrams of cholesterol a day while continuing to consume around 10 percent of your total calories from fat.

The Ingredients in Alcoholic Beverages

Most common source materials ... x   Less common or used in small amounts ... o

	Corn (a)	Barley (malt)	Rye	Wheat	Oats	Rice	Milo	Potato	Grape	Plum	Citrus	Apple	Pear	Apricot	Peach	Cherry	Berries	Carob	Hops	Juniper	Cinnamon	Mint	Misc. Herbs	Cactus	Milk	Chemicals	Egg	Beet	Cane	Yeast	Water
Whiskey — Straight																															
Corn	x	x	x	o	o	o	o																			o				x	x
Bourbon	x	x	x	o	o	o	o																			o				x	x
Malt	x	x	x	o	o	o	o																			o				x	x
Rye	x	x	x	o	o	o	o																			o				x	x
Wheat	x	x	o	x	o	o	o																			o				x	x
Whisky — Blended Straight																															
Corn	x	x	x	o	x	x	o																			o				x	x
Bourbon	x	x	x	o	x	x	o																			o				x	x
Malt	x	x	x	o	x	x	o																			o				x	x
Rye	x	x	x	o	x	x	o																			o				x	x
Rye-malt	x	x	x	o	x	x	o																			o				x	x
Wheat	x	x	x	x	x	x	o																			o				x	x
Whiskey																															
Blended	x	x	x	o	o	o	o	o	o	o	o	o	o	o	o	o	o	o								o		x	x	x	x
Light	x	x	x	o	o	o	o	o	o	o	o	o	o	o	o	o	o	o								o				x	x
Spirit	x	x	x	o	o	o	o	o	o	o	o															o		x	x	x	x
Canadian — Blended	x	x	x	x					x	x	o															o			x	x	x
Scotch — Unblended, all malt	o	x																								o		o	o	x	x
Scotch — Blended	x	x																								o		o	o	x	x
Irish — Unblended	x	x	x	x																						o			o	x	x
Irish — Blended	x	x	x	x	x				x	x	o															o		o	o	x	x
Alcohol																															
Grain	x	x	x	x	o	o	x																			o				x	x
Cane																										o			x	x	x
Fruit	o								x	x	x	x	x	x	x	x	x									o				x	x
Gin																															
Grain Spirits	x	x	x	o	o	o	x		x											x	o	o	x			o		o	o	x	x
Cane Spirits																				x	x	x	x			o			x	x	x
Flavored	x	x	x	x	x	x	x	x	x	x	x	x	x	x	x	x	x	x	x	x	x	x	x			o		x	x	x	x
Vodka																															
Domestic	x	x	x	x				x																		o		o	o	x	x
Imported, some	o	x						x																	o	o			x	x	x
Flavored	x	x	x	x	x	x	x	x	x	x	x	x	x	x	x	x	x	x	x	x	x	x	x			o		o	o	x	x
Rum																															
Domestic											x											o				o			x	x	x
Jamaican																										o			x	x	x
Miscellaneous																															
Akvavit			x					x			?											?				o		?	?	x	x
Saki						x																				o				x	x
Tequila																								x		o			x	x	x
Malt Beverages																															
Ale	x	x	o	o	o	x	o												x							x				x	x
Beer	x	x	o	o	o	x	o												x							x				x	x
Beer — Alcohol Free	x	x	o	o	o	x	o												x							x				x	x
Beer — Flavored	x	x	o	o	o	x	o		x	x									x							x				x	x
Wine																															
Grape	x								x																o	x	o	x	x	x	x

(a) Corn includes the grain entering the mash, the corn-steeped liquor upon which brewer's yeast is commonly grown and the corn sugar (dextrose) which is sometimes added to the manufacturing process. Items which claim to be made in California are required by law to be free of added sugars; however, corn and other sugars are often used to make the caramel that is often added.

This study was originally done in 1948 by Theron Randolph, MD. There have been several changes since then, especially the added use of allergy-causing chemicals — 75 are allowed in beer and 70 in wine. Unfortunately, the alcohol producers are very secretive and it is difficult to discover what the ingredients are. Expanded in 1991. Reprinted by permission of Dr. Randolph.

Chapter 8
Damaging Dairy Products

Dairy products are continuously promoted and have numerous health claims made for them. Most people have been told they need dairy products to be healthy. However, scientific studies tell a different story. These discoveries demonstrate a direct cause-and-effect relationship between dairy products and several diseases.

The following information can help you take an important step toward freeing yourself and your friends from the damaging misinformation surrounding dairy products. You will be empowered to improve your health and longevity.

People worry they will have a deficiency and become unhealthy if they do not eat dairy products. The calcium content of dairy products is used as their main selling feature.

A comprehensive bone calcium study was done by Dr. A. R. Walker. He studied native African women over 60 years old. The women had rarely if ever eaten dairy products and averaged only 300 milligrams of calcium a day from vegetables, yet none had calcium deficiencies or weak bones or teeth.

In contrast, young American women with no children, who eat the typical American diet heavy in dairy products with over 500 milligrams of calcium a day, suffer dangerous calcium loss from their bones, known as osteoporosis, and have weak teeth.

The more children a woman has, the more calcium she loses. The native women had no calcium deficiencies even though they had an average of nine children.

When some of the native women moved to cities and started eating dairy products and other high protein and processed foods similar to those eaten by most Americans, they also suffered significant calcium loss from their bones and teeth.

These native women were not biologically different from Americans; when they ate a damaging diet, they also developed weak bones and teeth. (*Clinical Science*, 1972, Vol 47.) People in Asia and South America who also eat a dairy-free, high-vegetable diet have solid bones and teeth.

In 1985, the dairy industry financed a study to convince the public that people who eat more dairy products assimilate more calcium. The study lasted two years and carefully measured the changes in 22 young women. The results surprised the dairy industry. Those who drank three additional glasses of milk a day lost twice as much calcium from their bones as did the study's control group.

Even the control group lost bone calcium while eating the high American level of dairy products. The dairy industry's own study revealed that dairy products do not build strong bones and actually cause calcium to be lost. (*American Journal of Clinical Nutrition*, 1985, Vol 41.)

The dairy industry now tries to diminish the importance of its own study. Fortunately, it was reviewed by Richard Mazess, PhD, who understood the study's important health message. (*American Journal of Clinical Nutrition*, 1985, Vol 42.)

The typical American is on a high-dairy diet, thus a high-calcium diet, and yet the average older American has weak, calcium-deficient bones. Over half the people in the world consume virtually no dairy products throughout their lives, yet have healthy bones in old age and no calcium deficiencies.

People lose calcium from their bones and other vital minerals from their entire bodies because the acid level of their blood becomes elevated. The body has to buffer the acid by giving up calcium from the bones and other important minerals from vital organs. High acid levels are caused by two major factors: excess protein in the diet and hidden or delayed allergic reactions. Dairy products are a major cause of both these problems.

Another reason dairy calcium is poorly retained in the bones is that most dairy products are high in phosphorus, and excess phosphorus causes demineralization. Vegetables are low in phosphorus and their calcium is easily assimilated. The original Eskimo diet was high in animal protein and phosphorus, and by the time most Eskimos were 45 years old, their bones were weak, brittle and calcium-depleted. This happened even though the Eskimos were consuming up to 2500 milligrams of calcium a day, which is more than three times the amount recommended by the traditional medical establishment.

People not eating dairy products and other allergy-causing foods, while avoiding a high protein diet, have strong bones and receive all the calcium they need from fresh vegetables.

Mothers' milk is low in calcium compared to cows' milk. A quart of mothers' milk has 300 milligrams of calcium, versus 1200 milligrams of calcium in a quart of cows' milk. Nature is telling us we need one fourth the calcium that calves need.

Even though cows' milk has four times the calcium of mothers' milk, it is not well assimilated. Infants actually retain more calcium in their bones when they drink an equal amount of mothers' milk.

There are a number of health problems caused by consuming excess calcium. It builds up in soft tissue throughout the body. This includes the arteries, where it adds to blockages and heart attacks. Calcium also makes arteries stiff and brittle, which leads to burst arteries and death. It also upsets cell function and heart function. Doctors try to reverse this with powerful drugs known as "calcium channel blockers."

Calcium builds up in the kidneys causing one of the most painful ailments humans suffer — kidney stones. The stones are made of calcium, and part of the traditional treatment is to stop eating dairy products. When people with kidney stones stay free of dairy products, they do fine. Most traditional doctors have missed the irony of recommending dairy products to most people and yet their kidney-stone patients are fine when they are free of dairy products and excess calcium.

The World Health Organization recommends that people eat 400 milligrams of calcium a day. The United States Government, after being pressured by the dairy industry, recommends 800 milligrams a day or more. Most Americans eat dairy products and thus are on a high-calcium diet. However, the majority of them over 60 years old still have weak bones and teeth. It is not the amount of calcium you eat which is most important to your bones and teeth, but the calcium you retain. Allergy-free meals which are moderate in protein make for strong bones. After a health-building start on breast milk, humans receive all the calcium they need from non-dairy foods.

Have you heard of any chimpanzees or gorillas with weak bones? These animals are very similar to humans and never eat dairy products, yet their bones are fine. Many veterinarians and pet owners have already caught on. Producers of quality dog and cat food have eliminated allergy-causing ingredients such as dairy products, wheat and soy.

The Impact of Dairy Products on Infants

Frank A. Oski, MD, Director of Pediatrics at Johns Hopkins University School of Medicine, led a team of scientists and medical doctors which completed several studies proving cows' milk causes severe damage to infants.

During the first two and a half years of life, infants go through their only period of rapid brain growth. Without sufficient iron, their brains do not grow to their full potential, and their opportunity for full brain growth is lost forever.

Dr. Oski found that most children consuming cows' milk suffer from internal bleeding along their digestive tracts. Even though the amount of bleeding is small, the loss of iron that is in the red blood cells is significant. The children's brains were not developing properly because they were drinking cows' milk. Dr. Oski has shown that mental capacity is permanently reduced if infants are fed dairy products and become iron deficient. (Dietary Iron: Birth to Two Years, Raven Press, 1989.)

Dr. Oski's research shows that children under two years old should not eat any dairy products, and all people would be healthier if they did not eat them. His research has been confirmed by scientists from around the world. His book, Don't Drink Your Milk, gives additional, well-documented evidence of the health damage caused by dairy products.

The ingredients in mothers' milk are very different from those in cows' milk, and human infants' nutritional needs are very different from calves' needs. Mothers' milk is part of the foundation of health necessary for a person's entire life.

Research done in England with 300 children, and published in the leading medical journal, The Lancet, in February 1992, discovered that infants fed mothers' milk "had a significantly higher IQ" compared to infants who were fed cows' milk. When the dairy-free children were eight years old they had IQs that were 10 percent higher than the children fed cows' milk. These children avoided iron losses as infants. Infants eating dairy products risk brain damage and continued blood and iron loss. Avoid infant products made with any dairy product.

A study done in Brazil compared cows' milk to mothers' milk. It showed that infant death rates went up over 11 times when children were fed cows' milk instead of mothers' milk. The healthiest babies were fed mothers' milk exclusively for a full year. (*The Lancet*, 1987, Aug 8.) Breast feeding is vital for infant health.

The medical literature is full of studies which demonstrate that cows' milk is the cause of a long list of ailments in infants and adults. Dairy industry pressure has kept this information buried and traditional medical doctors have been unaware accomplices.

A New Understanding of Allergy

The connection between cows' milk and allergy has been known for a long time. In 1936, scientists found that infants fed cows' milk had skin rashes (eczema) seven times more severe than those who were fed mothers' milk. The traditional type of allergy is called an acute allergy and affects only three percent of the population. Delayed allergic reactions are much more common and significantly impact over half of the population. This newly-understood delayed allergic reaction is the underlying cause of a broad range of symptoms.

Robert Zeiger, MD, PhD, at the Kaiser Medical Center in San Diego, headed a four-year study on the effect of cows' milk and other common allergy-causing foods on 103 pregnant women and their infants. The women avoided cows' milk, eggs and peanuts during their third trimester and while breast feeding. The infants had breast milk exclusively for the first six months. For the next six months, they had breast milk along with meals free of dairy products, eggs, peanuts, wheat, corn, soy, citrus and fish.

After 12 months, the health of these infants was superior in several areas to traditionally fed infants. Not all of these improvements can be attributed to eliminating cows' milk; however, it was one of the foods removed and milk often causes delayed food allergies. Unfortunately, most of the breast-fed infants started eating dairy products after one year, and their health problems increased and began to parallel those of the average child.

The traditional skin test for allergies was used in this study. This test is not capable of discovering delayed food allergies. However, the infants fed cows' milk every day at every meal had skin reactions to cows' milk 12 times more often compared to those not consuming cows' milk. (*Journal of Allergy*, 1989, July.) The more repetitiously a food is eaten, the more often allergic reactions and addictions develop to that food.

A similar study was recently completed at the Clinical Allergy Research Unit at St. Mary's Hospital in England. The doctors studied 120 infants to see if their health would be better if their mothers consumed no cows' milk, eggs, fish or nuts while breast feeding. In addition, the infants were kept free of dairy products, wheat, soy and oranges, and were exposed to reduced dust levels. After one year, only 14 percent of the infants on the program had observable allergies, compared to 40 percent in a traditionally fed control group. This study showed again that delayed food allergies are a major health problem and preventive care is effective.

The mothers in these two studies were tested and counseled only for acute allergies, not for delayed food allergies. Had the mothers and infants received specialized white blood cell testing and counseling for delayed food allergies, their health benefits would have been greater and would have continued throughout their lives. The immense potential of discovering and avoiding delayed food and chemical allergies has yet to be fully realized. This new understanding of allergy is the foundation of preventive care.

Colic causes severe abdominal pain and continual spitting up along with constant high-pitched crying. Colic often lasts for months and can cause malnutrition. Each year it causes suffering for over one million infants in the United States.

An ingenious study discovered the cause of infant colic. Damaging particles, called IgG antibodies, are made in the cows' body and pass with the cows' milk into the nursing mother. From there they pass in the mothers' breast milk to her infant. Thus, breast milk causes damage if the mother is eating dairy products. The breast milk stays contaminated for up to ten days from the mothers' last exposure to dairy products. (*Pediatrics*, 1991, April.)

This 1991 research helps explain part of the patient successes reported by Arthur Black, MD, in his landmark 1956 study, also published in *Pediatrics*. Dr. Black discovered the first white blood cell test for revealing delayed food allergies. White blood cells are killed by IgG antibody reactions and by several other types of allergic reactions.

This 1991 research also explains, for the first time, why twice the number of infants who are given cows' milk directly get colic, compared to those nursed by mothers who eat dairy products.

Some mothers' bodies filter out the damaging IgG cow antibodies and some do not.

Infants fed cows' milk are also twice as likely to die of Sudden Infant Death Syndrome. (Parish W: "Hypersensitivity to Milk and Sudden Death in Infancy," *The Lancet*, 1960, Vol 2 ; Coombs R, Holgate S: "Allergy and Cot Death: With Special Focus on Allergic Sensitivity to Cows' Milk and Anaphylaxis," *Clinical Experimental Allergy,* 1990, Vol 20.)

What a mother eats is passed, in part, to her infant, and some of what the cow eats is passed to the mother and then to the infant. This may cause the infant to have additional allergic reactions to the foods the cow ate.

It is common for people of all ages to have symptoms caused by dairy products without their knowing the reason. Delayed allergic reactions are the underlying cause of numerous ailments. They also are the cause of debilitating food addictions and make people more susceptible to infections. Delayed allergic reactions usually become worse as people become older.

Doctors who test for delayed food allergies have excellent results with their patients when they use accurate testing. Dairy products are recognized as one of the top three foods causing delayed allergic reactions. With accurate testing, these delayed reactions to dairy products can be clearly seen, through a microscope, killing white blood cells.

Numerous additional scientific studies confirm that infants, children and adults can suffer permanent damage from cows' milk. On May 15, 1992, the American Academy of Pediatrics made it unanimous: no cows' milk for infants under one year old. This is a good start, but this progress needs to be expanded to help people over one year old.

More than 45 years ago, Dr. Benjamin Spock wrote the all-time best-selling book designed to help mothers raise their children: *Baby and Child Care.* He recently acknowledged that cows' milk "causes intestinal blood loss, allergies, indigestion, and contributes to some cases of childhood diabetes. Human milk is the right one for babies." If he were to write his book today, lets hope he would change his recommendation that children should eat dairy products. Progress is being made, but there is a lot of damaging information in old and current books, articles and the media.

Misinformed doctors still pressure pregnant women and mothers to eat dairy products and thereby damage pregnant women, fetuses, mothers and nursing infants.

Juvenile-onset diabetes, also called insulin-dependent or type 1 diabetes, is a devastating disease. The pancreas is damaged, and even with the best medication, those afflicted live limited lives and die prematurely. In the United States alone, more than one and a half million people are suffering from this disease.

An extensive study to discover the cause of juvenile-onset diabetes was conducted by the University of Toronto. The doctors found that of 142 people with juvenile-onset diabetes, all 142 had an allergic reaction to dairy products, which had damaged their pancreases.

This occurs because the insulin-producing part of the pancreas has the same structure as a component in cows' milk. When the white blood cells of some infants discover cows' milk in the body, the cells attack and destroy the milk particles and then mistakenly destroy the insulin-producing parts of the pancreas after mis-identifying these parts as more cows' milk. The damage is irreversible. (*New England Journal of Medicine*, 1992, July 30.) These results have been confirmed by testing a group of 400 people.

A basic principle of preventive care is that a suspicious food should be avoided until it is proven safe. However, when several leading traditional doctors were asked about the high cause-and-effect relationship between dairy products and juvenile-onset diabetes, the typical reply was, "no mother should have her infant avoid cows' milk until more studies are done because cows' milk is so nutritious."

These doctors had not done their homework. Studies have already been done and clearly show that all the nutrients from cows' milk are fully supplied by many other foods, and that dairy products cause many additional serious health problems. In addition, the American Academy of Pediatrics had already warned doctors not to recommend cows' milk for infants because it causes internal bleeding and brain damage. Misinformed traditional doctors are still recommending dairy products and thus sentencing infants, children and adults to a lifetime of suffering.

The type of allergic reaction found to cause

juvenile-onset diabetes is the same damaging IgG reaction which causes colic, except with juvenile-onset diabetes the reaction starts in the human body instead of the cows'. This is one of the types of allergy exposed by the Prime Test. This reaction is very different from the one tested for by traditional allergists. The traditional type of allergic reaction is called IgE and causes an acute reaction rather than the delayed type revealed by the Prime Test.

The gold standard for infant growth is how an infant develops when drinking only mothers' milk, while the mother is avoiding dairy products and other allergy-causing foods. However, infants often gain weight faster on formula or cows' milk because of allergic swelling and excessive calories. Such rapid weight gain is one indication that breast milk substitutes are undesirable. If a pediatrician pushes a mother to use formula instead of mothers' milk, the mother should call the La Leche League for a referral to a doctor who is better informed. The La Leche League can be reached toll free at 1-800-La Leche.

If a mother is having trouble breast feeding, or needs help locating a healthy milk donor, or has adopted an infant, she can receive help from the La Leche League. If mothers' milk is not a possibility, select a dairy-free formula which does not cause delayed or acute allergic reactions. Formula-fed infants also need omega-3 oil, omega-6 oil and intestinal flora supplements (bifidus and acidophilus). All infants need frequent sunlight so they can produce vitamin D.

A large double-blind study demonstrated that 93 percent of the participants eliminated their migraine headaches by avoiding their delayed food allergies. The major problem was cows' milk and cheese. Other ailments which cleared up were: asthma, eczema, mouth ulcers, rhinitis, abdominal pain, diarrhea, flatulence, vaginal inflammation, aches in limbs, epilepsy, and behavior problems. (*The Lancet*, 1983, Oct 15.)

An important study on behavioral problems, including juvenile delinquency, was done by Alexander Schauss. He set out to see if the high sugar level in the American diet caused criminal behavior in young people. Although sugar does damage health, he found no correlation between sugar consumption and severe behavioral problems. However, he was surprised to discover a direct cause-and-effect relationship between drinking cows' milk and juvenile delinquency.

The children who had the most trouble drank about twice as much milk as a control group which was on the traditional American diet. Schauss was able to predict when a child in the control group was going to start getting into trouble by observing an increase in the child's milk consumption. (*Journal of Orthomolecular Psychiatry*, 1979, Sept.) Most children's behavior and health improve when they are free of all dairy products.

This discovery was later confirmed by a study done by the United States Department of Justice. It was found that 88 percent of a typical group of juvenile offenders had milk allergies. (*Journal of Behavioral Ecology*, 1981, March.)

A couple of the vitamins in milk are depleted when it is heated during pasteurization. However, all the beneficial nutrients in raw milk are abundantly supplied by a diet high in fresh vegetables. On rare occasions, certified raw milk does cause bacterial infections; but the major problem with certified raw milk is that it causes the same delayed allergy reactions and heart disease, stroke, cancer and diabetes as pasteurized milk.

Goats' milk also has damaging levels of fat, protein and the simple sugar, lactose. Like cows' milk, if goats' milk is consumed regularly, most people become allergic to it.

Doris Rapp, MD, is one of the nation's leading specialists in helping hyperactive children. She has conducted several double-blind studies testing hyperactive children to see if delayed food allergies are their problem. In one study, five out of five children tested had delayed allergic reactions to milk that caused their hyperactivity. When they remained free of all dairy products, four had excellent health, and one had good health. Dr. Rapp is consistently able to help children become free of hyperactive behavior without using Ritalin or other drugs. (*Journal of Learning Disabilities*, 1979, Nov.)

Presidential Medicine

The claim that dairy products promote health and growth is not supported by unbiased research. However, health damage caused by dairy products is well documented in numerous medical studies. Many serious ailments are caused fully or in part by eating dairy products. In addition, they are often a major cause of delayed food allergy symptoms.

High consumption of dairy calcium blocks the

assimilation of other important minerals. One important function of these minerals is to enable your muscles to work properly. If your heart muscle does not work properly, you develop irregular and rapid heart rates. Delayed food allergies and high-protein foods make this problem worse by drawing minerals out of your organs and bones.

Delayed allergic reactions to dairy products often upset the endocrine system, causing the thyroid gland to become under-active or over-active. These allergic reactions can also upset the heart rate.

Misinformed doctors allowed non-fat milk to be fed to President Bush while they gave him radioactive drugs to destroy his thyroid gland. His doctors gave him artificial thyroid medication to try to control his blood thyroid level and other drugs to control his irregular heart rate. Be wary of doctors who do not understand that many diseases are caused by delayed food and chemical allergies.

It would have been helpful for President Bush to know that his daily aerobic exercise reduced symptoms of delayed food allergies. Unfortunately, he was told to cut back on exercise. If he keeps eating dairy products and other damaging foods, he is likely to become easily fatigued and unhealthy. President Bush needs to discover his compatible foods, maybe even broccoli.

President Clinton is fortunate because he already knows he has allergies to dairy products and chocolate, plus some airborne reactions. It is important for him to add a food-allergy specialist to his personal health team so he will be able to do his job and not be held back by eating the wrong foods. He has invited Dean Ornish, MD, a specialist at using the 10–10–80 principle for preventing and reversing artery disease, to establish a new way of eating at the White House.

Using this part of The Quality Longevity Program is progress, but it does not include the delayed food allergy awareness; thus, President Clinton's health is likely to become worse.

The most frequent visible symptom of delayed food allergies is swelling or dark circles under the eyes. See how common delayed food allergies are by observing the people you meet over the next week, and by looking in the mirror. Other common symptoms are voice problems and physical addiction to ice cream.

People from all walks of life are hooked on dairy products. In early March 1993, the First Lady concluded that President Clinton's health would be better if he did not eat ice cream. Late at night the President got an overwhelming urge for ice cream and found that the refrigerator had been cleaned out. He concluded he needed ice cream and roared off with the Secrete Service men to find some. After searching around, the President ended up at a friend's house where he polished off a whole quart of vanilla.

Many people have trouble believing that dairy products are not needed to be healthy. This is because the dairy industry has been so effective at misinforming governments, nutritionists, doctors and the public. Scientific research demonstrates that dairy products cause numerous health problems, including delayed and acute food allergies.

*Cows' milk is for calves,
I never eat dairy products.*

Arnold Schwarzenegger
*Eight times Mr. Olympia, Five times Mr. Universe,
Actor and Health Consultant for President Bush*

My personal experience, while heading up a preventive care center during the 1980's, gave me the opportunity to see the damage caused by dairy products. We tested people for delayed food allergies by exposing a sample of their white blood cells to microscopic amounts of different foods. The testing and follow-up demonstrated that dairy products are one of the foods most damaging to white blood cells. Over 90 percent of the people we tested reacted by having their white blood cells killed by dairy products.

A double-blind study by Richard Panush, MD, uncovered one of the causes of arthritis. Some people experienced crippling joint pain when they consumed dairy products and were free of symptoms when they avoided them. (*Journal of the American Medical Association*, 1986, Aug 1.)

The lactase enzyme produced by our bodies breaks down the milk sugar, lactose. It is natural for the production of the lactase enzyme to stop after the age of four. When this happens it is mistakenly called a lactase deficiency. With the decline of the lactase enzyme and continued consumption of dairy products, there is a damaging build-up of undigested lactose sugar in the body, including in the lens of the eye. This is one of the causes of cataracts. (*Digestive Diseases and Sciences*, 1982, Vol 27.) Dairy industry ads boast that milk gives you energy from carbohydrates. What they do not tell you is that the carbohydrate is the health-damaging sugar, lactose.

Lactose and one of its components, galactose, have been discovered by doctors at Harvard to be part of the cause of ovarian cancer. This cancer is difficult to diagnose and is usually fatal. According to the American Cancer Society, in the United States in 1989 approximately 20,000 women were discovered to have ovarian cancer, and about 12,000 died. This cancer takes years to develop and the percentage of women who have it is increasing.

In high dairy-consumption countries like Denmark, six times as many women have ovarian cancers as in Japan. Japan was nearly dairy free until the end of World War Two.

When many women eat lactose, their level of a beneficial enzyme called transferase goes down, and the incidence of ovarian cancer goes up. Among dairy foods, yogurt and cottage cheese contain large amounts of lactose. (*The Lancet*, 1989, July 5.) Other researchers have shown a cause-and-effect relationship between eating lactose and infertility.

Living a life free from painful, recurring ailments caused by delayed food allergies is a good reason to avoid all dairy products. A second reason is to avoid and reverse deadly degenerative ailments, such as heart disease, stroke and kidney disease, by avoiding excess fat, protein and cholesterol.

*The most damaging foods
are dairy products.*

*Nathan Pritikin
Health Researcher and Author — 1915 to 1985*

Dairy Products and Contamination

The Center for Science In the Public Interest used a new, more accurate test and discovered that up to 51 percent of dairy products are contaminated with antibiotics or sulfa drugs. Dairy farms keep cows producing milk by injecting them with drugs. These drugs end up in the milk and are harmful to humans.

The Food and Drug Administration (FDA) recently rediscovered that dairy products are heavily contaminated with pesticides. Pesticides come from the foods eaten by cows and are concentrated in their milk. There were 19 different pesticides in 16 samples of butter. The most common pesticides found were BHC, Dieldrin,

Penta, Heptachlor, Octachlor, HCB and DDT. No one knows all the health problems caused by having pesticides in your body.

The FDA knows dairy products are contaminated by the medications given to cows and by toxic chemicals in the cows' food. However, its staff does not adequately inspect dairy products. There are 145,000 dairy farms producing milk in the United States. If the FDA tested only two percent each week, it would be inspecting 2900 dairy farms a week. The FDA claims it is doing a good job, but it tests only five dairy farms a week. And it tests only for penicillin residues.

The FDA's current milk inspection program allowed a dairy with defective equipment to put toxic levels of vitamin D into milk for more than two years before anyone figured out why so many people were becoming sick. The FDA's excuse was it did not have enough money for inspectors.

When people who have been consuming dairy products are accurately tested for drug and chemical residues, their blood is found to be contaminated with the same drugs and chemicals which are in the dairy products they have been eating. The damage this causes needs to be investigated.

On the average, Americans receive 24 percent of their pesticide residues from dairy products, 56 percent from meats, 10 percent from fruits and vegetables and 10 percent at home, work and from drinking water. Pesticides and toxic chemicals in dairy products are concentrated in high-fat products such as cheese and butter. If you are allergic to a particular pesticide, you can react by feeling sick when first exposed to it and again feel sick when the pesticide moves around in your body. Some of these pesticide residues remain in your cells and can cause continual symptoms. You can significantly reduce your level of pesticides by avoiding foods containing dairy products.

When cheese is made, a milky liquid called whey is left over. Cities complained because the dairy industry dumped whey down the drain, clogging up the sewers. This same allergy-causing whey is now used in the weight-loss industry's expensive meal replacements and in infant formulas. Whey is also manufactured into lactose.

No dairy product builds health or is safe for humans: not yogurt, cheese, cottage cheese, butter, cooked butter, lactose, whey, non-fat milk or foods made with milk products.

Are there any health benefits from eating dairy products? Many traditional medical doctors have their ulcer patients sipping milk throughout the day. This is called the Sippy diet, not because patients sip milk all day, but because it was started by Dr. Sippy more than 80 years ago.

A follow-up study was finally done to see how well this high-milk diet worked. Patients who sipped milk regularly had more stomach acid and more serious stomach ulcers. They also had up to six times as many heart attacks compared to patients treated without any dairy products. (*Circulation*, 1960, Vol 21.)

Some patients do feel better after drinking milk. One reason is they are physically addicted to dairy products, and drinking milk or eating another dairy product cuts off their withdrawal symptoms. One of the body's mechanisms which is involved in delayed food and chemical allergies is the same one involved in drug addictions. When you quit consuming dairy products, the withdrawal symptoms last for less than a week, and the symptoms and dairy-product cravings do not come back unless you eat something containing a trace of any dairy product.

Delayed milk allergies and addictions are made much worse by adding sugar to the dairy product. Ask anyone who gets started on a little sweetened yogurt or ice cream and has trouble stopping. This is a clue that the person is physically addicted to dairy products. Do you know any dairy addicts? Becoming free of food addictions often empowers people with drug addictions to break their drug habits.

Another problem with dairy products is they are a fertile ground for bacteria. *Consumers Reports* magazine found liquid dairy products had high levels of harmful bacteria and other bugs growing in them.

Over 20 percent of dairy cows are infected with the leukemia virus. The human connection has not been fully studied; however, chimpanzees and other animals fed contaminated cows' milk caught the virus and got leukemia. (*Science*, 1981, Vol 213.)

There is a new infectious agent called a "prion" that is entirely different from a virus or bacteria. A January, 1995 report in *Scientific American* explained that prions infect brain cells and are eventually fatal. Prions are very hard to detect. One way to become infected is to eat food from an animal that is contaminated.

Since the mid-1980s, more than 130,000 cattle have died in Great Britain from the prion infection called "mad cow disease." The scientists are hoping that those who eat beef and dairy products will not become infected.

Dairy Industry Propaganda

In order to keep people eating dairy products, the dairy industry continually thinks up new sales slogans. The dairy industry's motto was "Everybody Needs Milk." Because so many people are made sick by dairy products, the Federal Trade Commission declared the motto to be "false, misleading and deceptive." The dairy industry fought back but lost.

The United States Supreme Court ordered the dairy industry to stop deceiving the public. The dairy industry ignored the verdict and starting a massive ad campaign claiming "Milk Has Something for Everybody" and "Milk. It does a body good." This violation of the intent of the court order is still going on. This defiant and dishonest advertising is financed in part by government milk subsidies. Thus, our tax dollars are being used to promote milk sales, which in time cause an increase in our health costs.

Dividing foods into "Four Basic Food Groups" is another sales slogan. It was dreamed up in the 1940's and has no scientific basis. This slogan is still used by the dairy industry to indoctrinate children, traditional doctors, nutritionists, schools and government agencies. When people promote the "Four Basic Food Groups" or dairy products, you know they have been misled.

The federal government is trying to replace the "Four Basic Food Groups" with a new gimmick called the "Food Guide Pyramid." Because of dairy industry influence, dairy products are part of the new pyramid scheme. The dairy industry and the government suggest you eat dairy products two or three times a day. However, scientific studies show that non-dairy foods have all the fats, proteins, carbohydrates, vitamins, minerals and trace elements humans need. Your body fulfills all its needs from other foods and needs nothing from dairy products.

Stating the level of fat in food as a percentage of calories clearly identifies whether the food is health damaging. This approach was made the scientific standard more than 20 years ago by the health researcher, Nathan Pritikin. It is misleading to use the percent of total weight because most of the weight is often water. For example: "two percent" milk or yogurt is actually 30 percent fat when figured in calories; whole cows' milk is labeled 3.5 percent fat, but is actually 49 percent fat by calories; most cheese is around 75 percent fat by calories. Most dairy products are just concentrated milk and are excessive in fat and protein and contain the health-damaging milk sugar, lactose.

By using the percent-of-calories method, anyone can see if a food has around 10 percent of its calories from fat, or if it is excessive in fat. The dairy, meat and egg industries like to use ambiguous words like "reduced fat" or "low fat" and reveal their food's fat content as a percentage of the deadly 30 percent fat diet. This keeps people unaware of a food's actual fat content by calories. There are over a hundred scientific studies which demonstrate the optimum diet has about 10 percent of its calories from fat, 10 percent from protein and 80 percent from complex carbohydrates. This is how the 10–10–80 principle got its name.

The federal government tried to clear up the confusion. However, the dairy, meat and egg industries knew public awareness would reduce their sales. After these industries pressured the legislators, Congress decided in December of 1992 not to require the disclosure of the percent of fat by calories on labels. Instead, it allows ambiguous words like "low fat" and requires the grams of fat and the percent of a "standard" fat diet on the label. There are no warnings that the "standard" is based on the 30-percent-fat diet, the same one which causes heart disease and cancer. Without the percent of calories you do not know what you are buying.

The FDA and Department of Agriculture have made up permissive definitions for words like "low fat" and are requiring all food producers to follow them — all food producers except one. The dairy industry could not even meet the new loose definitions and was given a special exemption. They will be allowed to continue lying to the public by claiming that "two percent fat" dairy products are "low fat."

The raw political power of the dairy industry overwhelmed the most powerful legislative body in the world. The money spent on dairy products

is going to stay artificially high, as are health-care costs and the level of taxpayers' money going to dairy farmers.

Power tends to corrupt and absolute power corrupts absolutely.

Lord Acton
Historian and Author — 1834 to 1902

Dairy products comprise over 15 percent of the calories Americans eat, add an unnecessary 13 percent to the average food bill and add an unknown amount to medical bills, government spending and human suffering. Dairy products increase your weight while reducing your bank account and health.

In a recent study done by Dr. Cambell at Cornell University, it was shown that the dairy and meat industries heavily influence many of our congressmen by giving them millions of dollars each year. One of the ways these industries are paid back is by our legislators requiring the nation's school lunch programs to buy one billion dollars worth of dairy and meat products each year. Thus, informed parents who want the best for their children are pressured by politicians to feed their children damaging dairy products at school. Government awareness should be improved.

Food companies are not supposed to make false claims. Yet the FDA allows the dairy industry to make false claims about dairy products, and Congress helps subsidize false dairy advertisements with our tax money. The dairy industry gives more money to politicians than does any group except medical doctors.

The dairy industry is now using sexually provocative ads directed at children to try to maintain sales. TV ads imply that young boys will grow up big and strong, and every woman will want them, if they drink their milk. This approach is also used by the tobacco and alcohol industries. However, people are becoming aware of these attempts at brainwashing and are rejecting dairy products, tobacco and alcohol. Overall, dairy industry sales have been slowly declining for years. It is important to accelerate this decline.

It is amazing to see how often adds on television show milk drinkers as incompetent, stupid and desperate for more milk (addicted). It is depressing to realize that the dairy industry receives enough of our tax money as farm subsidies (welfare) to cover the costs of their adds.

The FDA is required by law to direct food companies to provide honest labels. However, the FDA has been manipulated by the dairy industry. Casein is a dairy product; but, in violation of its own principles, the FDA allows companies to put casein in products and still claim the product is dairy-free. This causes continual health problems for people with delayed food allergies who rely on labels to stay free of dairy products.

Dairy Products and the Environment

The earth's environment is severely damaged in the process of feeding cattle and producing dairy products. Cows eat large amounts of food to produce a small amount of milk. However, so much milk is produced, 280 quarts per person each year, that numerous natural resources are depleted and recreation and wildlife preserves are polluted. Cow excrement contaminates streams and drinking water.

In dairy-producing areas, the ground water has become overloaded with cow urine, and the contaminated water has flowed to cities far from the source. Scientists have no way of stopping this underground yellow tide, and vital drinking-water wells are becoming hopelessly contaminated.

The process which keeps cows producing milk creates an immense number of cattle, and this adds to environmental pollution. Eighty percent of the nation's water supply is used by agriculture, and half of that water is used to grow food for meat and dairy animals. Eighty percent of the cereal grains produced are used to feed animals to produce meat and milk.

John Robbins, of the Baskin-Robbins ice cream empire, has written a powerful book, *Diet for a New America,* which reveals the damage done to health and the environment by dairy products and meat.

Dairy products are items made primarily from milk. Eggs and mayonnaise cause several health problems; however, they are not dairy products.

Are Dairy Products Natural?

Scientists learn what is natural for humans to eat by studying what other mammals eat. Two important observations are: mammals in their natural environment never drink milk after infancy, and they never drink another mammal's milk.

For hundreds of thousands of years humans did well in a demanding environment without eating dairy products. Whenever you see the word "Natural" on a dairy product, someone is lying to you.

The History of Dairy Products

The tradition of eating dairy products started around 7000 years ago in India. The rulers found that their people had something to eat when the crops failed if dairy products were available. They began promoting dairy products and created rules requiring their people to eat them.

For a long time most people did not follow India's example and did not raise cattle or eat dairy products. However, during the dark ages in Europe, people began supplementing their diets with dairy products.

Even though dairy products did help fend off starvation, they were not consumed to any significant degree until recently because they were labor intensive to produce and easily infected with bacteria. During the late 1800's, the pasteurization process, developed for the wine industry, was added to milk production. This process killed most of the germs, and fewer people were made acutely ill by dairy products.

In the early 1900's, the wide use of ice, and later the invention of the refrigerator, dramatically increased the consumption of dairy products. The habits of Europeans and Americans have influenced people all over the world to eat dairy products.

In Japan, since 1940, the number of people who had ever eaten dairy products has changed from one percent to over ninety percent, with many now eating them repetitiously. As the consumption of dairy products has gone up, the Japanese have suffered an increase in the type of diseases caused by delayed allergic reactions to dairy products and other European and American foods.

Knowledgeable leaders in India, Europe and the United States have spoken out against dairy products for decades. Gandhi wrote, "I believe that in the limitless vegetable kingdom there is an effective substitute for milk, which, every medical man admits, has its drawbacks." If Gandhi were alive today, he would be happy to discover that there is no special nutrient in milk. Diets high in fresh vegetables supply all the necessary nutrients which are in dairy products, and vegetables do not have milk's damaging side affects.

One of England's most brilliant minds and prolific writers is Ashley Montagu. He is the author of more than 50 books on different subjects which have changed the thinking of educated people the world over. He wrote, "Cows' milk is no substitute for human milk. Cows' milk is splendid stuff — for little cows."

In the United States, the world-famous defender of the environment and founder of the Sierra Club, John Muir, wrote, "The butter-and-milk habit has seized most people; bread without butter or coffee without milk is an awful calamity, as if everything, before being put in our mouth, must first be held under a cow."

When John Muir wrote about people being seized by a habit, he was close to today's scientific understanding — people often become physically addicted to some foods as a part of the delayed food allergy reaction. If he were alive today, he would have discovered that, in addition to dairy products, wheat and coffee are physically addicting for many people. This helps to explain why these foods are so popular.

It seems ridiculous that a man,
especially in the midst of his pleasures,
should have to go beneath a cow like a calf
three times a day — never weaned.

Henry David Thoreau
Poet and Author — 1817 to 1862

People often experience some health improvements when they consume milk alternatives, if they also avoid all dairy products and have no delayed allergic reactions to the ingredients in the dairy replacement. Unfortunately, most of these replacements for milk products are made with allergy-causing foods like soy or cereal grains and are packaged in factories contaminated with milk powder from the production of other products.

Any dairy product can cause delayed allergic reactions, which in time cause numerous diseases. In addition, the fat, protein, cholesterol, lactose, calcium, chemicals and bacteria in dairy products have been scientifically shown to damage people's

health and shorten their lives. Improve your health and longevity by becoming free of all dairy products.

Dairy products have not been proven safe; in fact, they have been proven unsafe. The scientific evidence is clear — dairy products are unnecessary for health or growth, and they damage the health of infants, children and adults. The Physicians Committee for Responsible Medicine is conducting a national education campaign to help free Americans from dairy products by the year 2050. Why wait? Discover now how great you feel when you are free of dairy products.

Dairy Products and the National Budget

An example of the dairy industry's power can be seen by observing how the news media handled the American Academy of Pediatrics' announcement that it had changed its recommendation regarding cows' milk. The Academy sent out a news release to the major news sources. There should have been front-page articles announcing that "infants under one year old should not be given cows' milk." However, almost no mention was made of this major change. The political power of the dairy industry helps to explain why there is so little awareness of the damage caused by dairy products.

To keep the dairy industry happy, our elected representatives agree to buy, with our tax money, all the unwanted milk products the dairy industry can produce. These are the same dairy products which cause a broad range of health problems, damage the environment and waste everybody's money.

A feature on "60 Minutes" exposed the dairy industry's heavy influence on our government. The dairy industry gives large campaign donations to legislators and then receives immense amounts of our tax money as farm subsidies.

As of 1984, there were eighteen billion pounds of dairy products in storage, slowly rotting. This milk, cheese and butter cost our government several billion dollars to buy, and it costs billions of dollars more to store it in refrigerated buildings.

David Stockman, the first Budget Director for President Reagan, stated that giving billions of dollars to dairy farmers "is probably the single most worthless, lacking-in-merit program in the entire federal budget. We will have an adequate supply of milk whether we subsidize farmers or not." Stockman wanted to end the dairy subsidy program entirely. He presented the facts to President Reagan, but Reagan refused to upset the dairy industry.

Congress then came up with a "solution" to the dairy problem — kill 12 percent of the nation's cows. They paid farmers a lump sum to kill their cows and close their dairies for five years. To get more money, the farmers sold the dead cows to make into low-quality hamburger meat.

An example of how this worked is the case of the Magic Valley Dairy in Idaho. The owner was given ten million dollars to have 4,000 cows killed and was paid another two million dollars for the meat.

In two years our elected representatives spent over one and a half billion dollars of our tax money to kill cows. One of the results of the President's and Congress' cow-killing program was to flood the market with low-quality hamburger meat. This upset the cattlemen, so Congress agreed to buy half of the surplus. They bought four hundred million pounds of old cow meat at high prices and shipped it, at great cost, all over the world to our people in the military.

This massive killing of cows did bring about a temporary reduction in the amount of milk, cheese, butter and other dairy products going into surplus. However, by 1988, more cows had been put into production than had been killed earlier, and more milk was being produced than when the program started. This program turned out to be a total disaster for everyone except the dairy farmers and their favorite politicians.

Many dairy farmers saw this program as a signal to keep their cows and actually increase their herds because the President and the Congress were going to continue to buy everything the dairy industry could not sell to the public. The dairy industry realized it was going to be able to keep its hand in the taxpayer's pocket.

Stockman concluded that the President and Congress should get out of the dairy business. However, he knew this was unlikely to happen, because both the Republicans and Democrats are heavily influenced by dairy industry contributions.

Even the "60 Minutes" special brought about no change. Warehouses are still stuffed with rotting dairy products. Old dairy products are either dumped in landfills or given to the poor.

This giveaway is unfortunate, because these products cause health problems for the recipients, and it is then more difficult for them to find work when they are sick. Giving dairy products to poor people eventually increases the government's health care costs.

Pressure Against Progress

Another problem is that traditional medicine, medical insurance companies and state and federal agencies harass those who promote preventive care.

An example of one way this is done involved John McDougall, MD, in Hawaii. Dr. McDougall and his wife, Mary, wrote an excellent book called *The McDougall Plan*. They explained how important it was to have a very low fat, low cholesterol diet, free from all dairy products. They carefully documented the diseases caused by dairy products and how the high fat levels of dairy products are a major contributing factor for the development of breast cancer in women, prostate cancer in men and colon cancer in everyone.

Because of Dr. McDougall's efforts, Hawaii passed a law requiring doctors to give all breast cancer patients a pamphlet explaining different treatment options and how high-fat foods, like cows' milk, cause breast cancer. It is only logical to avoid the foods which cause an ailment while trying to cure it.

Shortly after Dr. McDougall's success with the state legislature, his malpractice insurance was not renewed — without cause. This is just one of the subtle ways in which health professionals who promote effective preventive care are harassed.

California state agencies started attacking preventive care providers after Governor Deukmejian took office in 1982. He had received large contributions from traditional doctors.

The preventive care centers I directed during the 1980's helped more than 8000 people with a broad range of symptoms become free of their delayed allergies and related ailments. At the centers, medical doctors prescribed the white blood cell test for discovering delayed food allergies, rather than the inaccurate skin test used by traditional allergists.

We combined, for the first time, several different health breakthroughs, and the results were unprecedented. Our clients became free of their symptoms and no longer had to take drugs or allergy injections. The traditional allergists could not compete, so they pressured other traditional doctors, insurance companies and state and federal bureaucrats to have us put out of business.

The Medical Board of California harassed us even though our clients were healthier than they had been in years. Our clients were happy and were enrolling others in our program. No one was being harmed except the traditional allergists, who were losing their patients.

Insurance companies were pressured to cut off reimbursements to people who wanted to use our program. False press releases sent out by traditional allergists and the Medical Board of California damaged our credibility. They followed this with harassment lawsuits which drained our resources. In time, we had to close.

We must free science from the grasp of politics.

William Clinton
Forty-second President of the United States

There are now 52 medical studies supporting white blood cell testing for delayed food allergies. There are six old negative studies, but they were done by traditional allergists who did not believe in delayed food allergies and did not understand the significance of the dead white blood cells they saw under their microscopes.

Another example of our government's misguided harassment involves Jonathan Wright, MD. He is respected as one of the top researchers who helps people with delayed food and chemical allergies.

Dr. Wright is also a leading expert on the use of vitamins, minerals and other supplements. He has taught for years how damaging dairy products are.

Dr. Wright has been in practice near Seattle, Washington for twenty years and has successfully helped more than 10,000 people. His patients were not complaining; the only complaints were from the traditional doctors who had lost their patients to his preventive care practice, and the bureaucrats the traditional doctors had manipulated.

On May 6, 1992, fifteen FDA agents and ten King County police officers broke into Dr. Wright's office with their guns drawn and held the nurses at gunpoint. After searching his office, the FDA agents confiscated his preservative-free vitamins.

The FDA knew in advance that Dr. Wright was not manufacturing illegal narcotic drugs, but misled the King County officers into believing otherwise so they would participate in the raid.

Something is seriously wrong when the FDA has the money, authority and teams of agents with nothing better to do than harass people who help patients with delayed food allergies, yet claims it does not have enough inspectors to test for toxic levels of contamination in dairy products.

This is the same FDA which allows prescription drug companies to run false ads and get by with dishonest research, but blocks others from giving information about alternative approaches to health and about specialized vitamins and supplements.

Big institutions, if unwatched and unchallenged,
make big mistakes. And when institutions
as powerful as drug manufacturers,
medical associations, hospitals,
insurance companies
and the Food and Drug Administration
make mistakes, the results are often suffering,
pain and death.

Ralph Nader
Consumer Advocate and Author

The FDA's efforts are aimed in the wrong direction. It needs to warn the public against unnecessary surgeries, health-wrecking procedures like breast implants, damaging prescription drugs, ineffective and dangerous traditional allergy testing and injections, pesticide-contaminated foods, and inherently damaging foods like dairy products.

Had the FDA hired Dr. Wright as a consultant 15 years ago, it would have known about the dangers of delayed chemical allergies. If the FDA had then done its job, chemical-filled breast implants would not have been allowed. In many other areas the FDA would be successful today, instead of failing to perform its legally-mandated duties.

Research has discovered 19 other attacks similar to the one on Dr. Wright during the Reagan and Bush administrations. This had not happened before. The FDA now spends its time and our tax dollars attacking doctors who recommend helpful supplements. This is happening while the overwhelming majority of dairy products, meat and traditional medical procedures go untested. It is urgent that the FDA be redesigned and redirected.

Any increase in the FDA's authority
over anything is a clear and
present danger to the nation's health.

Milton Friedman
Nobel Prize-winning Economist and Author

Why is the FDA and the Department of Agriculture failing the American public so completely? Industry groups are controlling our government. The dairy industry does not want you to know dairy products cause delayed allergic reactions in infants, children and adults. The prescription drug industry does not want you to know you can become allergic to the chemicals in over-the-counter and prescription drugs. The traditional allergists want to continue skin testing and giving shots for years rather than lose their patients to doctors who know how to test and counsel for delayed food and chemical allergies.

President Bush stated clearly what was needed in his inaugural address. "Government doesn't know best, parents know best...we offer a philosophy that puts faith in the individual, not the bureaucracy." What went wrong? Much of our government, particularly the FDA, lost direction under Presidents Reagan and Bush. The agencies went further under the influence of special interests like the dairy industry and traditional medicine and began attacking our right to chose for ourselves.

A movement has begun that is dedicated to stopping the FDA and other government agencies from attacking those who are practicing preventive care and to informing the public about the health damage caused by misinformed traditional doctors.

It is hoped that President Clinton and his team will correct the injustices of the past. Write to your representatives in the federal and state legislatures so they are aware of your desire to be free to choose the type of health care which works for you. In the future, vote for the person who will defend your right to select the type of health care you need.

Despite the health problems caused by dairy products, the FDA should not ban them. This would just alienate the public against the government and prolong the time it takes for people to become free from dairy products.

The FDA should conduct an extensive educational program to expose dairy products, like the one used for cigarettes. The information must be presented on television, in print and in schools so the public becomes aware of the health, environmental and financial damage caused by dairy products. This would include the following notice on all items containing dairy products:

Warning

Scientific studies have shown that dairy products cause or contribute to the following diseases: internal bleeding, iron deficiency, food allergies, food addictions, kidney stones, calcified arteries, calcified organs, weak bones and teeth, juvenile-onset diabetes, heart disease, cancer, infertility, colic, sudden infant death syndrome, pesticide overload, chemical overload and food poisoning.

The cost of this education program could be covered by discontinuing subsidies to the dairy industry and a health tax on dairy products. There would be money left over to help people who have already been damaged by dairy products. There would also be a monetary windfall for the public because of money saved on health care and not wasted on buying dairy products.

The Choice Is Yours

The smallest amount of any dairy product keeps delayed allergic reactions going and thus damages your health. Become entirely free of all dairy products and see how good you feel.

Most medical doctors have little understanding of the fundamentals of accurate nutrition, let alone the advanced approaches. Fortunately, many food-allergy specialists have done their homework and are experts at white blood cell testing and are able to help people with delayed food allergies.

Let the information you have gained about dairy products become a part of your health program. Then help your friends improve their health and enjoyment of life by sharing this information with them so they know the damage caused by delayed food allergies and dairy products.

Mammals in their natural environment
never drink milk after infancy,
and they never drink
another mammal's milk.

Chapter 9
Health Wrecking Foods and Chemicals

There are a few foods and chemicals which damage everyone's health. When people stay free of them, most are able to notice a significant improvement in their health. The foods and chemicals exposed in this chapter and the dairy products explained in the previous chapter are not natural for humans to eat. Until a few thousand years ago, people never ate these foods or chemicals. The consumption of these items has gone up dramatically over the last hundred years. Avoiding them is an important step along the path to great health.

Some people are sad when they find they are allergic to some of the foods they enjoy, until they become free of their health problems by avoiding them. This discovery and the following information makes it easier to stay free of these damaging foods and chemicals.

Coffee

Coffee contains one of the most powerful stimulant drugs known to man. The drug is caffeine, and it is commonly used to increase energy levels. Caffeine blocks the awareness of chronic fatigue which is one of the most common symptoms of delayed food allergies. Many find they have trouble functioning unless they have coffee, tea, chocolate or the so-called "soft drinks" that contain caffeine.

In time, many people become chronically fatigued as a result of their food and chemical allergies. When they were younger, many of these same foods and chemicals caused stimulation. However, a drug-addiction type of tolerance develops with time. They then think they have to keep consuming the offending item just to keep going. This often happens with coffee and other caffeinated drinks.

One of the ways caffeine changes the body is by stimulating the adrenal glands. In the short run, it gives people a boost. However, it exhausts the adrenal glands and upsets the rest of the endocrine system; this leads to chronic fatigue. People often try to attack the fatigue with more caffeine. However, even caffeine cannot continue to hide the symptoms of delayed allergic reactions.

Caffeine's powerful stimulant reaction upsets sleep that is needed for rest and is a requirement for mental health. In experiments where people have been kept awake for four or five days without any sleep, many develop paranoia, schizophrenia, manic depression and other common mental illnesses. In caffeine-sensitive people, even small amounts can cause lack of sound sleep. This can lead to emotional outbreaks and breakdowns.

Sheldon Hendler, MD, PhD and professor of medicine at the University of California at San Diego, explains that caffeine competes with the natural brain chemical, adenosine. This neurotransmitter acts in the brain by connecting to nerve cell receptors, and thus relaxes the brain. Caffeine blocks this process, causing the brain to malfunction and the person to become stimulated.

Because items with caffeine have been sold for so many years and unwittingly accepted as safe, they can be sold without prescription or health warnings. Caffeine is such a powerful drug, with so many damaging side effects, if companies tried today, for the first time, to have coffee, tea, or other caffeinated drinks approved by the FDA, they would probably be blocked.

Unfortunately, most psychiatrists do not know about delayed food and chemical allergies and their damaging affect on brain function. Instead they focus on talk therapy and encourage their patients to take damaging drugs. Doctors can start having real successes by freeing their patients from stimulating foods and chemicals. This enables people to enjoy quality sleep and avoid emotional problems.

Coffee has been shown to compound mental health problems by changing brain chemistry. A recent study demonstrated that when patients in mental institutions became free of coffee, the incidence of violent outbreaks dropped in half. Coffee and caffeine can also cause inappropriate behavior in people who are not mentally disturbed.

There are a number of ailments which the traditional medical establishment agree are caused by caffeine consumption. Caffeine has been shown to increase blood cholesterol levels. This may happen by stimulating the liver's production of cholesterol. People who drink five cups a day have twice as many heart attacks as people who are free of coffee and caffeine. Caffeine has also been shown to increase triglycerides, a blood fat that impairs circulation when it is elevated.

Coffee depletes mineral reserves from the body, including calcium from the bones. Other symptoms that are now recognized by scientists include sleeplessness, irritability, anxiety, depression, restlessness, nervousness, excitement, flushed face, excessive urination, constipation, heartburn, muscle twitching, and rambling thought and speech.

The stimulant effect of caffeine prevents people from recognizing the cause of their health problems. Allergic food and chemical reactions often cause them to become sleepy after meals. Many people drink coffee to keep going, not knowing they are hiding allergic reactions. It is better for them to improve their life-style and avoid the cause of fatigue.

Besides caffeine, there are several other harmful chemicals in coffee which damage health, some quite seriously. One study discovered that women who drink coffee regularly when pregnant are three times more likely to have a child with observable birth defects. It is unknown how much damage is done which is not observable at birth.

The beginning of damaging allergic reactions can be clearly seen by looking at white blood cells under the microscope after exposing them to a minute trace of coffee. These reactions include damage and death of the person's white blood cells.

This damaging stimulant drug blocks people's awareness of their food and chemical allergies. One of the reasons the public is not aware of this problem is that traditional allergists and most doctors do not understand delayed allergic reactions. In time, people end up much sicker because they masked their symptoms with coffee or caffeinated beverage. Even decaffeinated coffee contains damaging chemicals, and drinking it keeps the addictive process controlling your life.

One of the ways scientists measure the damage caused by a drug is by observing how severe the withdrawal symptoms are when the drug is avoided. Another way is how tempted people are to go back once they are through withdrawal. One reason heroin is uniformly condemned is because of the severity of the withdrawal symptoms and the difficulty in staying off the drug.

Many people are highly addicted to coffee, and when they quit they have painful withdrawal symptoms for a few days. If you are a regular coffee consumer, it is easy to test this for yourself. Stay free of coffee and all caffeinated beverages for a week. Withdrawal may cause symptoms that you have had before and possibly some new ones.

Many people who stop consuming caffeine experience withdrawal symptoms which include headaches, body aches, irritability, nervousness, inability to work effectively, nausea, depression and constipation, and cravings for caffeine, damaging foods, chemicals and drugs. In a few days you will clear from the allergic addictive reactions and feel much better. To experience the full benefits, it is also necessary to avoid the foods and chemicals to which you are allergic. One way to help free yourself from craving caffeinated drinks is to have a non-toxic herbal tea, such as linden flower or rosehips.

Each patient carries his own doctor inside him. We are at our best when we give the doctor who resides within us a chance to go to work.

Albert Schweitzer
French Philosopher and Nobel Laureate — 1875 to 1965

Eggs

Eggs have had a bad rap for several years but it is nothing compared to how bad eggs actually are.

The number of people with delayed allergic reactions to eggs is significant. Eggs are included in many products. For many people, eggs and chicken cause severe delayed allergic reactions.

The most damage caused by eating eggs is not chronic diseases caused by allergies but degenerative diseases caused by clogged arteries. The problem is the cholesterol content in the egg yolk. Most people are able to tolerate up to 80 milligrams of dietary cholesterol a day. The average egg yolk has around 200 milligrams of cholesterol.

Eighty percent of the population cannot assimilate all the cholesterol they eat. Their digestive tracts start being overwhelmed at 200 milligrams a day. If more is eaten, the cholesterol is not absorbed by the digestive tract and is excreted. The remaining twenty percent absorb most of the cholesterol they eat, and they often die at a younger age. One person out of 500 has a genetic defect which causes the liver to produce excessive amounts of cholesterol; their arteries are clogged by their early twenties. They have numerous heart attacks and usually die before age forty.

Most people are already eating over 200 milligrams of cholesterol a day. Even if they ate ten eggs a day, their blood cholesterol would not go up because they are already assimilating all the cholesterol they can absorb. It may actually go down a little because of natural fluctuations in blood cholesterol levels and variations in the test equipment.

The Standard American Diet (SAD) has around 500 milligrams of cholesterol a day. Eating 200 milligrams a day is enough to overwhelm our digestive system and cause premature death. If you have been eating over 80 milligrams of cholesterol a day for most of your life, it is a good idea to eat under 25 milligrams until your blood cholesterol level is under 150.

A double-blind study was done by Frank Sacks, MD, and associates at Harvard Medical School. Seventeen students avoided all dietary cholesterol, except from dairy, for three weeks. The students then added one egg a day to their diet while making no other changes. The most damaging type of blood cholesterol, the LDL type, went up 12 percent in just six weeks. This amount of change is known to cause heart disease and clogged arteries throughout the body. Even better results would be expected if the subjects had started from a lower cholesterol diet that was dairy free.

A companion study with 19 men and women, aged 14 to 54, went on for three months. They avoided eggs and several other cholesterol-containing foods. Their total blood cholesterol went down 22 percent. (*The Lancet*, 1984, March 24 / *Hypertension*, 1984, March.)

The National Egg Board advertises that eggs are not so big a problem as once thought because they have 22 percent less cholesterol (around 200 milligrams) than the previously inaccurately-measured 240 milligrams. Unfortunately, the American Heart Association believed the advertisements and increased its recommended weekly allotment of eggs from three to four. The safe, health building allotment is zero.

Besides the cholesterol problem with eggs, there is also a fat problem. Eggs have 65 percent of their calories in fat. Therefore, if you eat eggs you will significantly increase your dietary fat level, which also increases the risk of cancer.

Ironically, the one area where the egg industry claims eggs are good for us is also a problem. It claims that the egg is a good source of protein.

However, the American diet is already too high in protein. This causes a number of problems throughout the body, not the least of which is the leaching of essential minerals from the body. Low levels of essential minerals cause the immune system to malfunction. Eggs are a contributing factor to most peoples' excessive protein intake because they are 35 percent protein. Thus, the one ingredient in the egg claimed to be good for us is adding to our protein overload.

Because eggs yolks are a highly concentrated source of cholesterol and fat, they must be carefully avoided if you want to avoid a heart attack. If you have heart symptoms before you have the opportunity to put this information to work for you, find a doctor who specializes in reversing heart disease by using the 10–10–80 balance of fat, protein and carbohydrates. There are now specialists who use non-damaging therapies for reversing heart disease without surgery or damaging drugs.

Be careful to avoid the common mistake of going to a traditional doctor and being told you must have an angiogram. These x-rays always show some blockages if you have been eating the Standard American Diet. The doctors then show you the blocked arteries and tell you to take drugs, have balloon angioplasty or coronary-bypass surgery. In most cases this advice is likely to damage your health beyond repair or kill you.

Published studies show that people should not have coronary bypass surgery unless they are having constant chest pain that can not be relieved. Based on the medical establishment's own studies, the Rand Corporation reported that 44 percent of people who had coronary bypass surgery should not have had the operation. The cost of these unnecessary operations exceeds $1.4 billion a year and causes over 7000 deaths a year. This equals a waste of $4 million and 19 lives a day.

Where are the FDA and state regulators when they are needed? Could it be they are under the influence of traditional doctors?

Angiograms are often misleading and sometimes cause lasting damage. Balloon angioplasty is expensive, dangerous and does not provide long-term results. The 10–10–80 balance is rapidly effective, inexpensive and safe, and its benefits last.

Instead of checking into a hospital to have your

chest cut open and then find you need to make the same changes in your diet after the surgery, find a doctor who starts you on the right diet program so you will not need surgery. Heart surgery causes serious side affects and is a major factor in bankrupting the entire health care system.

The idea that heart disease is caused by stress has been further discredited in recent studies. A stressful job or life-style does not cause people to have heart attacks. The only emotional factor that caused any increase in heart problems was whether a person was hanging on to anger. Therefore, if you do not have chest pain or other heart symptoms, cheer up, forgive those who have made you angry, enjoy your challenging job, and eat the foods that make up the 10–10–80 balance of macronutrients, and the surgeons will never have an excuse to cut you open.

Eggs are often infected with disease-causing bacteria. This is now such a serious problem that the state of New Jersey, after 86 known deaths and an unknown number of people with attacks of the "stomach flu," made it illegal for restaurants to serve eggs unless the yolk is cooked solid.

Because of delayed allergies, heart disease, cancer, mineral loss and infections, eggs should be enjoyed only by chickens who want to have chicks.

Peanuts

Peanuts are another food which is highly promoted and heavily consumed.

Peanuts rank in the top dozen foods which cause delayed allergic reactions, and are one of the most addictive foods. This shows up when people decide to have a few peanuts and then have trouble stopping after eating several handfuls. They also cause acute food allergies. A few people die each year from acute reactions to peanut products used by chefs and food producers.

Peanuts contain 70 percent fat by calories. A small amount of peanut butter on a sandwich will make it over 30 percent fat. Vegetable oils increase the blood fat called triglyceride. When you have high triglycerides and high LDL cholesterol, you have the most potent producer of heart disease.

Studies were done with animals which never develop heart disease when they eat the foods on which they evolved. When they were fed cholesterol and different vegetable oils along with their natural foods, all the test animals developed clogged arteries (heart disease), and all of them developed clogged

arteries at the same rate, except for those given peanut oil. Peanut oil caused blockages to develop much faster than the other vegetable oils.

The reason for this has never been discovered, and it should be carefully researched. If these animals developed allergic inflammation in their arteries from peanuts, this could cause plaques to form at a higher rate. If this turns out to be true, we would have evidence that delayed allergic reactions help to accelerate cardiovascular disease.

Peanuts cause another type of damage important to know about. In 1957 a shipment of peanuts was fed to 50,000 turkeys in England. Within weeks all were dead. The autopsies disclosed the turkeys had died of liver cancer. When people die of liver cancer, its often thought to be caused by "normal" causes or bad luck. However, when farmers lose 50,000 turkeys, people start looking for a cause, and it was found. It was aflatoxin, a chemical excreted by a mold. This mold grows readily on peanuts, potatoes and cereal grains. Aflatoxin accumulates in animals which eat these foods, and it is not destroyed by cooking.

When people regularly eat foods containing aflatoxin, liver cancer is epidemic. Liver cancer is a minor killer of people in the United States but a major killer in African countries where peanuts and peanut oil are consumed commonly because they are inexpensive. There are areas in Africa where up to 24 percent of the people die from liver cancer, primarily caused by aflatoxin-contaminated peanuts. One study on peanut butter done by Consumers Union found that some jars from every manufacturer contained small amounts of aflatoxin.

It is sad to see children eating peanut butter after being told it is good for them. Peanuts should be sold with a warning on their label stating they are a major cause of delayed allergic reactions and a major contributor to heart disease, stroke and cancer.

Yeast

Eating yeast increases health problems because it causes delayed allergic reactions for most people. Avoid yeast by not consuming alcoholic beverages, bread, some vitamin products, flavorings, vinegar and other fermented products.

When people are not eating yeast, they can usually handle the small exposures which come from the air. When people eat yeast repetitiously, they often become allergic to it and then can be damaged continuously by the small amounts in the air.

There are about 10 different types of yeast which grow in the body and cause problems. The most common yeast is called Candida albicans.

Yeast is kept under control in our bodies by our white blood cells which eat the yeast. Delayed allergies reduce the white blood cell's ability to keep yeast from growing. Yeast begins to grow in the digestive tract. This makes delayed allergies worse and contributes to yeast infections throughout the body.

Infants are born with many of the same food allergies as their mothers. Because of years of eating allergy-causing foods and chemicals, eating too much sugar and taking antibiotics or birth control pills, most people have some internal yeast problems. There are several medications for reducing these yeast problems; however, in most cases, eating foods compatible with our white blood cells will enable the cells to bring yeast problems under control naturally.

People often feel poorly while their white blood cells are cleaning the excess yeast out of their bodies. This can extend the time it takes to feel good after going through withdrawal.

Avoiding delayed food and chemical allergies is the foundation of effective yeast reduction therapies and is the place to start.

Damaging Chemicals

There is a broad range of chemicals which damage people. Doctors and toxicologists are aware that a large exposure to a chemical can cause severe problems. They have missed the fact that it is possible to become allergic to a chemical and then to be continually damaged by minute exposures to that chemical. Therefore, a pesticide in a food that does no noticeable damage to most people can make some people sick if they have a delayed allergic reaction to that chemical.

The most common chemicals are those made from petroleum. Petroleum by-products include car and natural gas exhaust fumes, plastics, detergents, pesticides, and chemicals in the fertilizers used to grow foods. By reducing the amount of petroleum products in your life, you can significantly improve your health. If you have become allergic to certain chemicals, their removal can significantly improve your health.

Pesticides are on our foods and in our foods. They are sprayed in our homes, gardens, markets, restaurants and the workplace. Animal products have high levels of toxins because animals concentrate chemicals in their bodies from the foods they consume. Pesticides can cause us to be sick much of the time because they are in our blood and are being continually pumped throughout our bodies.

Chemicals can be a constant cause of irritation to your body and thereby contribute to cancer. However, a much larger cause of cancer is the eating of vegetable oils and animal fats which deprive your cells of oxygen.

Studies done in the United States show mothers' milk to be heavily contaminated with the same kinds of pesticides used in our foods, homes, restaurants and the workplace. This was discovered in 1976, but little has been done to warn women and teach them how to eat right. Woman need to clean out their bodies before becoming pregnant.

Traditional allergists do not believe in chemical allergies because they mistakenly believe there has to be a protein molecule present for there to be an allergic reaction. This is true only of IgE reactions. IgG and immune-complex reactions can happen without the involvement of any proteins. Thus, traditional allergists do not believe it is possible for a person to have an allergic reaction to cigarette smoke. Anyone who has delayed allergic reactions to cigarette smoke knows that traditional allergists have not done their homework.

We can become allergic to any food or chemical to which we are exposed repetitiously. Thus, we need to clean pesticides, cigarette smoke and car, jet and gas-appliance exhausts out of our lives as best we can.

One chemical which merits special mention is formaldehyde. Many people have heard about formaldehyde because it is the embalming fluid pumped into people after they die. However, formaldehyde accumulates in your body while you are alive. It often causes the smell which comes from new, inexpensive clothes. You notice it clearly when you go into stores which are filled with polyester fabric. It is also in the glue used in less expensive furniture and chip board. It has been replaced in carpets with other damaging chemicals.

Formaldehyde is one of the chemicals used in the construction of mobile homes which causes people to get sick with what is called "mobile home syndrome." Traditional allergists call the disease a syndrome because they do not understand that people can become allergic to formaldehyde.

Your health will be improved by removing formaldehyde from your environment. Many people are starting the embalming process before they die. Morticians are now finding that corpses do not deteriorate so rapidly as they used to. The reason for this is the high levels of formaldehyde, pesticides, preservatives and other health-damaging chemicals which have accumulated in people who did not clean up their environment and life style. Select carpets, clothes and furniture made without allergy-causing chemicals.

Ground water and water-delivery systems have become so contaminated with pesticides, gasoline, cow urine and multiple chemicals that tap water is not reliable for drinking. Because we absorb chemicals through our skin and our lungs, it is also helpful to filter shower and bath water.

Silicone-filled breast implants contain several other chemicals besides silicone. If plastic surgeons understood the problems caused by delayed chemical allergies, they would never have used silicone-filled or silicone-covered implants.

After a few years, some women become allergic to the outer silicone covering on saline implants. As of 1992, there are 2400 known cases of immune problems caused by saline-filled breast implants. Heart surgeons discovered years ago that the safest plastic to use in the body is Dacron. However, because of the dangers, no implants should be used unless there is a medical necessity.

The chemicals in artificial sweeteners cause several problems. The aspartame in many artificial sweeteners can cause delayed chemical allergies and physical addictions. When proper testing techniques are used, cancers have been caused in lab animals by artificial sweeteners.

Monosodium glutamate (MSG) is used as a flavor enhancer in several food items and by most Chinese restaurants. MSG is unique in how it affects us. It works as a stimulant on the taste buds and disguises bad tasting foods. That does not seem so bad, until you realize that you get the stimulation by damaging the nerve endings in the taste buds. When the nerve endings are inflamed, you get more sensation from the food. MSG goes on to damage nerves throughout your body, and when it reaches your brain cells it upsets brain function.

MSG can be put into your foods without your knowing it. The FDA will be changing the rules in the future but for now, avoid foods that have "hydrolyzed vegetable protein" on their label because it has MSG. Also check to make sure that ones with "natural flavor" do not include MSG.

Hair spray is a damaging combination of chemicals which causes allergic symptoms for the user and for people who inhale the surrounding air. Use safe lotions with hair styles that do not need to be sprayed. Also avoid spray perfumes and deodorants.

Other chemicals to avoid are those used in air deodorizers. These chemicals are difficult to notice because they have no smell themselves and are designed to block our sense of smell so that we can not smell what is in the air. They knock out our warning mechanism that tells us when damaging chemicals are present. Most taste and smell come from the same sensors; thus, air deodorizers diminish our ability to taste and enjoy the foods we eat.

With an in-depth awareness of how chemicals affect our bodies, we can improve our health and enjoyment of life. Some people's health is dramatically improved when they clean up their surroundings, because they have developed delayed allergic reactions to certain chemicals. Avoid unnecessary chemicals whenever you can.

Legal and Illegal Drugs

The common approach used by the traditional medical establishment is to give people drugs to suppress their symptoms instead of discovering and removing the underlying cause. Suppressing symptoms with drugs is dangerous because the underlying cause of the damage is not discovered and removed. Also, the drug approach is damaging due to known and unknown side effects of most medications. In addition, many people become allergic to the drug. This is especially true of medications designed to be taken every day for months or years.

A common example of this problem involves the giving of thyroid medication to people whose thyroid glands are underactive. It is much better to discover and remove what is causing the suppression of the thyroid gland. The cause is often delayed allergic reactions to foods and chemicals. To take thyroid drugs for any length of time often destabilizes the endocrine system further, and the person becomes allergic to medication. Other symptoms develop, and the problems multiply.

Thyroid problems are also serious when the

thyroid gland becomes overactive. Traditional medical doctors often destroy the entire thyroid gland with nuclear radiation and then commit the person to a lifetime of thyroid drug dependency. It is much better to discover what is causing the hyperactivity of the thyroid gland and then remove the cause.

The most common drugs prescribed for people with delayed food allergies are cortisone and steroids. These drugs dramatically reduce allergic inflammation; however, they seriously weaken the immune system. Six months or a year later, the people using them are reactive to so many foods and chemicals, it is hard to help them. It is even difficult to test them because their white blood cells fall apart before the cells can be placed on a microscope slide. Avoid all types of these drugs in skin creams, nose sprays, pills and injections.

Careful double-blind studies have shown that hyperactivity in children is caused by delayed food and chemical allergies in most cases. Because most people are not aware of this, many children are put on mind-altering drugs such as Ritalin. In some areas as many as 10 percent of the children are being drugged to "solve" their behavior problems. Follow-up studies have shown that when the children are older and taken off the drugs, a high percentage develop criminal behavior.

Children see their friends put on drugs for emotional problems. Later, when the children have emotional problems, they look for relief by taking illegal drugs instead of removing allergic foods and chemicals that upset the emotions. Delayed food and chemical allergies upset brain functions, and Ritalin changes brain functions. When Ritalin helps calm children, it is an indication that delayed allergies are the underlying problem.

*Some remedies are worse
than the diseases.*

Syrus Publilius
Syrian Author— First century BC

When most people started smoking tobacco, they did not realize they were taking a drug. It is hard to believe how long it took the medical establishment to recognize the damage caused by tobacco. Not until thirty years after Ernst Winder, MD, demonstrated that smokers had dramatically higher levels of lung cancer did the government begin its anti-smoking education program. During the first part of the 1980's, the president of the American Medical Association said smoking was not a significant problem. He was a smoker, and we now know that most smokers live in a fog of denial caused by their physical addiction.

The discovery that smoking is an addictive disease was made in England in 1942. Doctors had a group of smokers stop smoking for a few hours. These people became tense, irritable, pained by headaches and unable to function well, as they went through withdrawal. The smokers were given an injection of nicotine and they became pleasant, relaxed and symptom free. This addictive reaction was confirmed by scientists at Loma Linda University during the 1970's.

C. Everett Koop confirmed that smoking was addictive in the 1988 Surgeon General's Report. From the time the addictive nature of cigarettes and other tobacco products was discovered and the American government acknowledged it, more than 45 years had passed. It is common for traditional doctors and the government to be more than 40 years behind the scientific research. If you wait until the medical establishment and the government understand a problem, you will probably be 40 years behind the scientific breakthroughs.

If people smoke in the same building you are in, you are damaged to some degree if their smoke travels into your air. You are damaged more if you are an ex-smoker because smokers become highly allergic to smoke. Re-exposure causes discomfort and symptoms in ex-smokers, which is why they complain more than people who have never smoked. Smokers should smoke outside until they are able to quit.

It is important to stay free of second-hand smoke when you are quitting so that your addictions are not triggered. Think of how hard it would be for a heroin addict to become free of heroin if someone sprinkled heroin powder in the addict's food. It is often difficult to quit smoking because it is common for smokers, who do not understand the allergy/addiction problem, to contaminate the air.

When you look back and see how many people have been damaged and prematurely killed by cigarettes, you see the importance of more education about delayed allergic reactions, addictions and the right to clean air. By looking through a microscope, one can see the severe damage done to white blood cells after exposure to minute amounts of tobacco. Something is wrong when the government gives money to tobacco growers and spends money attacking people who help those with delayed allergic reactions to tobacco.

A recent study shows that the major reason women live longer than men is that more men smoke than women. Some of the progressive steps which need to be taken are: dramatically increasing education, raising taxes on tobacco products, greatly expanding non-smoking areas, stopping all tobacco advertising and requiring the tobacco industry to pay for the related health care problems of ex-smokers.

> *Whatever else you do,*
> *don't smoke.*
>
> *Yul Brynner*
> *Actor, Smoker and*
> *Lung cancer fatality — 1915 to 1985*

One illegal drug often thought to do little damage is marijuana. This is believed because there are few withdrawal symptoms when one uses marijuana. This comes about because marijuana's active ingredient, THC, is different from that of most other drugs. Instead of being water soluble like alcohol, THC, like DDT, is oil soluble. It ends up in the fat cells and does not leave the body rapidly the next day; thus, there are few withdrawal symptoms. The THC accumulates in our fat cells, and health deteriorates so long as it is retained there.

It is common for people who occasionally smoke marijuana to remain unhealthy. It can take over a month from the last exposure until a person's health improves because the THC is continually released from the person's fat cells.

Illegal drugs cause a broad range of complications. The problems are made worse because the drugs have to be obtained through criminal channels which damage the person's life by association.

There is a prescription drug that strengthens cells against delayed allergies called sodium cromolyn. Adrenal cortical extract reduces inflammation without causing significant side affects.

There are no drugs which are entirely safe. Be sure to read the warnings on the information sheet before you decide to take any prescription drug. If you have to take an antibiotic, be sure to start taking some dairy-free bifidus and other intestinal floras a few days after you finish the antibiotics.

Wheat

Wheat did not exist until about 12 thousand years ago. At that time a mutation developed when goat grass crossed with another grass similar to wheat, and wheat as we know it started to take over.

When you look at why so much wheat is consumed, several facts become apparent. Wheat grows readily where other crops cannot. It is inexpensive to produce and can be stored for years. Wheat's wholesale cost is around $.60 for a thousand calories compared to carrots at about $1.75; both retail for around $2.00 for a thousand calories. Meat and dairy products usually retail at over $3.00 per thousand calories when you include damage to the environment and taxpayer dollars that go for government price supports.

Food producers promote the consumption of wheat in all its forms because the raw material is very inexpensive, and thus they are able to mark up the price dramatically. People eat huge quantities of wheat because it is inexpensive, heavily promoted, and they think it is good for their health.

The allergic reacting antigens in wheat are more concentrated in the outer surface of the wheat, known as bran. The increased consumption of whole wheat products over the last forty years may help to explain the dramatic increase of delayed food allergy-caused ailments from asthma to eczema. Much of the food industry believes wheat is a wonder food, and it often uses one hundred percent whole wheat in its products.

The oil in whole wheat becomes rancid within a few days of milling. Rancid oils cause destructive free radicals which then travel through the body, damaging cells at random. The bran from all cereal grains becomes rancid and should be avoided whether you are allergic to it or not. Orientals eat white rice because brown rice becomes rancid easily. Rice bran also contains more allergens than the center of the grain.

When the original studies were done to see whether delayed food allergies contributed to mental problems, doctors took a group of schizophrenic and manic-depressive patients off all foods for a few days. They found that more than half of them became free of most of their symptoms within a week. The majority had their mental symptoms return when they ate wheat again. Dairy products were the second most mind-disrupting food.

Many of Sigmund Freud's ideas have been

found to be invalid. However, it is important to acknowledge that he began to change his own ideas shortly before he died. His final writings stated that the major cause of mental illness is probably upset brain chemistry rather than psychological factors. Recent studies have shown delayed allergic reactions upset brain chemistry.

Psychiatrists attempt to re-balance brain chemistry by using drugs, but the drugs often cause worse problems. William Howard Hay, MD, said that a properly functioning brain must be constantly bathed by a properly fed blood stream.

Over half of the hospital beds in the United States are used for people with mental illness because they are often committed for months or years. The annual cost is over $250 billion. Many of the homeless street people are emotionally unbalanced and are currently unable to find effective health care.

Many people discover they are addicted to wheat. To stay free of wheat takes long-term dedication to health and avoidance of denial. When people become free of wheat they discover a much higher level of health than they were ever aware of before, and are fully rewarded.

Wheat is also a problem for animals that do not eat it in their natural environment. Up-to-date formulas for dog and cat food are free of wheat, dairy and soy. When hogs are fed an all-corn diet, they are fairly healthy, but an all-wheat diet kills them.

A rarely mentioned problem with wheat is caused when wheat products are cooked. When wheat is heated until the outer surface is brown, a chemical is formed called benzo-a-pyrene. This chemical is known to be a cause of cancer in humans. Benzo-a-pyrene is in the smoke when tobacco is burned and is a major factor in how cigarettes cause lung cancer. Benzo-a-pyrene is formed when bread has a crust or is toasted as in a roll which has a browned surface.

One problem with wheat is caused by a misunderstanding about delayed allergic reactions. The body often becomes free of a food it is allergic to by rushing the food through your digestive tract. This reaction is one of the causes of diarrhea. Not being aware of this, a small group began selling people on drinking wheat grass juice, believing its damaging allergic reaction was a wonderful cleansing process. People who continue drinking wheat grass juice often find their health deteriorating. Their ability to admit they are

making a mistake is often blocked by the highly addictive nature of wheat. The way to become healthy is to avoid what you are allergic to.

Of all the damaging foods, none is more dangerous than wheat. Not only are many people allergic to wheat, but wheat is known to break down the inner lining of the digestive tract and create open, bloody sores. The part of wheat that causes this problem is called gluten. The book *Good Food Gluten Free* gives more documentation.

The small intestine is designed to filter selectively the broken down food particles through its membrane before they slowly enter into the circulation. If we have open sores along the inside of our small intestine, any food we eat will flood directly into our blood stream. When we have unfiltered food in our blood stream, our white blood cells will see it as a foreign invader. Our white blood cells are designed to attack foreign invaders. When our white blood cells attack the foods, our bodies are damaged in the battle. See the photograph of the broken-down intestinal lining on page 86.

There is an epidemic of delayed food allergies, and wheat may be one of the underlying causes of so many people's suffering. Read the labels carefully. You will find that there are now a number of new products on the market which are wheat free. Becoming free of wheat is an important step toward great health.

Hidden Advantages

When you avoid dairy products and the highly-allergic foods and chemicals explained in this chapter, along with the ones the Prime Test and your body indicate as damaging, you will not need stimulants to make it through the day. You will also sleep soundly and not need naps, and you will be free of the health and emotional roller coaster.

While you are rebuilding your health, it is important to develop good exercise, work and sleep habits. People often find that their health becomes much worse when they no longer have to get up each morning and do something important during the day. There is some unknown factor which causes people to be less healthy when they sleep in. When people lose their jobs or become sick for a while, it is important they find a regular activity until they recover. Otherwise, sleeping in and lack of activity will contribute significantly to their health problems.

Summary

The best way to help people reduce consumption of something unhealthy is to give them all the information and place a health tax on the item. This is working with cigarettes and is starting to work with alcohol, and would work with other unhealthy foods, drugs and chemicals.

What the government is doing with dairy products is the opposite. It gives us inaccurate information, and gives our tax dollars to the dairy industry.

The ancient Greek philosophy, "Nothing to Excess" is very different from the modern cliche "Everything in Moderation." Is there a moderate amount of tobacco or cocaine?

Your health will improve dramatically by completely avoiding delayed food and chemical allergies. Continuing to consume small amounts can prevent the benefits you are looking for.

Additional research is always wanted and more studies will be helpful. However, there are already enough high-quality studies available which demonstrate you can dramatically improve your health and longevity by avoiding dairy products, coffee, eggs, peanuts, yeast, damaging chemicals, legal and illegal drugs, and wheat.

*We are half dead
before we understand our disorder,
and half cured when we do.*

Charles Caleb Colton
Author, Gambler and Clergyman — 1780 to 1832

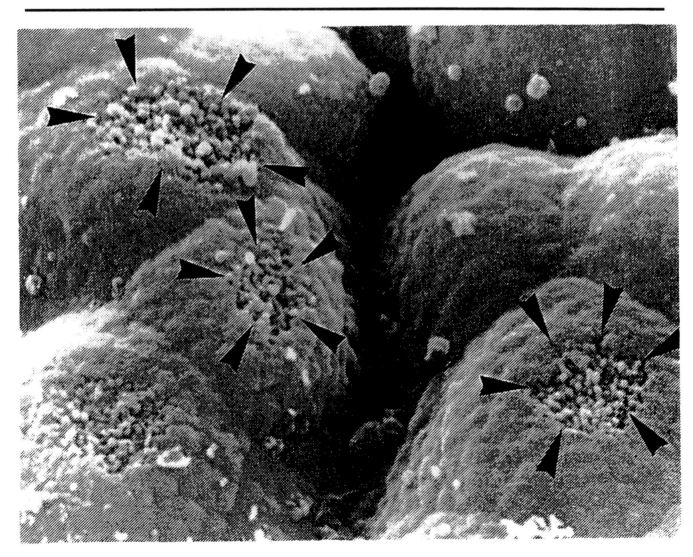

This photograph was taken through a microscope and shows damage done to the inner surface of the small intestine.

You are looking at the tips of the small villi, and you can see the surface tissue missing in the area surrounded by the pointers.

Chapter 10
Forty-Eight Ways to Optimize Your Health

The following information will help you achieve optimum health from your program when used in combination with your Prime Test results.

Some people become overwhelmed when they see all the different things they can do for their health. A much better way to look at the information is to approach each new insight as a step up a ladder that takes you to a higher level of health than you have enjoyed before.

Take advantage of each step and you will be rewarded by ever-improving health and a longer life. You will be spending so much less on your health care in the future that you will recover the cost of this program several times over. The more steps you take to help your health, the sooner you will feel well.

1. The first week on your new program can be very challenging. Many food allergies progress and become food addictions; therefore, you are likely to experience some withdrawal symptoms when you stop eating your reactive foods. Acknowledge your progress and reward yourself with your favorite nurturing activities.

2. Rapid weight loss is common as the allergic swelling goes down throughout your body. If you are overweight, be happy; if you are underweight, do not worry — you will be losing water and some fat, not muscle tissue. Keep a daily log of your weight and your symptoms.

3. Remember that one cause of delayed food allergies is eating the same foods every day. Other health and weight loss programs have people eating the same foods day after day. They also have people eating foods without knowing whether the person is allergic to them. Shortly after these types of programs become popular, reports of people getting sick start showing up in the press. Now you know why. With the passage of time, the liquid diets, the repetitious nutrition plans and other incomplete health programs fail.

4. Most people with food and chemical allergies find it helpful to share their progress and new insights with people who understand the importance of food and chemical allergies. Help the people around you to understand your program so they will be helpful and supportive.

5. Be creative and have fun with your meals. Eat in a comfortable and relaxed setting. Use your favorite dishes and glasses. Celebrate the splendor of your new health.

6. It helps to relax or meditate, with your eyes closed, for one minute before each meal. After meals, both digestion and overall health are significantly improved by going for a brisk, continuous walk for 20 minutes or more.

7. Whenever possible, avoid canned food. When using frozen foods, rinse before cooking and steam lightly. Remember — fresh is best. Eat as many raw foods as you are comfortable with, gradually increasing the amount. Chew thoroughly.

8. Use organically grown foods as much as possible. Our bodies have a buildup of pesticides, chemicals and toxic metals. It takes time to detoxify; by using niacin, exercise and saunas, you can speed up the process. Carefully clean all foods before eating. Wash and then soak legumes overnight before cooking.

9. Avoid over-cooking your fresh vegetables. "Yams," sweet potatoes and regular potatoes can turn into simple carbohydrates by baking. Peel, slice and steam them instead. Over-cooked vegetables have less nutritional value.

10. Cook in stainless steel, glass or ceramic cookware. Aluminum cookware and containers contaminate your food. Aluminum is found in the brain cells of people who have lost brain function and may contribute to senility and Alzheimer's disease. Avoid all aluminum consumption. Check for it in antacids, baking powders, cosmetics, toiletries, toothpastes, deodorants, etc. Even zinc oxide can cause problems when used as a deodorant.

11. Do not sleep with your car. Cars outgas allergy-causing chemicals and should not be parked in garages which are connected to the house. If this can not be avoided, seal the walls and doors and vent the garage well. Avoid diesel cars and trucks whenever possible.

12. It helps to remember that the healthiest groups of people in the world do not consume

dairy products. These people have solid bones all their lives and receive all the calcium the human body needs from fresh vegetables. When you look at nature you see that no other mammal consumes milk after infancy and no other mammal consumes another mammal's milk.

13. Women who are planning to have a child are dramatically benefited by this health program and so are their children. It is important for your child's health and for yours to breast feed for at least the first nine months, without any other foods added. It then works well to start adding a small amount of organically grown fresh vegetables to your child's diet along with your milk. Watch how your child reacts as you introduce one food at a time. Most children are born allergic to some of the foods their mother is allergic to. In addition, children can become allergic to the foods they eat before their bodies are ready for them.

It is important for you and your child's health to avoid your allergic foods while you are pregnant or nursing If you are not ready to make the commitment to breast-feed properly, wait until you are ready before you have a child. It is helpful to use the new approaches for preparing for child birth and for delivery.

The United States is the last country to circumcise male infants for previously believed health benefits. Even here the rate has dropped to under 48 percent. The foreskin is important and should be operated on only if it is defective.

14. It is helpful to avoid most brands of toothpaste. They are a chemical soup likely to cause delayed allergic reactions. Fortunately, the best tooth cleaning and gum-helping materials are compatible with your immune system. Brushing your teeth with baking soda, salt and diluted hydrogen peroxide is best for your teeth and gums and will save you money.

Mix four parts baking soda with one part salt and then combine with diluted hydrogen peroxide (mix three percent hydrogen peroxide with an equal amount of water to get one and one and a half percent hydrogen peroxide). Wet your tooth brush in the hydrogen peroxide solution and then dip lightly in baking soda/salt powder. The Interplak toothbrush works better than a regular tooth brush. The Sonicare toothbrush works even better. Follow by using a Water Pik type cleaner with the same diluted one and one half percent hydrogen peroxide. Then hold some of the hydrogen peroxide in your mouth for three minutes to kill additional damaging organisms.

Once a week, use a regular tooth brush with a little powdered pumice and the diluted hydrogen peroxide to remove stains and keep your teeth whiter. Regular tooth paste has abrasives in it and will wear down your enamel if used everyday. Some hardware stores have powdered pumice. Flossing after meals is also very important.

15. Bleeding gums after brushing is one of the signs of periodontal disease. You can see the blood when you rinse out your mouth. Sick gums are the major cause of tooth loss and tear down your overall health. Over 60 percent of adults have gum problems. A 1990 report by the American Academy of Periodontalogy states that the root of the problem is an immune system disorder; specifically, a deficiency and abnormality of white blood cells.

The type of white blood cell involved is the same one studied during the Prime Test. Save your gums, teeth and overall health by brushing properly, flossing, having your teeth cleaned twice a year and staying on your new health program.

16. Avoid silver fillings; they are actually over 25 percent mercury and release mercury vapors into your body. If you have silver fillings — also known as amalgam fillings — have them removed by a dentist who understands how mercury damages the immune system. Be sure your dentist uses rubber dams and an oxygen nose cup when removing your silver fillings. There are now low-cost replacements which are the same color as your teeth. One of these composite materials is Herculite. If the cavity is large, you may need to use gold.

Make sure your fillings and crowns are in excellent condition. If one leaks, the inflammation under it can keep you sick. Avoid root canal therapy — even when done properly they leak toxins and bacteria into the body. Read *Root Canal Cover-up* by George Meinig, DDS. Order the book by phone (805) 646-2865. Replace root-infected teeth with bridges or implants.

17. Full-spectrum light is important for

health. Some of the light that enters your eyes sends stimulation to your endocrine glands. The type of light our endocrine system needs is ultraviolet light — the same type of light that dark glasses are designed to block out. If you wear dark glasses, regular glasses or hard contact lenses, you are not receiving all the light your endocrine system needs. Wear dark glasses as little as possible and go for walks without your glasses or contacts when the sun is out. See page 173 for more details.

18. Store leftovers in glass or ceramic jars rather than plastic. Avoid Tupperware or other soft plastic products; they leak chemicals into your food.

19. The first step in proper digestion takes place in the mouth. It is important to chew each bite until it is fully broken down. This adds important digestive enzymes. You can only enjoy the good flavors when the food is in your mouth. There are no teeth or taste buds in your stomach.

20. Do your best to avoid fruit juices and vegetable juices. If you occasionally drink juices, dilute them with clean water. Do not exceed six ounces of fruit juice or eight ounces of fruit at any one time. Eat fruit in its natural form.

21. Alcoholic beverages create a long list of major health problems. In addition, they all have yeast residues in them. It may help you to stay free of alcohol by remembering that alcohol is made by yeast breaking down cereal grains or grapes into carbon dioxide and alcohol. Most beverages contain chemical additives. Enjoy high quality, wonderful tasting water.

22. Have properly filtered water, clean spring water or distilled water readily available at all times for drinking and be sure to cook with it. To be properly filtered, water must go through two types of filters, reverse osmosis and activated charcoal. Do not drink tap water or water purchased in opaque plastic bottles. Drink little or no water with meals; it impairs digestion. It is very helpful for adults to drink twelve, eight ounce glasses of water, throughout the day.

23. One of the major ways we get damaging chemicals into our bodies, other than eating them in our foods, is by inhaling them or absorbing them through our skin. You may have to move to an area which has clean air before you will become fully well. It is important to take the chemicals out of the water before you shower in it. This can be done by putting an activated charcoal filter above the shower head.

24. It strengthens the immune system to finish a warm shower with up to one half minute of cool or cold water. Start carefully with cool and build up to cold.

25. Cooking with gas is harmful because of the fumes from the burners and pilot lights. Use electric ranges or hot plates.

26. Electromagnetic fields have been shown to cause problems for some people. Therefore, avoid living near high-voltage lines and remove all electric motors from your bedroom. Do not use electric blankets. If you have a water bed, connect the heater to a timer so that it is only heating when you are not in bed. The bed will cool slightly during the night. The slight cooling actually helps you to sleep better. Limit the amount of time you spend watching television or using a computer with a cathode-ray tube.

27. Eat snacks one hour before or after meals and be very careful not to eat snacks or meals within one hour of taking a nap or going to bed. Snacks may be helpful, but are not mandatory. It is important to eat three equal-sized meals a day. The general rule is, "Eat only when you are hungry and sleep on an empty stomach."

28. Be careful of cereal grains. They are one of the major causes of allergy problems. If you eat cereal grains, be sure you space them out on a four-day rotation. If you eat rice on Monday, do not eat it again until Friday.

29. Keep a journal of your reactions. After checking with your counselor and waiting two weeks, you can begin adding variety to your menu and experimenting with different foods. If you are still having some problems, your counselor will explain how you can re-test to confirm a food the Prime Test said was compatible.

30. Delayed food allergies fluctuate. After you have gone off a reactive food for at least two weeks and then have a test meal of that food, you may not have a reaction; however, it may react the second or third time you try the food. Stay in touch with your body.

31. Special selection of the materials in your environment and careful cleaning is important. Clean the air in your car, home and at work with activated-charcoal filters and negative-ion generators. Avoid carpets which have an odor. Do not fumigate your home or live in one that has been sprayed or fumigated during the last year. Termites can be removed with liquid nitrogen or electrical impulses. There are also safe ways to eliminate other insects. Be aware that government officials are often controlled by farmers, and thus people end up getting sprayed instead of farmers' doing a proper job of controlling insects with non-chemical methods.

32. Most people react to some degree to dust, dust mites and dust-mite droppings. Do not use a humidifier because moist air causes dust mites to multiply rapidly.

Regular filter-type vacuum cleaners are a problem because they blow the dust-mite droppings through the bag and into the air. They end up in your mouth, nose and lungs. It was believed that the best type of vacuum cleaner was one that filtered the debris through water, as the Rainbow model does. However, recent tests have shown that cat danders and many other particles are not removed by the water. Also, the Rainbow and nearly all other vacuums cleaners do not suck the debris out of the lower levels of the carpet. Thus, as you walk around on your carpets, the dirt keeps billowing out of the lower levels and into your mouth, nose and lungs.

The best approach is to have a powerful central vacuuming system with a rotary brush. Next best is to have a Eureka Excalibur or World Vac with hard case. Also wear a 3M mask (#8540) while vacuuming with the windows open.

33. Special cleaning solutions should be used for washing clothes. Never use detergents or fabric softeners. Never use detergents or spot-removing chemicals when washing dishes. One cleaning liquid to test is Shaklee's Basic-H. Choose the soap you use on your body with similar care. Avoid clothes that have chemicals in them. Polyester is treated with formaldehyde. Pure wool and silk are compatible with most people. Pure cotton is the safest. Wash new clothes twice before you wear them.

34. When selecting a dry-cleaner, find one that uses Valclene solvent made by Du Pont. Other solvents have been shown to cause cancer and are harder on the immune system. Air out your clothes before you wear them.

35. There are several important supplements specially made for people with food and chemical allergies. Besides vitamins and minerals, there are glandular extracts and many other items which are helpful. Be sure to use products free of the items you are allergic to. Repetitious use of any item can cause you to develop a delayed allergic reaction to it.

36. As important as supplements are, they will be of no lasting help if you go back to eating improperly. Nothing can overcome the damage caused when you eat excess fat and cholesterol or foods you are allergic to.

37. Many people have low level infections caused by the yeast called Candida. When delayed food allergies become worse, yeast infections can become a major problem. It is important to avoid too many simple carbohydrates (sugars and fruits) because they help the yeast to grow.

38. Intestinal parasites have become very common. It is valuable to get special tests to discover if they are causing problems for you.

39. Cortisone and steroid medications are hard on your body. You feel or look better in the short run but have more symptoms and allergies in the future. Even small amounts of over-the-counter cortisone creams are very damaging.

Women often find the steroid type birth control pills make their delayed food and chemical allergies worse. The contraceptive called Depo Provera is effective and reduces premenstrual problems but often reduces interest in sex. Norplant may work for some women. IUD's can cause infections after years of use. Tubal ligations for women are effective, safe and sometimes reversible. Vasectomies for men often cause an immune reaction to develop against their own sperm and this damages overall health.

Monitoring body temperature helps women know when they are fertile. The Billings Method of natural birth control uses vaginal mucus as a clear sign of fertility. This method has been carefully studied and found safe, reliable and economical. The book, *The Billings Method* by Evelyn Billings, is very helpful.

40. Recent studies on people who eat no red meat, fish or fowl showed they had much healthier white blood cells. Their white blood cells attacked and killed cancer cells at twice the rate of those on the Standard American Diet.

41. It makes no sense to avoid the foods you are allergic to and become free of your day-to-day aches and pains while continuing to eat the foods that cause the silent killers such as heart disease, stroke, weak bones and cancer. Most people have spent their lives eating too much animal fat, vegetable oil, cholesterol and protein. By dramatically reducing these food ingredients, you will start to clean out your body and add years to your life. This is a long process; however, as time goes by, you will feel better and better.

42. Several animal studies have shown that by reducing calories, ailments go down and life expectancy goes up. Research shows the most important ingredient to reduce is protein. Eating less also helps people who want to lose weight.

43. The following wisdom helps people stay on their new health program: "What looks like aging in older people is not true aging — it is the result of a lifetime of eating the wrong foods."

44. The best health program is about 75 percent what you put in your body and about 25 percent aerobic exercise with weight training.

45. Most people find it very helpful to use the services of a counselor who specializes in food and chemical allergies and also knows how important it is to eat the right percentages of fat, protein and carbohydrate. This makes it easier to incorporate these improvements.

Be sure to keep in touch with your doctor so you receive the support you need to make your program successful and more rewarding. It will take some time to reverse all the damage of years of improper eating; however, it happens when you stay on the right path.

46. The program you are starting is the best approach for preventing ailments. And, it is important to remember that the best approach for preventing an ailment should be used whenever treating an ailment. Use supplements carefully; it is common to become allergic to the materials they are made from. Your body uses a little vitamin C and zinc whenever it

knits two cells back together. If you are going to have surgery, take four grams of Ester-C and 50 milligrams of zinc every day for two weeks before and after the operation. For colds and the flu, slowly dissolve 24 milligrams of zinc under your tongue every two hours.

47. Many people, including doctors, are not aware of the existence or importance of delayed food and chemical allergies. You are benefiting from the most advanced health program available. When you are on the leading edge, it is hard to get all the support and understanding you would like. Do not let well-meaning friends or traditional doctors talk you out of your new, correct path to great health.

48. The foundation of health is eating foods which are compatible with your white blood cells and the rest of your body while avoiding excess fat, protein, cholesterol, sugar and damaging chemicals. Enjoy regular aerobic and strength exercises, work and relationships. Be careful about getting caught up in all the different types of fine tuning and ignoring the fundamentals.

After carefully eating your compatible foods for one month, your health will probably be much improved, and you will be at an important crossroad. Many people continue eating well and become even healthier. Some people slip back, and their symptoms return so they go back to their compatible foods. Occasionally people slip back and their symptoms do not return; however, if the symptoms do return, the person knows how to become well again. Some people find it helpful to get re-tested.

Whatever path you take, you will always have a powerful awareness that you can take advantage of all the rest of your life. Your life will be healthier and longer because of your commitment and work during the first month of your new health program. The more you do for your health, the better you will feel and the more freedom you will have in your life.

There are two great joys that come with your new health program. The first is you feeling wonderful, the second is being able to help your friends and loved ones improve their health. Obtain information from your doctor which will help you enroll your friends into beginning The Quality Longevity Program.

Shared Experiences

My family has used The Quality Longevity Program for more than five years. My son is a world-class athlete, and the white blood cell test and the resulting nutritional program have been beneficial.

The regime is very good, and many people have been helped by the program.

Jack Knorpp, Santa Ana, California

I wish to express my deep appreciation for the marvelous benefits I have received through your program and the white blood cell test. I have followed the program for more than two months, and am becoming healthier each day. So many of my health problems have vanished it's hard to believe they were caused by delayed food allergies, but I have the proof.

I have suffered for two years from chronic bladder problems and have never been totally free of infection in spite of taking antibiotics. Now, I feel I am cured; I have been free of antibiotics and free of infection for more than six weeks. My weight is normal now, the swelling and severe fluid retention has disappeared. The stricture, heaviness and pain has gone from my legs. There were days when it was almost too painful to walk. Now I feel normal. I am 72 years old but have a youthful appearance and renewed ambition. I am surprising my family and friends by my appearance, my renewed ambition and vigor. One of my friends remarked the other day, "You must have found a new youth pill." This statement is not so far-fetched; we really have found a most beneficial program — a medical breakthrough.

Iola I. Berg, Lynnwood, Washington.

Perhaps the most significant and most healthful change that occurred for me is the alteration of my eating habits and the elimination of harmful foods which are every-day dieting choices for many people. The program taught me a different and more nourishing way of taking care of myself. I feel great.

Louise M. Atty, Registered Nurse
Brea, California

Since childhood I have been troubled with hay fever, asthma, itchy eyes and severe sinus headaches. I was labeled by my family and friends as always being lazy.

I had to take anti-histamines to relieve my symptoms. They did help temporarily, but the side effects were terrible. I was always tired and irritable.

Before I heard about The Quality Longevity Program, I had given up hope of finding a solution to my health problems. In just one week of being on the program, I felt like a new person. My sinus headaches disappeared, the congestion in my lungs cleared up as did the itchy eyes, and my energy level increased. Last but not least was the weight loss I wasn't expecting.

An additional benefit is that I can now be around cats and dogs which I never could do before without getting so ill that I would have to spend the next day in bed.

I am so excited now because I never knew one could feel so good!

Nancy Ross Berg, Pasadena, California

I want to thank you for helping me feel better. I had been suffering for years with mood swings, irritability, fatigue, bloating, stuffy nose, plus other symptoms. In spite of seeing several doctors and taking pills, I wasn't getting much relief. At times, I was so irritable that my best friends didn't want to be with me; I was so depressed.

After attending your seminar, I was hopeful these health problems could be relieved by finding out which foods I should eat. I became more aware of how I felt after meals and could see that some foods made me sleepy or irritable. Sometimes it was difficult for me to concentrate on my job.

The Quality Longevity Program enabled me to clear up some of my symptoms within the first week, including the fatigue and swelling. After a few months of monitoring my reactions, I began to see a change. As the months passed, my symptoms lessened; some completely disappeared.

Now that I have used the program for years, I clearly feel better, work better and relate better when eating my compatible foods. When I don't, my symptoms come back. The program has also helped me to give birth to and nurse a healthy girl.

I am writing to you in appreciation and I hope other women and mothers will gain this awareness and stop suffering.

Valerie Watkins, Mother
Temecula, California

Chapter 11

Understanding Allergies: The Science, History and Politics of Allergy Testing for Foods and Chemicals

Introduction

A comprehensive understanding of the different types of allergy reactions provides the best opportunity for a major improvement in people's health and a significant reduction in health care costs.

There is a hidden war being waged by traditional allergists against several different groups of health professionals. These alternative groups use a comprehensive understanding of food and chemical allergies. This "turf war" has been going on in the United States for over 40 years and people everywhere have been kept in the dark about a better approach to their health problems.

The awareness that food allergies are a major health problem is being crippled by a very narrow definition of the word "allergy." Traditional allergists define allergy as only acute reactions which are caused by just one mechanism. This type of reaction is caused primarily by airborne antigens. A second, broader definition of allergy defines allergies as altered reactions and are usually caused by foods and chemicals. One definition limits the field of allergy to acute reactions — the second definition expands the field to include acute and altered or delayed reactions.

The broader definition of allergy is understood by a growing number of people in the medical and scientific communities as well as the public. This type of reaction causes damage in one person but not in others and is not limited to one mechanism. This definition includes food and chemical allergies which are hidden or delayed. Delayed food allergies are sometimes called hidden food allergies, food sensitivities or food intolerances.

Traditional allergists believe that less than three percent of the population has food allergies. This is because their narrow definition of allergies includes only acute reactions and leaves out hidden or delayed reactions. However, food-allergy scientists have shown that over 50 percent of the general population has significant health problems caused by delayed food and chemical allergies. For people with significant health problems, the percentage affected by delayed food allergies is often over 90 percent.

There are now several ways of testing people for food and chemical allergies, but most of these techniques miss many of the reactive foods and chemicals. The optimum first step for helping people with a broad range of health problems is for them to have a blood test which uses their white blood cells, followed up with comprehensive nutritional counseling.

After you look at the evidence presented in this report, you will see that the six negative articles on white blood cell testing were done by traditional allergists who used the narrow definition of allergy and did not believe in delayed food and chemical allergies. In addition, they had no experience working with patients with health problems caused by delayed allergies. These traditional allergists had been losing patients to doctors who were using white blood cell testing.

These six negative studies were used by traditional allergists to persuade insurance companies to stop reimbursing their policy holders for delayed allergy testing. These allergists also used the negative studies to pressure state and federal agencies to harass people who use food and chemical allergy testing to help people remove their symptoms. Sadly, their strategy has worked well. Many people are now unable to obtain this type of effective health care for their problems.

The overwhelming majority of doctors are unaware that there are 60 positive studies and reports which support white blood cell testing and this evidence has been arbitrarily disregarded

---

This chapter was originally part of a presentation to the California State Legislature that was designed to increase the awareness of improved approaches for health care.

and covered-up by traditional allergists.

Of the 60 positive studies and reports, nine were published in medical journals before the cytotoxic test was developed in 1956. Since then a total of 42 studies supporting the white blood cell test were published in medical journals, many peer reviewed, all editorial board reviewed. There are at least nine additional supportive papers in other health publications.

Of the six negative studies, one reported on no white blood cell reactions to pollens. White blood cells do not usually react to pollens, and thus, there is no problem with the first study. Five were done after the first white blood cell test for food reactions was reported in 1956. Of these five negative studies, all were done by traditional allergists and every one reported observing white blood cell destruction by reactions with foods, depending on the patient. Thus, these negative studies also support the principle underlying the white blood cell test. Therefore, after careful analysis, there are no negative studies.

The authors of these five so called negative studies did not know at the time they did their studies that killing white blood cells with food reactions causes many allergy and other symptoms. These five studies are the entire foundation of the traditional allergists constant attack against white blood cell testing.

Had the information which follows been available earlier, the traditional allergists' strategy would have been exposed. This would have helped the public and health care professionals to be more aware of an important advancement in health care and better understand preventive care. The following information helps reverse the negative propaganda and thereby increases the availability of effective health care.

As important as it is to find a cure for each disease, it is far more important to prevent disease. The best cures still leave people coming down with different diseases. Also, most cures cause some damage and are often expensive. Using preventive care principles enables one to avoid most ailments. If an ailment does become a problem, it is possible to regain health faster by avoiding delayed allergic reactions. Major health problems are being solved by using this approach; however, the public is not being informed about this breakthrough.

By 1991 there were 42 positive studies done by

doctors and reported in medical journals that are peer reviewed or editorial board reviewed which confirm the value of white blood cell testing for delayed food allergies. All 42 of these positive studies were done by doctors who had been performing the test for years and were continually obtaining significant health improvements for their patients.

In contrast, all five negative studies were done using the original cytotoxic test and were conducted by traditional allergists who had been relying on their type of skin test for years. They used the cytotoxic test with only one group of patients. Even though all these allergists saw white blood cells being killed by reactions with foods, they concluded these reactions were of no significance. (These 47 studies are identified by a period after their number, starting on page 114.)

There is now abundant scientific information on how delayed food and chemical allergies cause a broad range of ailments. People need this information so they can choose the type of health care which works for them.

History

The knowledge that delayed food reactions are the underlying cause of a broad range of health problems began around 400 BC with the Greek physician Hippocrates. He wrote in great detail about food reactions and how they caused a broad range of common ailments. He noticed that when some people ate certain foods they would have a severe, fast-acting reaction, causing a skin rash or trouble breathing. However, he also noticed many people had delayed reactions which created several different types of symptoms. These delayed reactions are now called delayed food allergies, hidden food allergies, food intolerances or food sensitivities.

Hippocrates noticed these hidden, delayed reactions would often show up when some people stopped eating a food they had been eating regularly. He also noticed symptoms when they ate more of a particular food in a day than they were used to. This area of his work has turned out to be the most brilliant. However, one problem he was not able to solve was how to test people accurately to discover which foods were actually causing the damaging reactions.

After Hippocrates died, much of his

knowledge about food reactions was lost. The medical establishment began treating symptoms with herbs, drugs or surgeries instead of discovering and removing the underlying causes of the symptoms.

The awareness of how important the right foods are for health blossomed again around 1200 AD with Maimonides. He was the physician to the Egyptian royal family and believed that people with symptoms and ailments should first be helped by trying different foods before experimenting with any other approach. His wisdom is still valuable for us today.

Little knowledge was added to how foods can cause ailments until 1905, when Francis Hare, MD, in Australia, wrote a book titled *The Food Factor In Disease*. He observed that a broad range of common ailments went away when cereal grains were avoided. Unfortunately, the concept of allergy had not been developed yet and he did not understand what was going on.

Hippocrates's discovery that delayed food reactions cause many of the most painful ailments was still lost. For generations this has caused untold suffering and ever-growing medical costs.

The word "allergy" was first coined in 1906 by Clemens von Pirquet, MD. He specified that allergy means altered reaction. The field of allergy grew rapidly during the first 25 years of the twentieth century. However, a major problem began around 1920 when several European doctors demanded the word "allergy" be redefined to mean only acute reactions. Many American doctors objected and pointed out that this narrow definition of allergy was not consistent with what they were observing with their patients.

Arthur F. Coca, MD, the founder and editor of the *Journal of Immunology*, led the battle to retain the broader definition of the word "allergy." Unfortunately, he lost. In 1926 the limited definition of allergy was accepted by most doctors on both sides of the Atlantic. During the 1960's, this narrow definition of allergies was further promoted by the discovery of an immune particle produced by the body and found in the blood. They called the particle Immunoglobulin E, and abbreviated it to IgE. Unfortunately, after the discovery of IgE, most doctors stopped looking for other mechanisms which cause allergic reactions.

However, doctors helping patients suffering from delayed food and chemical allergies do understand there is more than one antibody and there are other mechanisms causing allergies. They continue to use the original, comprehensive definition of allergy.

These doctors can demonstrate how allergies to foods, drugs and environmental chemicals usually do not involve IgE reactions or any type of antigen or antibody. Instead, they have discovered that the reactions are caused by immune complexes, prostaglandins and other mechanisms that have yet to be fully understood.

These aware doctors also demonstrate that many reactions are not detectable by such approaches as skin tests, IgE tests and the other procedures employed by traditional allergists.

The doctors with this new, comprehensive knowledge about the cause of health problems are commonly able to help patients who have symptoms which do not show up for hours or days after exposure. These delayed allergies are often the cause of the most common, recurring symptoms.

In the United States there was a rebirth of the awareness of delayed food allergies around 1928. It started in California with Albert Rowe, MD. He rediscovered that delayed food allergies cause a broad range of ailments. However, like Hippocrates, he was unable to figure out a practical way to test accurately which foods were causing people's health problems. He tested by using elimination diets and by trial and error.

The differences of medical opinion about the correct definition of allergy and whether food and chemical allergies are common has led to a division between the traditional allergists and the doctors who believe in the comprehensive definition of allergy. These comprehensive doctors are known as food allergy specialists or Clinical Ecologists and practice Environmental Medicine. Clinical Ecology is the study of how our health is affected by our environment, especially by foods and chemicals.

The history of the research done in the field of non-IgE, delayed food and chemical allergies has recently been documented in detail by Theron G. Randolph, MD, in his book *Environmental Medicine: Beginnings and Bibliographies of Clinical Ecology,* published in 1987 by Clinical Ecology Publications, Fort Collins, Colorado, (708) 844-9898.

It is important to know that when Clinical Ecologists use the word "allergy," they are not using the limited IgE definition of allergy used by traditional allergists. The Clinical Ecologists define allergy by stating that it is an altered reaction to a food, chemical, mold, pollen or other substance that damages some people but not others.

Delayed food allergies are also called non-IgE food allergies and food addictions, in addition to hidden food allergies, food intolerances and food sensitivities. These different names are used to try to get around the problems caused by two separate groups of doctors having different definitions for the word "allergy." These problems would be solved and people's health would be improved if all doctors used the original and complete definition of allergy, which is "altered reactivity." Altered reactivity is also the definition the public understands.

People who are suffering with health problems want the right to choose the approach which will help them become well rapidly and at the lowest cost. The broad, comprehensive definition of allergy makes this possible.

A delayed food allergy testing method was not discovered until 1950, when Dr. Randolph began fasting his patients and then "challenge testing" them with each food. This method required the person to eat no food at all and drink only properly filtered water or clean spring water until they became symptom free. This usually took about five days. After the fast the person would test three foods per day by eating one at each meal. This would continue for 25 days. This method was helpful because their symptoms recurred when they reintroduced the foods to which they were allergic. There was then no doubt about the cause of their health problems.

This cause-and-effect demonstration of delayed food allergies helped people continue to stay free of their damaging foods. However, some reactions are delayed by a day or more. Therefore, it is often difficult to identify the foods which are causing people's health problems. In addition, sometimes reactions from allergic foods would be missed. Numerous other complications would occur because of reactions to pesticides in the foods or chemicals in the air. Because of these and other problems, the fasting and food-challenge testing approach is about 70 percent accurate.

For food-challenge testing to be accurate and safe, it had to be done after a fast and in a specially cleaned and modified hospital. Also, when people test a food and experience a reaction, their health is further damaged and they feel significant discomfort during the testing. Fasting often leaves people more reactive in the future. This approach took about one month in a specially designed hospital to test around 60 foods and the cost was over $15,000.

A better approach for testing was needed that would be safe, inexpensive and reliable. A blood test would solve these problems because it would cause no harm or discomfort to the person and it would save time because several items could be tested from one blood sample. A blood test would also reduce costs and could be more accurate and objective.

Research on a blood test for allergies started about 75 years ago. Published medical studies first appeared in 1917 explaining a blood test which used white blood cells to reveal various allergic reactions [1,2]. (The bracketed numbers refer to medical studies and reports listed chronologically, starting on page 114.)

In 1936, it was first discovered that food allergies lower a person's white blood cell count. (Vaughn, WT: "The leucopenic index as a diagnostic method in the study of food allergy" *J Lab Clin Med* 1936; 21:1278-1288.)

A later discovery by George Ulett, MD, found that shortly after a delayed food allergy reaction, the white blood cell level in the person's blood goes up sharply as part of an alarm reaction. Several hours later the white blood cell level returns to a chronically depressed level [20].

The first usable white blood cell test for delayed food allergies was developed by Arthur P. Black, MD. In the early 1950's he went to

Europe and gained insights which helped him to develop a new test. He named the procedure the cytotoxic test. "Cyto" is the Greek word for cell and "toxic" means to poison. This test enables people to find out what their delayed allergic reactions are from a small blood sample instead of fasting and food testing or the painful, time consuming and inaccurate skin tests.

With the original cytotoxic test or the newer Prime Test, a technician looks through a microscope and identifies a reaction by seeing which foods damage or kill a person's white blood cells. Dr. Black's work was published in 1956 [10]. Unfortunately, he died shortly after his research was published.

His research on the cytotoxic test was continued and expanded by William Bryan, MD, and his wife, Marian Bryan. They saved his breakthrough for future generations. The Bryans made numerous improvements to the cytotoxic test, and it began to be used throughout the United States, Europe and Australia [11,15,16,17,23].

In August of 1991, I finished a thorough review of the medical literature and uncovered 66 studies and reports on the use of white blood cell tests to determine food allergies. These are all actual studies or reports — not opinion papers. Of these 66 studies and reports, 60 of them are positive (52 in medical journals and 8 in health journals), and six are, in varying degrees, negative. Thus, 90 percent of the studies and reports are positive and supportive of the efficacy of white blood cell testing.

Previous reviews of the literature by traditional allergists located only 25 studies, and some reviews relied on fewer than 15 studies for their negative conclusions.

The researchers who performed the 60 positive studies and reports concluded that this way of testing has significant value and clear efficacy. They demonstrated that the information gained is able to help patients overcome many of their health problems. In contrast, the negative studies came to the wrong conclusion because of errors in study design, materials, procedures and misunderstandings about the results.

The positive papers demonstrated that patients' health improved when the tests were done properly and patients stopped eating the foods which caused their symptoms. These beneficial results were obtained even though the materials and procedures used in the positive studies were primitive when compared to today's standards. In the last few years, there have been numerous improvements in white blood cell testing; however, the successes of the positive studies were obtained without any of these improvements.

A few traditional allergists are still trying to discredit the positive studies by stating they were not published in peer-review journals. A peer-review journal is one which sends submitted studies to those working in the related field for their approval before publishing.

Some traditional allergists, in their attempt to discredit the cytotoxic test, have testified under oath that the major studies supporting the cytotoxic test were not in peer-review journals. In fact, the top peer-review journals did publish major studies; examples are: *Allergy* [37,51,53]; *Ear, Nose & Throat Journal* [25,27,46]; *American Journal of Medicine* [54] and the *Journal of Nutritional Medicine* [60]. Some of the positive reports were not peer reviewed. However, the majority of the recent, major positive studies were published in peer-review journals. In contrast, the two most recent negative studies were published in journals which were not peer reviewed at the time they were published [65,66].

The 60 positive reports and studies have several things in common. First, the doctors involved had considerable experience in helping people with delayed food allergies. Second, they did not limit their definition of allergy to IgE-type reactions. Third, they had considerable experience with the type of test on which they were reporting. These important fundamentals were missing in each of the negative studies.

The conclusions of the positive studies are in general agreement. First, white blood cell testing is of value for discovering non-IgE food allergies. Second, the studies indicate that white blood cell testing can be used for detecting the underlying cause of a broad range of ailments not currently recognized as being caused by allergic reactions. Third, the test has significant value as a regular part of an effective practice designed to help people become free of their symptoms.

Negative Studies

A study which might be considered negative was done in 1949 by William Franklin, MD. This study was performed before the cytotoxic test was discovered, and it used different procedures. The seven patients selected had IgE-type allergic reactions such as positive skin tests for ragweed. They suffered from "ragweed hay fever" or "ragweed asthma." It was not known, at the time this study was done, that white blood cell tests are not effective for discovering rapid-onset IgE-type allergic reactions.

This paper is not a true negative study related to cytotoxic testing or other white blood cell testing because different procedures were used, and patients with acute airborne allergies were selected. This study was included for background information to help the reader understand why traditional allergists have had such trouble understanding a blood test that gives different results from their skin test for acute allergies.

One statement Dr. Franklin made about allergies is very valuable and would not be understood until many years later. He opened his study with the following words: "The cells of various tissues are of extreme importance in hypersensitivity. The difference between allergic and non-allergic individuals must fundamentally arise in the cells" [61].

The second negative study related to cytotoxic testing was headed by Van Vleck Chambers, MD, in 1958. There were numerous procedural errors. First, they did not use pyrogen-free water. Pyrogens are the minute parts of cells left over when you sterilize water. These particles upset the results. Second, the antigens were metered out with a toothpick instead of with an accurate $3,000 gram scale. In addition, no effort was made to calibrate the antigens. Third, they used Vaseline-ringed slides which leak and were later found to cause poor reproducibility. Fourth, they did not clean and coat the glass slides properly. Uncoated glass kills white blood cells. This mistake seriously damaged the results.

Besides these procedural errors, there was a fundamental error of study design. Dr.

Chambers selected patients who had "clear-cut clinical sensitivities to foods, animal danders, or pollen ...." White blood cell testing is not designed to discover these clear-cut IgE-type reactions. The white blood cell test is designed to discover delayed, non-IgE reactions.

The negative conclusions of this study are inaccurate because of the numerous procedural errors listed above, in addition to the fundamental mistake of choosing the wrong type of patients for the study.

A statement Dr. Chambers made in the opening paragraph of his study exposes the reason for the numerous unfounded attacks and five negative studies on the white blood cell test discovered by Dr. Black. He wrote, "Since the simplicity and accuracy claimed for the test and its convenience so far as the patient is concerned are so great, it was felt that, if Black's work could be corroborated, conventional skin testing would soon become an obsolete procedure" [62]. White blood cell tests dramatically reduce the number of people who go to traditional allergists.

The third negative study was done in 1975 by Phil Lieberman, MD and associates. It had serious flaws and there were procedural errors. First, serum dilutions were made with water instead of pyrogen-free saline. Second, they used Vaseline-ringed slides that were later found to damage reproducibility. Third, the antigen dilutions used in this study were later found to give inaccurate results.

The authors are to be credited for correcting one of the errors of the previous negative study. They did clean and coat the slides.

Besides the procedural errors, the basic design of this paper was flawed. The authors tested IgE-reacting patients (also called atopic patients) with the cytotoxic test, and thus the doctors were unable to obtain a correlation with their skin testing. There is not *supposed* to be a correlation with their skin testing. The cytotoxic test measures hidden or delayed food allergies, not rapid-acting IgE allergies. White blood cell tests are designed to discover the types of allergies that do not show up on skin tests.

In this study the delayed food allergy reactions were called "false positives." The authors did not realize they had discovered non-IgE, delayed food allergies. To call the cytotoxic test reactions false positives because they were missed by the skin test overlooks the fact that the traditional skin test is not able to test for delayed food and chemical allergies.

The authors did include a few people with delayed food allergy symptoms; i.e., "headache, fatigue, dyspnea, maculopapular rash, nasal congestion and diarrhea."

Even with the improper study design and defective procedures, 20 percent of the patients who used the results eliminated some of their symptoms. No explanation was given for these successes. It is unfortunate the authors did not know how to properly use the information from the cytotoxic test and help all the patients.

Most of the criticisms in Lieberman's study are based on the cytotoxic test's not giving the same information as the skin test. The study states, "The test had little diagnostic accuracy in the evaluation of atopic patients with well-established allergic reactions to foods." The fact that the test discovers allergies other than the ones that are the obvious atopic or skin type allergies is actually one of the major advantages of the white blood cell test.

There is reason to suspect that this study was rushed into print without careful peer review. One of the procedures said to have been used was placing liquid antigens on the slides and then setting cover slips over the antigens to let them dry. This would have been impossible because the slides would not dry with the cover slips on them. In addition, once the cover slips were placed on the Vaseline rings, they could not have been removed. This would have prevented the authors from adding the white blood cells and thus performing the test.

The authors admitted in the body of the study that their technicians did not have the necessary skills to obtain reproducible results. The authors wrote, "There was very little concordance between examiners when the same slide was examined by two people." In addition, the technicians did not have the materials necessary to make test kits which could give reproducible results. Also, they were supervised by doctors who did not understand non-IgE, delayed food allergies.

The authors who performed this study did acknowledge their negative bias and the bias

of most traditional allergists. In the opening section of their report they wrote, "Although the validity of the cytotoxic food test has remained in doubt, it continues to be used in the evaluation of food allergies."

Because of the serious defects in their study, it is a mistake to use it to challenge the efficacy of the cytotoxic test [63].

The fourth negative study was done in 1976 and was led by Thomas E. Benson, MD. There were serious problems with this study even though he thought he had learned how to do the cytotoxic test by visiting Marian Bryan.

The procedural errors were fewer than in previous studies; however, there were some serious mistakes. First, to dilute the antigens, they used sterile distilled water instead of pyrogen-free water. Second, they used antigen dilutions that were later discovered to cause errors. Third, they washed the slides in tap water instead of distilled water. Fourth, they used Vaseline-ringed slides which were later found to cause irregularities. Fifth, for diluting the serum, they used sterile distilled water instead of pyrogen-free saline. Sixth, they did not grade the readings properly.

They also made the same error as previous negative authors in the design of their study. They chose atopic patients (those with acute skin reactions) instead of people with chronic food-allergy symptoms.

Even with the above errors, the Benson group was able to achieve 86 percent reproducibility in one group of patients and 100 percent reproducibility when testing certain foods. With one patient they were also able to achieve 100 percent reproducibility.

These results are significantly better than those obtained with skin tests. The accuracy for the skin test is about 25 percent for IgE allergies and zero percent for non-IgE, delayed food allergies. The authors acknowledged, "The results of this study with a limited population of patients demonstrated that the test has a significant degree of reproducibility by these methods...."

They were using the skin test as a standard; thus, they falsely believed the cytotoxic test gave a high percentage of false positives. They were discovering delayed food allergies and did not realize it.

The authors acknowledged they did not understand the mechanism of the cytotoxic test. They concluded the test had no value because it did not match their clinical experience. Their experience was limited to the skin test and IgE blood tests.

Because they learned some of the procedures from Marian Bryan, they had fewer procedural errors than in the previous negative studies and thus obtained fairly good reproducibility. However, they still made mistakes in their procedure, and the basic design of their study was flawed.

Their negative conclusions are unsupported because of their errors and lack of understanding of the mechanism of non-IgE, delayed food allergies [64].

The fifth negative study was done in 1978 by William P. King, MD. It was a comparison study which demonstrated that the cytotoxic test and a non-traditional skin test gave different results. Both tests are of value, but are designed to test for different reactions. However, the author was not aware of this at the time he performed his study. The author dismissed them both because he only understood and believed in IgE allergies.

This study had several procedural errors and serious problems with the basic design. Also, the author did not follow through and use the information to counsel his patients [65].

The sixth negative study related to cytotoxic testing was done in 1980 by Carl W. Lehman, MD. It also had procedural errors. First, he used the wrong blood anticoagulant. Second, he used water instead of pyrogen-free saline for diluting the serum. Third, he used the problem-causing Vaseline-ringed glass slides. Forth, he used antigen dilutions that were later found to give inaccurate results.

Even though Dr. Lehman made procedural errors and his technicians lacked experience, the author obtained good reproducibility. He wrote, "The cytotoxic tests were exact duplicate results 79.9% of the time and an additional 18.3% of the cases varied by only one degree of reactivity." This totals 98 percent reproducibility. Dr. Lehman concluded, "I regard 1% of variance 98% of the time as quite acceptable reproducibility."

One reason for his negative conclusion about the cytotoxic test is that the test results varied with time. This is actually evidence that the test was working, because delayed food allergy reactions do change with time. The study is also invalid because he added a variable by giving his patients sublingual food drops while trying to evaluate their cytotoxic tests.

The doctor did not know how to counsel his patients after he obtained their test results; thus, he missed the opportunity to watch his patients become free of their symptoms. However, the doctor's reproducible results are important because they help confirm the efficacy of the cytotoxic test [66].

When read carefully, two of the six negative studies actually contain positive information supporting the cytotoxic test [64,66]. They showed that the white blood cell tests had very good reproducibility, nearly 80 percent, even though they used the original cytotoxic test. The authors of these two studies did a better job in following procedures; however, their technicians had little experience.

Unfortunately, the doctors heading up these two studies did not believe in or understand the importance of non-IgE food allergy reactions. Also, the doctors were critical because they did not understand how reactions that damage white blood cells could cause symptoms. In addition, they had no experience working with patients who had the non-IgE type of delayed food allergies. The doctors did not follow through with their patients; therefore, they never observed them become free of their symptoms.

The negative conclusions of these papers, which are all over ten years old, can now be seen as invalid. However, the reproducibility of the cytotoxic test demonstrated in two studies could actually change them from being considered negative studies into being positive studies for white blood cell testing.

One negative study on blood testing was done before the cytotoxic test was discovered and therefore is not directly relevant [61]. Another negative study was a comparison study of two different types of tests with no way of telling which was better [65].

Four of the six negative papers were done between 1975 and 1980 [63,64,65,66]. This corresponds to the period of time when the American Academy of Allergy and Immunology and the California Medical Association increased their campaign against food allergy specialists, Clinical Ecologists, the cytotoxic test and any approach to allergies which reduced the number of patients relying on traditional doctors. No negative studies have been published since 1980. Besides the 13 positive studies and reports published between 1975 and 1980, there have been 27 additional positive studies and reports published between 1980 and August 1991 — each one further demonstrating the efficacy and value of white blood cell testing for delayed food allergies.

There are several reasons traditional allergists had trouble performing and understanding the original cytotoxic test. First, it takes months of practice, after successfully completing an extensive training course, to develop the skills necessary to make the test kits accurately. Neither the traditional allergists nor their staff members had this necessary background. Second, most criticized the cytotoxic test because some of the results change within weeks. Delayed food allergies are different from IgE allergies; some do change within weeks. Thus, the changes seen when using the white blood cell test are actually an indication the test is working properly and reflecting what is happening in the body. This is one of the advantages of white blood cell testing: you can see improvements in a short period of time. The third complaint some traditional allergists make against the cytotoxic test comes about because they believe it reports that more foods are reactive than actually are. In fact, these reactions are real. This is one reason why the white blood cell test is so valuable and other tests are inadequate.

The damaging reactions to white blood cells are not difficult to see by people who have had special training with a microscope. In addition, the reactions are different for different people. This rules out any possibility that the reactions are inherent when you place white blood cells with food antigens.

The white blood cells were reported being killed in both the positive papers and the negative papers. No valid reason was given in the negative papers to explain *why* white blood cells were observed being killed. In addition, the observations and conclusions of the positive studies were never explained away. Also, the traditional allergists with negative studies were unable to explain why people became free of the health problems reported in the positive studies when they avoided the foods which were killing their white blood cells.

The observation that white blood cells die when exposed to non-IgE allergic-reacting foods and chemicals has since been rediscovered several times. There is no legitimate argument that the reaction does not exist. However, many traditional allergists still claim that the deadly reaction which kills a person's white blood cells does not exist. Others claim the reaction does not have any real meaning and cannot cause symptoms.

A review of the evidence suggests that some of the traditional allergists designed and performed their negative studies to make the white blood cell test appear worthless.

A few years after these negative studies were published, scientists discovered the mechanisms of how food reactions kill white blood cells and how dead white blood cells cause a broad range of symptoms in the body. They discovered that white blood cells are damaged by several different mechanisms, including immune complexes and the newly discovered IgG reactions.

Traditional allergists believe that all allergies are caused by IgE reactions. Because white blood cells are not damaged by IgE reactions, traditional allergists have not accepted the reality of delayed food allergies or the value of white blood cell testing.

Dead white blood cells create symptoms by releasing powerful digestive enzymes from inside their bodies when they die. The enzymes then cause inflammation and other symptoms in different areas throughout our bodies. The list of ailments which are now known to be caused by reactions that kill white blood cells is extensive and varied. Many of the most common and most painful ailments, including physical and mental problems, can be reduced or eliminated when people avoid their delayed food and chemical allergies.

Summary of the Negative Studies

When looking at the six negative studies, it can be seen that five have technical and design errors which are now obvious and thus their conclusions are invalid. The one additional negative study was a comparison of two testing procedures in which the author did not know how to evaluate the different results.

It is important to note that two of the negative studies on the cytotoxic test actually demonstrated good reproducibility — something that cannot be accomplished with the skin test used by traditional allergists.

The negative studies had several things in common. First, they were done by doctors who did not understand delayed food allergies. Second, none of the doctors who did these negative studies had any previous experience with the cytotoxic test. Third, the doctors were negative about the cytotoxic test before they did their studies. Fourth, they often did not choose patients to work with who had delayed food allergy symptoms. Fifth, they did not follow through properly with their patients to see if the test results were of value. Sixth, the doctors had office practices dependent on skin testing and weekly allergy injections.

There have been numerous improvements in the original cytotoxic test. Unfortunately, none of these improvements were used in any of the published medical studies. The new techniques would have enhanced the successes of the positive studies and could have changed the outcome of the negative studies. Even without the new improvements, when 60 medical studies and reports are positive out of a total of 66, the positive-to-negative ratio is ten to one in favor of white blood cell testing. There is a greater preponderance of evidence supporting the efficacy of white blood cell testing than for most medical procedures now being used in the field of allergy.

If there were one or two published studies supporting white blood cell testing and five or six against it, there might be some question about its value. However, with 60 published studies demonstrating the value of this type of allergy test and only six that are negative,

there is no valid argument against the value of this primary screening test for delayed food and chemical allergies. The evidence is even more overwhelming when you evaluate the defects in the six negative studies.

The first nine positive studies were done before the cytotoxic test was discovered; however, they support the principle of white blood cell testing. In addition, 100 percent of the modern studies — those performed since 1980 — have been positive. Several of these positive studies have explained in detail why white blood cell testing is so helpful for several different ailments. These recent studies now include three new types of white blood cell tests which support the principle of the original cytotoxic test and come to the same basic conclusion — white blood cell testing is a valuable tool for helping people improve their health.

Even though the last negative study was published in 1980, most traditional allergists continue to argue that the white blood cell test should be used only for experimental purposes. They are trying to persuade the insurance companies to label the test "experimental," because they know that if they are successful, the insurance companies will cut off reimbursements for the test. When this has happened in the past, it has put the traditional allergists' competitors out of business and left patients suffering with nowhere to go but back to the traditional allergists. This perpetuates suffering and escalates health-care costs.

The negative studies related to cytotoxic testing were done so long ago and with so many errors that they are now obsolete and irrelevant by today's standards.

The original cytotoxic test did have some problems, including the difficulty in properly making the kits for performing the test. However, because there were problems with the Model A Ford does not mean the government should now confiscate your car. The doctors who are trying to block the availability of white blood cell testing are like the buggy makers who tried to keep cars off the road.

Traditional Allergy Approaches

There is little evidence that traditional allergy injections based on traditional skin tests — also known as the scratch test or prick test — give much relief from airborne allergies. They give little or no help for most food allergies because the skin test only works for IgE reactions and it is unusual to have food allergies that are caused by IgE reactions.

The lack of value of skin testing and IgE testing was demonstrated by a large, well-controlled double-blind study. The study also demonstrated that the food-challenge technique for testing hidden, delayed food allergies enabled 93 percent of 88 patients to become free of their migraine headaches. The patients also became free of several other symptoms at the same time.

The food-challenge testing technique used in this study took approximately one month for each of the young people who were being helped. When the skin test was used on the same people, the results would have enabled less than three percent to become free of their headaches. When the IgE blood test was done on the patients, it also failed to give valuable results, with zero percent being helped by the traditional allergist's other testing techniques.

This study, the largest and most successful ever done on migraine headaches, clearly demonstrates that delayed food and chemical allergies are the major cause of migraine headaches. The study also demonstrates that the traditional allergy approaches do not work for detecting delayed food or chemical allergies. These results have never been successfully discredited.

This study was peer-reviewed and published in one of the world's leading medical journals, and its results have been confirmed by other studies. (Soothhill JF, Egger J, Wilson J, Carter CM, Turner MW: "Is migraine food allergy? A double-blind controlled trial of oligoantigenic diet treatment" *The Lancet* 1983: October 15.)

The white blood cell test technology has now been developed to the point where it is possible to obtain results similar to those of the food challenge technique used in the study described above. This brings about significant reductions in cost and time, without discomfort or damage to the patient.

There have been numerous other studies showing that traditional skin testing does not reveal delayed food allergies. Even when done properly, it often does not accurately reveal *acute* allergies. The newer studies done on skin testing show it is inaccurate and dangerous with little — if any — benefit coming from prolonged allergy injections. This skin test causes damage to the skin, creates reactions in the body, and leads to years of allergy injections and patient suffering. This approach gives little or no help to most people. Traditional allergists continue to use these old approaches on patients even though they have little or no valid scientific basis.

The traditional approach to allergies involves skin testing which is then followed by "allergy injections." The goal of this method is to numb people to whatever is damaging them by giving them regular injections of the damaging substance. The traditional allergists start with weak doses and then make them stronger and stronger in the hope that the person will become numb to the allergic substance. This desensitization technique does not work well and is very expensive. It takes years of injections given once or twice a week. The cost is often several thousand dollars.

This approach grew out of homeopathic techniques in the early 1940's. It does not work for most people with acute allergies and often makes delayed allergies worse.

It is enlightening to discover how traditional allergy injections have been handled in England. There, the government has to pay for health care procedures, and thus it has researched what works and what does not work.

After a thorough study of the traditional allergist's approach, the British Committee on Safety of Medicine ruled in 1986 to ban traditional allergists from doing allergy injections in their offices. They did this because the allergy injections did not work well, and there was a large number of severe allergic reactions to the injections, including several deaths.

In England, traditional allergy injections are now limited to emergency care facilities which have special staff standing by. However, in England there are no restrictions placed on white blood cell testing for delayed allergic reactions, and this approach has continued to grow in usage while allergy injections have nearly come to an end.

What has happened during the same period in

the United States is the exact opposite. Traditional allergists were able to enroll a number of unsuspecting government agencies and insurance companies to harass people doing white blood cell testing. It is now difficult to find accurate testing for delayed food and chemical allergies. Allergy injections continue to be the main source of income for traditional allergists.

Most people are damaged to some degree by the skin tests and traditional allergy injections. These types of allergy injections go on for years, cost thousands of dollars and can cause severe reactions and, in rare cases, death. (Lockey R: "Fatalities from immunotherapy and skin testing" *J Allergy Clinical Immunology* 1987; 79(8):660-677.)

Doing more of what doesn't work,
doesn't work.

I am not aware of many traditional allergists who have used their traditional allergy injections on themselves for any length of time. However, most food allergy specialists use the results of their testing to improve their own diets and to remove chemicals from their environments.

Modern white blood cell testing has a higher percentage of positive medical studies over the last ten years than do the traditional allergy approaches. In addition, white blood cell testing has a solid scientific basis.

There is no reliable evidence that anyone was ever harmed by having a white blood cell test and then using the nutritional counseling that is based on the information gained from the test. This is not true for the approaches used by traditional allergists. Aspirin causes far more problems than white blood cell testing.

Suffering from migraine headaches is widespread and they regularly cause severe pain. The traditional treatments only mask the problem and can cause crippling side affects. The Center for Disease Control reported that from 1980 to 1989 the number of people suffering with chronic migraine headaches increased nearly 60 percent. It admitted it had no idea why there had been such a sharp increase. Delayed food and chemical allergies which cause migraine headaches and numerous other symptoms are common and becoming worse because traditional doctors are fighting the awareness rather than supporting appropriate testing, treatment and research.

The migraine headache epidemic gives some insight into how common are delayed food and chemical allergies in the younger generations. Traditional allergists are still claiming delayed food allergies and white blood cell reactions do not exist.

Traditional allergy approaches have been used extensively from 1980 to 1990. During this time the cases of asthma have nearly doubled, and asthma-caused deaths have gone up dramatically. People are weakened by traditional allergy drugs, and many become allergic to the drugs. This causes some people to become more allergic and develop asthma. White blood cell testing and related counseling relieves these health problems without causing new problems.

Traditional allergists are the self-proclaimed "experts" for the entire field of allergy and call themselves "board-certified allergists," after they certify themselves. The label "board-certified" is only meaningful when the board understands the subject. How ironic this is when you realize that traditional allergists work only with people's acute reactions and these reactions are involved in such a small percentage of the overall allergy problem.

The professional society for the traditional allergists, called The American Academy of Allergy and Immunology, works like a trade union. This group and its numerous related groups are working to restrict the field of allergy and the public's awareness of delayed food and chemical allergies. This group and some of its members have actively pressured insurance companies to stop payments to people for delayed allergy testing. When a group interferes with reimbursements to a competitor, it is in violation of state and federal anti-trust laws.

There are additional problems with the traditional allergists' approach to allergy. A major cause of becoming allergic to foods and chemicals is repetitious exposure. The traditional treatment for allergies is weekly injections of an extract of the foods, pollens or whatever the person is allergic to. After a few years of repetitious injections many people become more reactive, their symptoms are worse, and they have to stop the injections. Others show no improvement. Although a few are helped, many feel better because of the cyclical nature of allergies.

One reason traditional allergy injections are continued is because they are lucrative. Much of the money has been used to block the needed challenge to the traditional approach of testing and treating allergies. Large amounts of money have been used by traditional allergists to discredit the cytotoxic test.

A comprehensive white blood cell test, with the necessary counseling, costs between $500 and $1000 depending on the severity of the problems and the number of foods involved. This one-time cost is often all that is needed to enable patients to avoid their health problems.

At approximately $18.00 an injection, traditional allergy approaches often cost the patient over $2000 the first year and over $1000 per year after that. This does not include the money charged by the doctor, or the cost and suffering caused by the drugs and surgery which often are tried after the allergy injections fail. The injections cost the allergist less than 50 cents to make.

Consumers Reports magazine did a report titled "The Shot Doctors" in February of 1988 which explained that allergy shots (injections) are ineffective, often cause allergic reactions and "in very rare cases, such reactions can be fatal."

They interviewed a former president of the American Academy of Allergy and Immunology about the profitably of allergy shots. He promoted their approach to allergy by stating, "When you put a patient on shots, you've got an annuity for life." He also said that prescribing allergy drugs requires patients to keep coming in only once or twice a year for life and "that reduces my income considerably."

In the same article, another traditional "board-certified" allergist acknowledged that over 80 percent of the traditional allergist's diagnostic effort is based on the history questions they ask their patients — people who also do not understand delayed allergies. The uninformed leading the blind.

Because traditional allergists do not accurately test for food and chemical allergies, and continually treat symptoms, they have the ultimate get-rich-quick scheme. You can see why traditional allergists try to discredit people who provide a blood test which enables patients to become aware of what to eat and thus not need to keep coming back every week.

It is best to discover in the beginning what is causing a health problem and remove the cause, rather than trying to cover up the symptoms with allergy injections, drugs and surgery. When you look at the difference in the costs explained above, you can see why most traditional allergists have been slow to change.

The poorly designed, negative studies done in an apparent attempt to defend the old approach to allergies have damaged the reputation of an important test for helping people discover which foods and chemicals they need to avoid. The white blood cell test is the best for helping people eliminate the cause of their symptoms in the least possible time at the lowest cost.

White blood cell testing has no negative side effects, unlike traditional allergy drugs, surgeries and prolonged allergy injections. People sharing their personal successes, and health professionals increasing their use of alternative medicine, preventive care and environmental medicine, have caused a dramatic increase in the use of effective health care. This progress decreases health care costs whenever it is used.

A new area of research being pursued in medicine today is called "outcomes research." It is the study of how well different approaches work. The results have shown that traditional allergy approaches do not work well, or at all. These include skin testing, desensitizing injections and the use of cortisone creams, pills or injections.

Outcomes research has also shown that coronary bypass surgery and other surgical or drug approaches do not work well, and that correct diet changes do work. It is sad how long ineffective procedures continue to be used, when they do not work and cause serious damage and financial waste.

Outcomes research should have been a regular part of medicine for the last hundred years. This type of research will awaken the medical establishment to the value of testing for delayed food and chemical allergies, and to the value of a diet which is around 10 percent fat and 80 milligrams of cholesterol. This type of research would also have prevented the problems caused by breast implants.

Most traditional allergists continue to limit themselves to treating airborne allergies such as dust, mold, dander and pollen. They do help some people with insect bite allergies. However, they are unable to help people with the most common type of allergy problems — the delayed food and chemical allergies. Allergists often put people on one of the most damaging of drugs — cortisone. Their patients experience short periods of feeling better, while their overall health continues to decline. Patients can be permanently damaged, and are then often difficult to help when they do find a doctor who understands delayed food and chemical allergies.

Traditional allergists continue to use obsolete approaches while suppressing the truth about new approaches. In no other field of medicine do doctors with so little knowledge claim to have so many answers.

When most people with typical allergy problems stop eating foods damaging to their white blood cells, they no longer need to take drugs, have surgery or receive traditional allergy injections.

Part of the unnecessary controversy about white blood cell testing comes about because the test demonstrates that the type of skin testing used by traditional allergists has no value for discovering non-IgE, delayed food and chemical allergic reactions. As this awareness of the facts grows, it becomes a threat to the income of traditional allergists. Not surprisingly, many traditional allergists are adamant in their denial of the value of white blood cell testing and the accompanying diet. However, patients who take the test and follow the program become better because their total allergic load is dramatically reduced.

Underlying the controversy is a turf fight waged by the traditional allergists who are trying to hang on to their patients. This is ironic: if traditional allergists accepted the reality of white blood cell testing and delayed food and chemical allergies, their practices would start growing instead of shrinking.

For traditional allergists to argue against the reality of delayed food and chemical allergies, and to suppress the white blood cell test, is illogical. It is the same as if nutritional counselors believed only in vitamin C and denied the existence of any of the other vitamins and tried to suppress the use of tests for other vitamin deficiencies.

Because so much money and political power have been accumulated over the years by traditional allergists, it is now difficult to find a doctor who knows the truth about white blood cell testing. When patients do locate a doctor who has this knowledge, they are able to improve their health and become free of their unnecessary suffering.

In 1983, several centers opened throughout the United States to provide cytotoxic testing and help fill the void in health care caused in part by traditional allergists. Unfortunately, the owners had little understanding of the test or of delayed food allergies. They used the original version of the cytotoxic test and had trouble obtaining accurate results. Also, many did not work with doctors and thereby made this new awareness an easy target for the traditional allergists.

Without having the latest research available to them, some state and federal agencies made incorrect decisions during the mid-1980's to harass centers doing cytotoxic testing. This happened because the regulators relied on the six negative studies supplied to them by the traditional allergists. This caused them to come to the wrong conclusions about the value of cytotoxic testing.

During that time, several knowledgeable doctors and successful health centers were harassed by various misinformed state bureaucrats for helping people improve their health with the help of the cytotoxic test. However, in the early 1980's the test received an unbiased hearing in Maryland and was judged by a court to be of value and in no way harmful to patients.

Over the years, the awareness of the importance of delayed food allergies and Environmental Medicine has continued to grow. From its beginnings with Dr. Theron Randolph and four of his fellow physicians in 1965, there are now more than 500 physicians who practice Environmental Medicine and belong to the

American Academy of Environmental Medicine. There are more than 2,000 additional physicians who practice many of the therapies. There are similar groups of significant size in Canada, Australia and Europe.

In the United States, the ear, nose and throat physicians have a specialty in allergy. They have almost entirely abandoned the traditional allergy treatments because they have discovered these treatments cause damage and don't work. This group adds another 2,000 physicians.

The Pan American Allergy Society and the American College of Advancement in Medicine also have several thousand members, many of whom help people with non-IgE, delayed food and chemical allergies.

A large percentage of the doctors who practice Orthomolecular Medicine test their patients for delayed food and chemical allergies.

Numerous other professional health practitioners have been using Environmental Medicine approaches for years. Many doctors of chiropractic, probably more than 2,000, are using this awareness. There are also untold numbers of naturopaths, nutritional consultants and other health professionals who use this information regularly.

The total number of health professionals in the United States helping people with delayed food and chemical allergies, sensitivities and intolerances is over 8,000. This is about double the current number of traditional allergists.

The number of traditional allergists has been dwindling since the late 1970's and especially during the 1980's when white blood cell testing was readily available and popular.

Unfortunately, white blood cell testing is hard to find today because the traditional allergists are still waging a very powerful negative propaganda campaign against improved allergy testing. This campaign is still influencing some government agencies and insurance companies.

The problems caused by traditional allergists are made worse by about a dozen who spend their time and make much of their money working for health insurance companies. They testify against patients who are trying to collect on their insurance.

These doctors also influence state and federal governments to file lawsuits against competing doctors and then collect huge sums of taxpayers' money for testifying in these cases.

These prosecuting doctors have been very effective in obtaining university positions and controlling the courses taught to medical students. From their positions of influence, they manipulate news reports and write articles which promote themselves as "quack busters." In reality, they are promoting obsolete approaches to health care which turn out to be the most common type of quackery.

They damage doctors practicing preventive care, alternative medicine and environmental medicine by manipulating review boards or administrative judges. The review boards and hearings are staffed by traditional doctors who are often using obsolete approaches. This has happened without there ever having been an honest examination of the scientific studies.

Quacks who are not traditional doctors cause such a small part of the health problems in this country it would be hard to measure. The quackery done by traditional doctors causes about 10 percent of the admissions to hospitals. It is likely that over 25 percent of the nation's health problems are caused by traditional doctors using traditional approaches which do not work and damage patients. The current attacks on "quacks" is a smoke screen to hide the overwhelming majority of "quacks" — traditional doctors practicing approaches which do not work. How ironic — those who think they are "quack busters" are actually "quack defenders."

When the self-ordained "quack busters" are exposed and discredited, superior approaches to health care will flourish.

What often happens today is that a person with delayed food allergies (the non-IgE type) goes to a traditional "board-certified" allergist and receives skin tests and then treatments for acute allergies for years with no help for the real problem. These people often end up on prescription drugs in an attempt to treat their symptoms.

Traditional allergists are making judgments about an area where they have no training and are out of their element. People with health problems need to be able to find doctors who are trained in preventive care, environmental medicine and the related specialities.

Doris Rapp, MD, did an extensive review of the medical literature and found numerous key studies on how delayed food and chemical allergies cause some of the major chronic ailments. Most of the studies were in peer-review journals, and some were done double blind. The report revealed that for arthritis there were six studies; asthma, three; autism, three; chemical sensitivities, twelve; colitis, two; Crohn's disease, one; delinquency, four; eczema, two; epilepsy, four; fatigue, two; gynecologic problems, two; hyperactivity, twenty one; immune dysfunction, sixteen; irritable bowel, three; migraine headache, six; nephrosis, six; otitis, six; psychological dysfunction, two; Tourette's syndrome, one; vascular disease, fourteen.

She also located general studies on how delayed food and chemical allergies cause symptoms. These include twenty six positive double-blind studies, seven single-blind studies and ten non-blind studies.

Freedom from Disease

Starting with Dr. Arthur Black's landmark study on white blood cell testing for delayed food allergies, the following ailments have been shown to be reduced or eliminated by using the white blood cell test and resulting counseling. Numbers relate to listed studies.

Notice how many of these ailments are the ones traditional medicine is unable to treat effectively: infant colic and failure to gain weight, allergic dermatitis, urticaria, eczema, erythema, intense itching, hay fever, chronic sinusitis, severe pain [10], swelling, itching, increase of mucus, gastrointestinal problems, arthritic pain, ulcerations, neurologic complaints [16], alcohol addiction [19], hearing impairment [22], vertigo, loss of hearing, pruritus, nervous stomach [25], minimal brain dysfunction [33], central nervous system disorders [34], secretory otitis media [37,47], irritability, restlessness, insomnia, migraine headaches, nausea, vomiting, edema, diarrhea, cardiovascular symptoms, palpitations, tension-fatigue syndrome, general malaise, muscle aches, mild headache [44], bronchial asthma [54], irritable bowel syndrome [59].

A more complete listing of ailments relieved or eliminated can be found in hundreds of additional, peer-reviewed medical studies

published on delayed food and chemical allergies.

In chapter 8, it was explained how infant colic is caused by delayed allergic reactions to IgG antibodies produced in the cows' body and carried in cows' milk to the mother eating dairy products and then carried in mothers' milk to the infant, causing colic. How many unusual ways do the type of reactions revealed by Dr. Black's test affect our bodies?

Most ailments currently baffling traditional medicine have delayed allergic reactions as a big part of the cause. Pre-conception counseling using the Prime Test is the key to the first generation of truly healthy children.

Do we want continued suffering and unnecessary medical costs caused by restricting the modern awareness of food and chemical allergies and the use of white blood cell testing?

One of the discoveries Dr. Theron Randolph made years ago can be very helpful today. He found that most of the people he tested with delayed food allergies had become physically addicted to some of the foods they were allergic to.

When his patients went off of the foods they were allergic to, they went through classical withdrawal symptoms — pain and discomfort in different areas of their bodies, plus numerous emotional symptoms. These included denying foods were a problem and craving the items they were allergic to. These cravings accelerate from foods to anything they think may relieve their symptoms.

People would become free of their withdrawal symptoms and other health complaints in about five days. People in this clear state who then consumed a food they were allergic to and addicted to had an accelerated return of their symptoms. This fast and food-challenge procedure is one way to test for delayed food allergies and addictions.

In daily life people are often going in and out of discomfort and cravings. Research has shown that when people are addicted to one item they often progress to other addictive items. When you combine this knowledge with the understanding of food addictions, it helps to explain why so many people digress into taking legal and illegal drugs to relieve their symptoms and cravings. In many cases, food addictions lead to drug addictions because people try to relieve food allergy stress and withdrawal symptoms by taking stress-relieving drugs.

This food factor in drug addictions has been carefully researched and presented in Dr. Randolph's medical paper titled, "Specific Adaptation," published in the medical journal *Annals of Allergy* in 1978. This, and additional information, is presented in his book, *An Alternative Approach To Allergies*. The book was published by Harper and Row in hardcover in 1980 and in paper back in 1990.

The problems we are having with illegal drugs will not be solved until the public, the medical community and the government are aware that many drug addictions start with food addictions.

Awareness of delayed food allergies and resulting food addictions helps to explain why over 90 percent of people who succeed in losing excess weight gain it back, and more. If the weight-loss diet is not free from the individual's addictive foods, the person will have trouble staying on the diet program. This is also true for staying on diets to reverse heart disease.

Severe mental problems are one of the areas where traditional psychiatry has failed miserably. Over half of the hospital beds in the United States are occupied by people with psychological problems.

Dr. Randolph has explained in detail in his medical articles and books the cause-and-effect relationship between delayed food and chemical allergies and numerous types of mental problems. This new understanding is also explained in the book *Brain Allergies: The Psychonutrient Connection* by William H. Philpott, MD, and Dwight Kalita, PhD, and in numerous medical studies.

To this day, most psychiatrists unsuccessfully treat mentally disturbed patients with drugs and talk-therapy instead of removing the major cause of much of the problem — delayed food and chemical allergies.

There is an important study in progress to see if avoiding foods which damage white blood cells will help AIDS patients live longer. In the Spring of 1984, Russell Jaffe, MD, PhD, began a study with 19 patients, all having AIDS symptoms. All were so ill none was expected to live for more than six months. Dr. Jaffe gave each patient a delayed food allergy test that uses the white blood cell known as the basophil. He then helped them change their diets and gave them special vitamins and supportive counseling. As of June, 1991, sixteen of the nineteen patients are still alive and doing fairly well. This is the longest-running and most successful AIDS study to date. (*East West Journal*; 1986, September.)

This study is being done without adequate financing and detailed follow up. Furthermore, the white blood cell used, the basophil, is not sensitive enough to give comprehensive results. However, the study is a guiding light to help find one of the tools to help stop a disease which, according to government estimates, will otherwise sentence 30 million people worldwide to death by the year 2000. In addition, the economic drain on those without the disease will be economically crippling.

Other helpful AIDS programs include some diet improvements as part of the treatment. Often, the compatible foods are determined by guessing. Delayed food and chemical allergy testing and the resulting immune-system supporting diet is an important part of any treatment program for AIDS.

Is there any valid reason to prevent an AIDS patient from having the best information and an effective diet program designed to support the immune system?

A recent study discovered that when non-smokers are exposed to secondhand cigarette smoke, their white blood cells are damaged. In addition, the damaged cells cause a chain reaction which includes breakdown of the walls of the arteries, clogging of the arteries and related degenerative diseases.

This research further demonstrates that white blood cells are damaged by non-IgE delayed allergic reactions, and thus adds to the extensive evidence which supports the principle underlying the white blood cell test for discovering delayed allergies and addictions.

In addition to the clear cause-and-effect relationship between white blood cell reactions and numerous chronic ailments documented in this report, there is now an established link between delayed allergic reactions and coronary artery disease. (Anderson R: "Passive smoking by humans sensitizes circulating neutrophils" *American Review of Respiratory Disease* 1991; 144:570.)

It is well known that white blood cells attack and kill viruses, bacteria and cancer cells throughout the body. However, no research has been done to discover if infections and cancer would be reduced or eliminated by diets free of foods which kill white blood cells. This is one important area where research and treatment should be funded.

Most ailments are relieved to some degree and many are eliminated by the diet improvements suggested by the white blood cell test. There are no negative side affects. People have the right to see how well this program works for them.

One additional way to test for ailment-causing reactions is by putting a food solution under the tongue or injecting it under the skin. This approach enables the doctor to work out a "neutralizing dose" of a food and thereby help patients who have so many reactions they are not able to avoid their allergic foods. This method is called "provocative neutralization testing and treatment."

This approach helps with both physical and emotional ailments. These techniques sometimes miss reactions, are costly, and cause some damage to the patient; however, these tests can provide valuable information when done properly. By using white blood cell testing before using the above-mentioned provocative neutralization testing, patients' reactions can be neutralized to their known allergy causing foods. They are relieved of their symptoms more rapidly, with less discomfort to the patient, while significantly reducing the overall costs of treatments.

White blood cell testing has also been shown to work with domestic animals. Veterinarians are having good results with dogs and cats [45].

In the early 1960's, the knowledge that people were having delayed allergic reactions to pesticides and other chemicals began with one of Dr. Randolph's discoveries. For many people, avoiding their reactive foods is not enough. They also need to avoid pesticides and chemicals to which they are allergic. White blood cell testing discovers their reactive

chemicals without making the patient more reactive as a result of the testing process.

An article in the August, 1989 issue of *Scientific American*, titled "Alternatives to Animals in Toxicity Testing," explains how a "new" test makes it possible to discover which cosmetics and other chemicals can be found compatible for humans by placing them with animal body cells rather than subjecting the animals to suffering. The white blood cell test for finding compatible foods and chemicals has been available for humans for over two decades.

Do not expect much help from the traditional medical establishment and the government in the near future. They are still feeding our astronauts steak, eggs, dairy products and orange-flavored sugar water, and wondering why half of them are getting sick when they are in space. They call the problem "space sickness." However, the symptoms are typical of delayed food allergies. This type of reaction is known by delayed food allergy specialists to become worse at high altitudes.

New Tests

During the last few years, three new testing methods, developed independently of each other, support the principle of white blood cell testing. Each test demonstrates that measuring a person's white blood cells reacting with foods and chemicals enables the doctor to discover what is causing the patient's suffering.

One of these new methods is a test developed in France by Dr. Jacques Bienveniste. This test uses the white blood cell known as the basophil. The test determines which drugs are compatible with each critically ill patient, thus avoiding allergic reactions to medications. Anesthesiologists are also using this test to select the most compatible drug to use before surgery. Patients do better because they have fewer reactions to their medications. This test is being used in several developed countries, but is blocked from use in the [43].

Dr. Bienveniste directs the largest allergy research laboratory in the world. His team of more than 60 scientists and doctors has been studying the different approaches to allergies and allergy testing. In his presentation in 1988 at the annual meeting of the American Academy of Environmental Medicine, Dr. Bienveniste stated that the future of allergy testing was going to focus upon the cells.

Modern European allergists no longer believe in the 1920's idea that allergies are only acute reactions caused by IgE antibodies. Ironically, their predecessors convinced the American allergists that the narrow definition was correct. Unfortunately, many traditional American allergists are still fighting for the narrow definition of allergy. They keep wondering why other doctors have stopped referring patients to them and why their share of the patient market keeps falling.

The second new method for food allergy testing is the autocytotoxicity test developed by W. K. Podleski, MD. His work demonstrates that white blood cell reactions to foods are one of the major causes of asthma. This test works on the same principle as the cytotoxic test [51,53,54].

The third test was developed by Mark Pasula and is called the ALCAT. This test measures the death of white blood cells by using a cell counter before and after each reaction. The number of white blood cells killed by a food gives some indication of the foods that are reactive. This type of cytotoxic test is a modification of Dr. Franklin's 1949 test [61].

The ALCAT misses some reactions and does not test for some of the changes to white blood cells. Although this test is more expensive, it does confirm the principle of the cytotoxic test [56,57,58,60].

In addition to these three new tests which use the white blood cells, there are now other blood tests available which show some of the mechanisms which damage white blood cells. These include the IgG RAST test, the IgG MAST test, and the ELISA test. However, a significant problem with these tests is that they miss many of a person's allergic foods. However, they confirm that other reactions are happening in the body to foods and chemicals besides the traditional IgE reactions.

These new tests are limited because they test for only one factor — the IgG reaction. Over 40 percent of the people who have severe delayed food allergies do not have IgG reactions to any significant degree. However, these tests are of some value and they confirm the need

for an improved white blood cell test.

Most traditional allergists are not only fighting against the above-mentioned new white blood cell tests, they are also resisting the new antibody tests for delayed food allergies. In fact, they are against any testing for delayed food allergies. They have staked their professional reputations on their claim that there are no delayed food allergies; yet all these tests demonstrate that traditional allergists are wrong.

A study in the September, 1988, issue of *Otolaryngology — Head and Neck Surgery* by John H. Boyles, Jr., MD, and others, investigated the use of IgE and IgG tests for detecting food allergies. According to Dr. Boyles, this double-blind study found that neither the IgE test nor the IgG test was adequate for helping people with delayed food allergies. In his study, fewer than half of the delayed food allergy reactions were caused by IgG reactions; the remainder were caused by other mechanisms. This further demonstrates the need for the Prime Test.

More than 50 years after the discovery of the IgE blood particle involved in acute allergies, several other blood particles have been discovered. These new particles are involved in other types of allergic reactions. These have been named IgA, IgD, IgG and IgM. Besides these mechanisms, there are immune complexes, prostaglandins and other mechanisms that have yet to be discovered. These new discoveries confirm the accuracy of Dr. van Pirquet's, Dr. Coca's, Dr. Randolph's and the Clinical Ecologists' original definition for the word allergy — "altered reaction."

One of the great values of white blood cell testing is that it can reveal delayed allergic reactions caused by several different mechanisms. However, the white blood cell test does not disclose IgE reactions and will miss an IgE reactive food unless it is also reactive by some other mechanism. This fact has caused most traditional allergists to be critical of the cytotoxic test. Not detecting the unusual IgE food reaction is seldom a problem because people already know which food causes their IgE reaction, because the discomfort shows up rapidly.

There is another type of allergic reaction

which damages red blood cells. It is not very often seen compared to the white blood cell reaction. The test for red blood cell reactions is based on the same basic principle underlying the white blood cell test. (Mayron L, Kaplan E, Interlandi J: "Induction of Antibody-Mediated RBC Lysis by Food Extracts" *Ann Allergy* 1977; 38:323-338.)

Several additional positive studies on white blood cell testing have been presented at medical conventions and were well received. Some were given awards. However, the authors were unable to get their studies published.

Part of the problem is that most allergy medical journals are controlled by traditional allergists and are financially supported by drug company advertisements. Peer-review journals in other scientific fields do not usually sell space for advertisements. White blood cell tests are a problem for drug companies. Once people find out which foods they are reactive to and stop eating them, their need for drugs is dramatically reduced or eliminated.

There are several studies which support the scientific principle of the white blood cell test by demonstrating change in white blood cells inside the body.

One of the most interesting was done by David W. Eggleston, DDS. His study demonstrated that the white blood cells called T4-lymphocytes were lower in some people with amalgam fillings or nickel crowns. When these were removed, the white blood cell counts went up in some people but not in others. He then replaced the amalgam fillings or nickel crowns in their mouths to see if their white blood cell count went down again. It did.

This study actually demonstrated allergic reactions to mercury and nickel. About one third of the patients had non-IgE allergic reactions to amalgam and nickel dental materials. These reactions lower white blood cell counts in the body in sensitive patients and not in others. This supports the white blood cell test principle by observing changes in white blood cells after an allergic reaction.

Amalgams, also known as silver fillings, are actually 20 to 50 percent mercury. Each time people with silver fillings chew their food, a small amount of mercury gas is released.

The mercury accumulates in body and brain cells and can cause malfunctions.

Besides causing allergic reactions, nickel corrodes and is a known carcinogen. Therefore, neither mercury nor nickel should be used in the mouth. (Eggleston DW: "Effect of Dental Amalgam and Nickel Alloys on T4-lymphocytes: Preliminary report" *The Journal of Prosthetic Dentistry*, May 1984, Volume 51 Number 3.)

Magazine and newspaper articles written about cytotoxic testing made it very popular during the early 1980's and a significant improvement in public health followed. Unfortunately, this progress is being suppressed by traditional allergists' influence over insurance companies, public media and state and federal governments. These allergists also control the spending of most allergy research funds and the allergy departments of universities.

Traditional allergists still argue, while ignoring the positive scientific evidence, that the types of allergies disclosed by white blood cell testing do not exist. In fact, there are several hundred carefully done, peer reviewed, published medical studies which clearly demonstrate that non-IgE delayed food allergies are the major underlying cause of many of the most common health problems.

There are more than three hundred published medical articles by Dr. Randolph. In addition, there are 26 double-blind studies published in the leading medical journals which support the conclusion that delayed food allergies are the main cause of many common health problems.

When people go to the average doctor, delayed food allergies are overlooked. However, awareness is growing. Credit for the growing interest in delayed food and chemical allergies within the scientific community goes primarily to the Clinical Ecologists and to pressure from a better-informed public.

Medical and Popular Books

Besides the 60 positive medical studies and reports published on white blood cell testing, there are thirteen popular books and one medical textbook which explain the value of the white blood cell testing and the importance of delayed food and chemical allergies.

The medical textbook *Clinical Ecology* was edited by Lawrence D. Dickey, MD. In chapter 47, William Bryan, MD, and his wife, Marian Bryan, wrote the following about the cytotoxic test: "After fifteen years of use on almost five thousand patients...many and even some spectacular cures have been accomplished. Others using the test have verified these observations which re-emphasize the importance of making specific diagnosis of allergy to food and of its subtle effects on many diseases of unknown etiology.

"The authors now consider the test as both practical and dependable both in allergy and as a factor affecting the immune status of many patients.... By direct microscopic observation of the action of serum and food extracts on the activity and viability of the neutrophilic leukocytes, an objective and reliable test for food allergy may be achieved.... The reason for bringing this to the attention of otorhinolaryngologists, allergists and other physicians is that, as yet, there is no other way of diagnosing multiple specific food allergies which play such important roles in the obscure etiologies of many symptoms and diseases among which are many of our therapeutic failures." Published in 1976 by Charles C. Thomas, $60.00.

The first popular book was *The Food Connection* by psychiatrists David Sheinkin, MD, Michael Schacter, MD, and Richard Hutton. This 1979 book compares many different methods of testing for food allergies. The authors wrote that, "Cytotoxic testing demands a minimal amount of time and effort by the patient...is efficient...perfectly safe (no pain or harm to the patient)...reactions are relatively objective, can be repeated if necessary with little hardship for the patient...the test picks up some latent food sensitivities that are sometimes missed by other types of tests." Published by the Bobbs-Merrill Company, $10.00.

In the book, *Dr. Wright's Book of Nutritional Therapy*, Jonathan V. Wright, MD, wrote that "Some physicians use cytotoxic testing. In this test, white blood cells are exposed to food antigen solutions and disintegrate more readily if there is an allergy. When done by well trained individuals, this

test may be very helpful." Published in 1979 by Rodale Press, $18.00.

In 1980 I wrote the first edition of *Quality Longevity*. A highlight is "Discovering compatible foods by using an accurate white blood cell test for delayed food allergies is the first step toward removing the cause of a broad range of symptoms. Also, selecting foods which are low in fat, moderate in protein and high in complex carbohydrates will enable you to improve your health further and become free of additional symptoms. It is now possible to enjoy good health continually and fully live a much longer life.

"A clean environment, in combination with aerobic and strength exercise, is necessary to regain and maintain health. Taking supplements to fulfill your unique vitamin and mineral requirements should begin after your compatible foods are identified.

"The Quality Longevity Program brings together, for the first time, the correct parts of the best health approaches. The combined effect of these breakthroughs enables you to become free of most allergic symptoms and degenerative ailments. You will be able to exceed greatly the average levels of health and longevity." Published by Advanced Health Center, $28.00.

The book, *Food Additives and Hyperactive Children,* was published in 1980 by Dr. C. Keith Conners. It includes a positive, double-blind study using the cytotoxic test. Dr. Conners concludes, "The test predicts which foods will show allergic response...is both reliable and valid." Published by Plenum, $29.50.

In the book, *Brain Allergies: The Psycho-nutrient Connection,* by psychiatrist William H. Philpott, MD, and Dwight K. Kalita, PhD, Dr. Philpott wrote that the cytotoxic test is one test which should be used because it gives "...microscopic evidence of the blood reacting to foods, chemicals, and inhalants..." He also wrote that "...insulin-dependent juvenile diabetics cannot be fasted. In those cases...the initial reliance of reactivity to a food or substance comes from the intradermal serial-dilution provocative test supplemented by information from the cytotoxic test...." Published in 1980 by Keith Publishing Inc., $15.00, paperback, $12.95.

The Nutritional Outline for the Professional

was written in 1983 by urologist James F. Balch, Jr., MD, and Phyllis A. Balch, NC. They summarized their study of different types of allergy testing by concluding, "A cytotoxic test is the best method to identify your allergies..." Published by Good Things Naturally, $15.00. In their new book, *Prescription for Natural Healing,* they recommend Advanced Health Center's test kits.

The Food Sensitivity Diet by Doug Kaufmann and Racquel Skolnik was published in 1984. They wrote "By far, the easiest way to isolate food sensitivities is by taking the Cytotoxic test. This test requires a small blood sample prepared and then placed on slides. Each of your slides is preinoculated with a different food substance and then placed under a microscope and observed by a technician. The technician can observe some of these food substances killing your white blood cells...." Published by Freundlich Books, $15.95. In paperback by Paper Jacks, $3.95.

Robert Buist, PhD, wrote *Food Intolerance* in 1984. His PhD is in medicinal chemistry and pharmacology. When writing about the cytotoxic test, he relates, "The other advantages of the test are the minimal time required and the lack of discomfort for the patient. This is especially important when testing psychiatric patients. It is also safe and objective." Published in Australia by Harper and Row and in the United States by Prism Press, $7.95.

The Allergy Connection by Barbara Paterson was published in 1985 in England. She reports on Dr. Downing's successes using the cytotoxic test: "Dr. Downing also considers that cytotoxic testing offers a possible solution to those who, for one reason or another, are unable to embark on elimination diets...the accuracy of cytotoxic testing varies, but averages 80%..." Published by Thorsons Publishers Inc., $8.95.

A popular book titled *Clinical Ecology* was published in England in 1985. The book was written by Dr. George T. Lewith and Dr. Julian N. Kenyon. After mentioning the difficulties and costs associated with the cytotoxic test, they state, "The correlation between food and/or chemical avoidance and clinical improvement is high for cytotoxic testing.... It is, however, less expensive than the RAST and much more clinically useful." Published in England by Thorsons Publishers, $7.95.

In his 1985 book, *Dr. Berger's Immune Power Diet,* Stuart M. Berger, MD, wrote, "Cytotoxic testing is a valuable tool in screening patients for food sensitivities. The test can be done quickly in the laboratory using only one blood sample from each patient, so there is no unnecessary evoking of possible allergic reactions. The test uses a drop of blood which is then exposed to various food extracts; by observing the patient's white blood cells' reactions to different food extracts, hundreds of foods can be tested quickly and efficiently for their immune-toxic potential. I have had superb results using this test to evaluate thousands of patients." Published by New American Library, $14.95.

In 1988 Robert Atkins, MD, wrote *Dr. Atkins' Health Revolution.* After working with several thousand patients he concludes, "With a good technician, the results of the cytotoxic test can be quite accurate and reproducible. The test has the advantage of being less expensive than most of the others; therefore, it is readily applicable for routine testing." Published by Houghton Mifflin Company, $18.95.

The Complete Guide to Food Allergy and Intolerance was published in England in 1990 by Jonathan Brostoff, MA, DM, FRCP, DSc and Linda Gamlin. Dr. Brostoff is a consulting physician in allergy at the Middlesex Hospital Medical School. While pointing out some of the problems experienced with the original cytotoxic test, the doctor writes, "Scientific appraisals of the cytotoxic test show that food extracts do sometimes affect the white blood cells...a recent study under carefully controlled conditions produced 65-70 per cent accuracy." Published by Bloomsbury Publishing, London, England, $12.00.

A summary and conclusion comes after the following listing of published medical studies.

Scientific Studies on White Blood Cell Testing from 1917 through August 1991

The following chronological list of published medical studies identifies research which has been suppressed, ignored or misrepresented by most traditional allergists. This list is based on the work of several researchers and is believed to be complete. It includes actual studies and reports.

Studies known not to have been peer reviewed are noted. The others are peer reviewed or are older studies done when that was not considered necessary. Historically, the reviewing was done by the editorial board or the editor.

In the past, it was possible to have a paper published which was not in the best financial interest of traditional medical doctors or drug companies which advertised in the journal. This is no longer the case because every article is now reviewed by a committee called the "peer-review board" before it can be published.

This stifling of new information by traditional medical doctors is rampant. However, it also happens in other sciences. A paper in *Scientific American* by Geoffrey Burbridge, professor of physics at the University of California, San Diego, clearly summarized the problem. He wrote, "Those of us who have been around long enough know that the peer review and the refereeing of papers have become a form of censorship."

It is interesting that all of the positive studies were done by people who had experience with white blood cell testing, while all the negative studies were done by people who relied on traditional allergy testing and had no previous experience with white blood cell testing.

The following list does not include opinion papers. The opinion papers on white blood cell testing were done by people who have no experience with the test but used selected comments from these studies and reports.

If you know of any additional studies or reports, please send the references or a copy of them to Mark Lovendale at 34146 Selva Road, Suite 200, Monarch Beach, California, 92629. Phone (714) 661-4001.

Total Positive Studies — 60

1 Pappenheimer AM: Experimental studies upon lymphocytes. The action of immune sera upon lymphocytes and small thymus cells. J Experimental Med 1917; 26:163.

2 Pappenheimer AM: Experimental studies upon lymphocytes. J Experimental Med 1917; 25:633-650.

3 Cromwell HW, Centeno JA: The reaction of the white blood cells to specific precipitates. Journal Immunology 1929; 17:53.

4 Squier TL, Lee HJ: Lysis in vitro of sensitized leukocytes by ragweed antigen. J Allergy 1947; 18:156-163.

5 Favor CB, et al: Factors affecting the in vitro cytolysis of white blood cells by tuberculin. American Review of Tuberculosis 1949; 60:212-222.

6 Waksman BH: Significance of complement in tuberculin cytolysis. Fed Proc 1951; 10:423.

7 Pettay O: Preliminary report on the use of in vitro leukocytolysis as a test in allergy. (Abstract) Scandinavian J Clinical Laboratory Investigation 1952; 4:77.

8 Waksman BH: Specific white cell lysis produced by combination of rabbit antiserum to purified protein (ovalbumin, bovine gamma globulin) with homologous antigen: the role of the nonprecipitating antibody. Immunology 1953; 70:331-334.

9 Hartman JD, Hock WC: Changes in blood leucocytes resulting from antigen antibody reactions. American J Psychology 1955; 183:214-220.

10. Black AP: A new diagnostic method of allergic disease. Pediatrics 1956; 17:716-724.

11. Bryan WTK, Bryan MP: The application of in vitro cytotoxic reactions to clinical diagnosis of food allergy. (non-peer) Laryngoscope 1960; 70:810-824.

12. McEwen LM: A method for the maintenance of leucocytes in their globular form. J Physiology 1966; 184:3-5.

13. Speirs, RS: The action of antigen upon hypersensitive cells. Ann New York Academy Science 1964; 113:819-824.

14. Ruddle NH, Waksman BH: Cytotoxicity mediated by soluble antigen and lymphocytes in delayed hypersensitivity. J Exp Medicine Dec 1968; 128.

15. Bryan WTK, Bryan MP: Cytotoxic reactions and the diagnosis of food allergy. Laryngoscope 1969; 79:1453-1472.

16. Bryan WTK, Bryan MP: Cytotoxic reactions in the diagnosis of food allergy. Otolaryngologic Clinics of North America 1971; 4:523-534.

17. Bryan WTK, Bryan MP: Clinical examples of resolution and some idiopathic and other chronic diseases by careful allergic management. Laryngoscope 1972; 82:1231-1238.

18. Baker SP: Allergic respiratory tract disease. Medical J Australia 1973; 1:126-127.

19. Ulett GA, Perry SG: Cytotoxic food testing in alcoholics. Quart J Studies Alcoholism 1974; 35:930-942.

20. Ulett GA, Perry SG: Cytotoxic food testing and leukocyte increase as an index to food sensitivity. (non-peer) Ann Allergy 1974; 33:23-32.

21. Ulett GA, Perry SG: Cytotoxic testing and leukocyte increase as an index to food sensitivity. II. Coffee and tobacco. Ann Allergy 1975; 34:150-160.

22. Hughes EC: Chemically defined diet in the diagnosis and management of allergy or food intolerances. I. With a group of sensorineural hearing impaired. Trans Am Acad Ophthalmol and Otolaryngol Allergy 1975; 15:60-71.

23. Bryan WTK, Bryan MP: Diagnosis of food allergy by cytotoxic reactions. Trans Am Soc Ophthalmol and Otolaryngol Allergy 1976; 15:14-23.

24. Bickmore JT: Leukocyte test for food allergies: its application toward clinical practice. Trans Am Soc Ophthalmol Otolaryngol Allergy 1976; 16:101-108.

25. Updegraff TR: Food allergy and cytotoxic tests. Ear Nose Throat J 1977; 56:450-459. Also Trans Am Soc Ophthalmol and Otolaryngol Allergy 1977; 16:48-64.

26. Hughes EC: Chemically defined diet in the diagnosis of food sensitivities. II. With a panel of seriously sensitive patients. Trans Am Soc Ophthalmol Otolaryngol Allergy 1977; 17:43-65.

27. Boyles JH: The validity of using the cytotoxic food test in clinical allergy. Ear Nose Throat J 1977; 56:35-43.

28. Duncan RB, Duncan TD: Otolaryngeal allergy in Wellington 1971-1975. New Zealand Med J 1977; 85:45-52.

29. Oehling A, Martin-Gil D, Jerez J, Subira ML: In vitro diagnosis of food allergy. Allergol Immunopathol (Madr.) 1978; 6:153-161.

30. Rubin JL, Griffiths RW, Hill HR: Allergen-induced depression of neutrophil chemotaxis in allergic individuals. J Allergy Clin Immunol 1978; 62:301-308.

31. Hughes EC: Use of a chemically defined diet in the diagnosis of food sensitively and the determination of offending foods. Ann Allergy 1978; 40:393-398.

32. Hughes EC, Gottschalk GH: Comparison of cytotoxic test for food sensitivities with food challenge experience: effect of sample timing. Trans Am Acad Ophthalmol Otolaryngol Allergy 1978; 18:39-51.

33. Hughes EC, Oettinger L, Johnson F, Gottschalk GH: Case report: A chemically defined diet in diagnosis and management of food sensitivity in minimal brain dysfunction. Ann Allergy 1979; 42:174-176.

34. Ulett GA: Food allergy: Cytotoxic testing and the central nervous system. Psychiatric J Univ Ottawa 1980; 5:100-108.

35. Stavish GE: The clinical aspects of the cytotoxic test. (non-peer) The Bion 1980.

36. Holopaninen E, Palva T, Stenberg P, Backman A, Legti H, Huokonen J: Cytotoxic leukocyte reaction. Acta Otolaryngol 1980; 89:222-226.

37. Ruokonen J, Holopainenen E, Palva T, Backman A: Secretory otitis media and allergy with special reference to the cytotoxic leucocyte test. Allergy 1981; 36:59-68.

38. Ruokonen J: Reactions in the cytotoxic leucocyte test. Allergol Immunopathol (Madr.) 1981; 9:281-288.

39. Hopkins JM, Tomlinson VS, Jenkins RM: Variation in response to cytotoxicity of cigarette smoke. Br Med J 1981; 283:1209-1211.

40. West WG: Food sensitivities through the cytotoxic test. The Bion 1981.

41. Stavish GE: Clinical application of cytotoxic test as it relates to comprehensive ecological investigation. The Bion 1981.

42. Stromp MA: The beauty of the cytotoxic test. Preventative Medicine Forum Fall 1981.

43. Bienveniste J: The human basophil degranulation test as an in vitro method for diagnosis of allergies. Clinica Allergy 1981; 11:1-11.

44. Trevino RJ: Immunologic mechanisms in the production of food sensitivities. Laryngoscope 1981; 91:1913-1936.

45. Cheung G, Plechner AJ: Diagnosis of canine and feline food sensitivities; a new method. J Anim Health Technol 1982; 5:20-25.

46. Hughes EC, Gottschalk GH, Kaufmann D: Effect of time of blood sampling on in vitro tests for food sensitivities. Ear Nose

Throat J 1982; 61:81-87.

47. Ruokonen J, Paganus A, Lehti H: Elimination diets in the treatment of secretory otitis media. Int J Pediatr Otorhinolaryngol 1982; 4:39-46.

48 King I: The cytotoxic test, uncovering hidden food allergies. Inter J Holistic Health & Medicine 1983; 2:30-32

49 Hopkins JM, Gorecka D: Tough cells and old age. Lancet 1983; ii:1170-1173.

50. Palva T, Legtinen T, Malmberg H: Separation of granulocytes for the cytotoxic leucocyte test. Laryngoscope 1983; 93:242-244.

51. Podleski WK: Cytodestructive mechanisms provoked by food antigens. II. Antibody-dependent allergic autocytotoxicity. Allergy 1985; 40:166-172.

52. Cheraskin E, Allen J, Zavik J: The psychotherapeutic implications of cytotoxic testing. J Orthomolecular Psychiatry 1985; 14:128-135.

53. Podleski WK: Cytodestructive mechanisms provoked by antigens. I. Direct, allergic autocytotoxicity. Allergy 1985; 40:157-165.

54. Podleski WK: Spontaneous allergic autocytotoxicity in bronchial asthma associated with food allergy. American J Medicine 1986; 81:437-442.

55 Lovendale M: Nurses help doctors find the missing diagnosis. (non-peer) California Nursing Today May 1986.

56. Fell PJ, Brostoff J, Pasula MJ: High correlation of the ALCAT test results with double blind challenge (DBC) in food sensitivity. Ann Allergy 1989; 62:253.

57. Sandberg DH, Pasula MJ: A comparison of the ALCAT test for food reactions amongst two population sub-groups. Ann Allergy 1989; 62:271.

58. Pasula MJ: A possible new whole blood assay for delayed hypersensitivity reaction. AMT CE Supp July 1988; 178-179.

59. Jackson JA, Riordan HD, Neatherly S: Comparison of two cytotoxic food sensitivity tests. American Clinical Laboratory March 1991; 20-21.

60. Fell P, Soulsby S, Brostoff J: Cellular responses to food in irritable bowel syndrome. An investigation of the ALCAT test. J Nutritional Medicine 1991; 2:143-149.

Total Negative Studies — 6

61 Franklin W, Lowell FC: Failure of ragweed pollen extract to destroy white cells from ragweed-sensitive patients. J Allergy 1949; 20:375-377.

62. Chambers VV, Hudson BH, Glaser J: A study of the reactions of human polymorphonuclearleucocytes to various allergens. J Allergy 1958; 29:93-102.

63. Lieberman P, Crawford L, Bjelland J, C(a)nnell B, Rice M: Controlled study of the cytotoxic food test. JAMA 1975; 231:728-730.

64. Benson TE, Arkins JA: Cytotoxic testing for food allergy: evaluation of reproducibility and correlation. J Allergy Clin Immuno 1976; 58:471-476.

65. King WP: Testing for food allergy: a statistical comparison of cytotoxic and intracutaneous tests. (non-peer) Laryngoscope 1978; 88:1649-1659.

66. Lehman CW: The leucocytic food allergy test: a study of its reliability and reproducibility. Effect of diet and sublingual food drops on this test. (non-peer) Ann Allergy 1980; 45:150-158.

Summary

The positive studies and papers were done by doctors and preventive care specialists who understand the importance of the original definition of allergy. They had used the cytotoxic test for an extended length of time, so they became accomplished in the performance of the test before they did their study or wrote their reports.

The negative studies were done by traditional allergists who use the limited IgE definition of allergy. They test their patients with skin tests and treat them with years of allergy injections. These negative studies were all done by doctors who had not used the cytotoxic test before and had no experience in making the kits or performing the test. Their studies are simply reports on their first try to perform a complex procedure. It is noteworthy that two studies with negative conclusions obtained good reproducibility (something that cannot be obtained with traditional skin tests). Because the cytotoxic test threatens the traditional allergist's practices and beliefs about what allergies are, it is not hard to see why they did not understand the results they were receiving from the test.

Numerous ailments are causing painful suffering for millions of people. Rapidly growing medical costs are bankrupting people, businesses, insurance companies and the nation. Both logic and compassion cry out for the wide use of a cost-effective and accurate white blood cell test and the improved diets which follow.

Most of the traditional approaches, such as drugs, surgeries and allergy injections, harm people and destroy their life savings. Allergy tests, other than white blood cell testing, miss many delayed allergic reactions. An accurate white blood cell test is the most effective, cost efficient way to discover delayed food and chemical allergies. These are two of the reasons why traditional allergists dislike it.

According to the *Journal of Allergy and Applied Immunology*, allergic reactions are probably the most frequently unrecognized cause of illness in the United States.

John H. Boyles, Jr., MD, is a past president of the Otolaryngology Allergy Academy and the American Academy of Environmental Medicine. He is the author of a peer-reviewed study, published in a leading medical journal, which used white blood cell testing for discovering delayed food allergies [27]. The study concluded, "We believe the results of this study unequivocally validate the use of the cytotoxic test as a clinical tool."

The approach which combines modern white blood cell testing and the individualized diet which follows, removes the underlying causes of most symptoms, reduces medical costs and does not harm people.

By comprehending this information, you have gained a better understanding of allergy than most traditional allergists have.

Conclusion

For a peer-reviewed article to carry any weight in a scientific argument, it has to be done properly and must be reviewed by peers knowledgeable about the subject. Four of the six negative studies were published in peer-reviewed journals; however, the doctors doing the peer reviewing were, as demonstrated by

the errors in the six studies, not qualified to review non-IgE, delayed food and chemical allergy studies.

Traditional allergists have nearly forced white blood cell testing for delayed food allergies off the market by claiming: first, that there are no peer-reviewed studies supporting the test; second, that there are six peer-reviewed negative studies; third, that the negative studies were done properly and accurately peer-reviewed; forth, that the majority of the scientific studies are negative on the test. All four claims have been demonstrated to be false by the preceding evidence. The traditional allergists have been able to get away with their claims because they have not been exposed until now.

Scientific decisions must be based on four basic principles: first, the accuracy of the information; second, the amount of information; third, how current the information is; and fourth, what actually works. Based on all four of these principles, overwhelming scientific evidence supports the conclusion that the efficacy of white blood cell testing has been proven.

Four major changes have taken place in the last few years. First, there have been 27 consecutive, new research studies and reports all supporting white blood cell testing since the last negative study was published in 1980. Second, for the first time, the 60 positive medical studies and reports are located and documented. Third, the defects of the six negative studies are disclosed. Fourth, there are now three new and different tests which are based on the same principle as the cytotoxic test which have demonstrated efficacy. Because of this scientific evidence, the value of white blood cell testing should be acknowledged by all insurance companies and by state and federal agencies.

When one carefully reviews all the known scientific studies and books on white blood cell testing and delayed food allergies, the conclusion is clear: whenever the researchers understood food allergies and were experienced with white blood cell testing, they concluded that the test is of significant value. However, if the doctors did not understand delayed food and chemical allergies, they were negative about the value of the white blood cell test.

Dr. Arthur Black's 1956 discovery of the

first white blood cell test for food allergies started a new era in allergy testing. This test increased the awareness of food and chemical allergies. His original work has now been confirmed 59 times in published studies and reports over the past 35 years. In addition, there are now three new types of white blood cell tests described in peer-reviewed medical journals which confirm the validity of the principles underlying white blood cell testing for hidden or delayed allergic reactions [43,54,56].

White blood cell testing has been found effective for more than 250 thousand patients over the last quarter century. This has happened without anyone being harmed. The people who took the white blood cell test and used the resulting information have been helped for life.

In the final analysis, it makes no sense to eat a food that kills your white blood cells. The white blood cell reaction is important to test for in order to provide accurate nutritional counseling.

There are 52 studies in medical journals which support the efficacy of the white blood cell test. The six studies with negative conclusions contain supportive data in them or are hopelessly flawed.

White blood cell testing has been used for more than 30 years as a valuable tool for doctors to use regularly for screening patients diagnosed as having delayed food and chemical allergies. Preventive care which includes white blood cell testing will dramatically reduce the amount of money insurance companies will have to pay out and thereby reduce insurance premiums.

In the past, when health breakthroughs have occurred, the traditional medical establishment has usually taken about 50 years before the new idea has been accepted and widely used. If history repeats itself, the use of the white blood cell test for delayed food allergies will become the widely used approach around the year 2000.

*You will observe with concern
how long a useful truth
may be known and exist, before it is
generally received and practiced on.*

*Benjamin Franklin
Scientist, Author and A Founding Father
of the United States — 1706 to 1790*

The white blood cell test works for people of all ages without causing any damage. In Finland the test is used to discover what infants should start eating after breast feeding so they have a healthier life. By using a small amount of blood from the umbilical cord, it is possible to discover the foods the infant was born allergic to. Mothers then know what to eat when they are nursing and which foods to feed their child when nursing is phased out.

The white blood cell test is also used to test for delayed allergic reactions to life-threatening chemicals and drugs. No traditional allergy tests work for testing people for reactions to the food preservative, sodium bisulfite. When traditional allergists test people for allergic reactions to this chemical, they put them in a hospital's intensive care unit and then give them the chemical. If they get a reaction, the doctors then try to revive them. Because this type of testing is dangerous, painful, and expensive, it is usually avoided. Several people have died because they did not know they were allergic to this chemical. A white blood cell test solves these testing problems and costs less than one percent of what the traditional allergists charge.

People are damaged by not having access to the type of health care that will enable them to become free of their suffering. The progress of scientific health care is crippled by the continued suppression of the knowledge of delayed food allergies and of the white blood cell test.

Insurance companies need to fulfill their commitments to their customers and pay their claims promptly. Unfortunately, some insurance companies are trying to get out of their commitments by claiming the cytotoxic test is not thoroughly proven and is only for investigational use.

Delayed food and chemical allergies are multifaceted, and no single test is the only one to use. There is no gold standard. White blood cell testing followed by challenge testing is the best approach. Both types of testing should be used for optimum results.

When people understand how diverse delayed food allergies are, they realize why traditional elimination diets fail. It is impossible to guess accurately which foods are needed for an allergy-free diet. You need the information from an accurate white blood cell test.

White blood cell testing is the optimum first step for helping people begin to benefit from true preventive care. This will dramatically reduce medical costs. One side effect of this is that many traditional allergists will be out of work. However, food allergy specialists who practice environmental medicine and preventive care will be in great demand.

The demand is growing because the American approach to health, diet and the polluted environment has been weakening the immune system. If people are unaware of delayed food allergies, they often become reactive to more foods, and some become allergic to minute amounts of chemicals. This type of environmental illness can be very debilitating for people. It is also a major financial burden for employers, insurance companies and the government.

In the 1988 *Surgeon General's Report On Nutrition And Health*, C. Everett Koop, MD, wrote, "Qualified health professionals should advise persons with food allergies and intolerances on the diagnosis of these conditions and on the use of diets that exclude foods and food substances that induce symptoms."

During the administration of Governor Jerry Brown, California was known as the leading state in supporting improved approaches for health care. Other states and the federal government often followed California's positive lead.

This dramatically changed in 1982 when Governor Deukmejian took over. He removed the previous health care administrators and reversed the direction of the state's health care system. Prior to his administration, the California state government was supporting preventive care and alternative health approaches, including white blood cell testing for delayed food and chemical allergies. This reversal of direction was done without the awareness of most of the people in California or the rest of the United States.

Governor Deukmejian and his appointees attacked preventive care approaches and supported only the older, traditional health care approaches of his backers. When the legislature tried to reverse this negative shift by unanimously passing corrective legislation, the Governor prided himself on vetoing the improvements.

Because other states and the federal government continued to follow California, Governor Deukmejian's changes have damaged health care throughout the country. He left office in 1990, and there is now an opportunity to right the wrongs of his administration.

Major breakthroughs are now changing the way medicine will be practiced in the future. One important change involves the California Medical Association.

The California Medical Association (CMA) is a powerful professional association that works as a trade union for its members. However, the CMA represents only 30 percent of the medical doctors in California and thus, a very small percentage of all the different health care professionals. The CMA has been a leader in the battle against the Clinical Ecologists and approaches to allergies that are different from its own.

The CMA's "Position Statement" against the cytotoxic test has been influential across the United States. A few states' regulatory agencies used this "Position Statement" as their basis for attacking cytotoxic testing. Also, many insurance companies used the CMA "Position Statement" as an excuse to cut off payments to their policy holders.

A major breakthrough occurred in December of 1989 when the CMA was called before the California State Assembly to testify about the need for new legislation. Pressured by antitrust lawsuits, including one I filed, the CMA withdrew its "Position Statement" against delayed food allergy procedures.

In 1979, Barbara Solomon, MD, was challenged by a few traditional allergists for using the cytotoxic test to discover delayed food allergies. These doctors persuaded the state of Maryland to block her from competing with them. After an in-depth review, her way of practicing medicine was found acceptable and she was allowed to continue using the cytotoxic test to help her patients.

In New York state, Warren Levin, MD, was challenged for using the cytotoxic test and other alternative therapies. Again, a state was misadvised to pursue one of its own preventive-care physicians. The state used as its highly paid witnesses, the leading self-proclaimed "experts" on fighting alternative therapies (the same people who instigated the challenge in the first place). In 1994, after a careful scientific analysis of the facts, the state's own Board of Regents concluded that the state's license committee and its "experts" had erred. Dr. Levin was exonerated and continues to help his patients with alternative therapies, including the Prime Test.

Testing for delayed food allergies is the foundation of accurate preventative care. Historically, food allergy specialists have been 20 or more years ahead of traditional medicine in recognizing the causes of numerous health problems.

Dr. Theron Randolph discovered the delayed allergy problem caused by indoor air pollution and the pesticides in our foods over 30 years ago. He was the first to explain that these pollution problems are made much worse for some people because they became allergic to the chemicals.

The Clinical Ecology approaches to health care are so far ahead of traditional medicine that traditional doctors do not understand or recognize Clinical Ecology and Environmental Medicine. Because this area is not taught in medical schools, most doctors stay in the dark, unless they read and understand the appropriate medical journals and attend conventions sponsored by the American Academy of Environmental Medicine and similar medical societies.

The pain and suffering caused by traditional medical approaches is massive, but hard to measure. However, the unnecessary financial drain caused by traditional medicine is easy to measure. Using the medical industry's own figures, we see that from 1960 to 1990, a day in the hospital climbed from $32 to $820; a trip to the doctor jumped from $5 to $50; traditional doctor's annual income went from $35,000 to over $225,000; and the number of doctors per 100,000 people went from 133 to 252. Health care took 5.3 percent of the Gross National Product in 1960; in 1990 it took 12.2 percent. To make matters worse, average health levels have gone down over the last 30 years.

One of the most glaring examples of how sick the system is involves Denton Cooley, MD. He was featured on the cover of *Forbes* magazine on May 25, 1992. In 1989 he made $9,000,000 doing heart surgeries. Most of those surgeries were coronary bypass operations, an operation which is ineffective and very dangerous. Nationally, around 5 percent of patients die from the operation. In addition, this operation does not solve the problem: only the 10 percent fat diet solves the problem.

Dr. Cooley performed up to 17 operations a day and was paid $4,000 for each one. Heart surgeons are paid by insurance companies, and this increases everyone's health insurance costs. The total cost of this ineffective operation averages over $20,000. The total cost should be less than $5,000, and in almost all cases the operation should not be done until it is seen if the person's problem is solved by using the 10–10–80 program for a year.

Neither the FDA nor any other government agency does anything to stop this damage to the public. Government agencies instead attack people who explain how the proper type of preventive care will prevent and reverse heart disease.

The problems caused by coronary bypass surgery have become worse since 1989. There are now so many doctors doing the surgery that the total costs — as well as damage — have gone up. This has cut into Dr. Cooley's assembly-line operation: he now does "only" eight operations a day and his income in 1991 dropped to $3,600,000.

The most important change to make in the health care system in the United States is to emphasize preventive care. Health care costs in 1992 were over $800 billion, which is $3000 for every man, woman and child in the country. That equals 13.4 percent of gross national product compared to 7 percent in Japan. In addition, there are nearly $300 billion going for legal costs related to traditional medicine compared to a negligible amount in Japan. Total health care costs in the United States were $74 billion in 1970. Businesses alone paid $186 billion for health care in 1990, which is more than they made in after-tax profits.

You pay when you go to a doctor and your income is less because your employer has given what could have been your money to health insurance companies. Also, when you buy something, some of the cost of the health insurance paid by the manufacturer for his employees is included in the price of the product.

The American health care system is collapsing. Part of the solution is breaking the monopoly held by traditional doctors and thereby allowing for freedom of choice by the individual.

Every $1 spent with doctors practicing alternative medicine and preventive care can save you $50 and sometimes more than $1,000. Even though their approach is cost effective, alternative doctors have trouble collecting the money due them from insurance companies. At the same time, they have to spend large sums of money defending themselves from attacks by state and federal agencies under the influence of traditional doctors.

Americans are having trouble competing with foreign producers. A major reason for this is that American products contain extra costs; one is the high medical costs of the employees. Several hundred dollars are added to the cost of each car produced in the United States because of the high cost of health care for the people who develop, produce and market the car.

According to General Motors, there is more cost in each car for employee's health care than for steel. Americans often buy foreign products because they are a better value. Other countries have far lower health care costs included in the price of their products because their health care system is more effective.

The health care costs added to American cars and other products make them less competitive in international markets. This contributes to our negative trade balances and recessions.

The major reason for overwhelming health care costs in the United States is the reliance on traditional medicine, including excessive and unnecessary drugs and surgery. In addition, there are many doctors who make over $2000 a day for doing procedures which do not work. Nearly 20 percent of heart surgeons earn over $600,000 a year. Based on their typical three-day work week, that equals $4000 a day. The Japanese health care system does not reward its doctors so foolishly. Also, the traditional Japanese are healthier because they eat differently.

If everyone took advantage of preventive care principles, employee health care costs would probably be under 25 percent of what they are today. Until the medical/pharmaceutical/health insurance industry monopoly is exposed and broken, preventive care advocates will continue to be harassed and their approaches declared invalid. Unless people become aware and demand a fundamental change, there will be a continuous decline in the average health level and medical costs will continue to increase, destroying our ability to compete with other nations.

Health care costs are growing so rapidly that if the necessary changes are not made now, in 20 years, over half of all the money you make will go to traditional doctors, drug companies, hospitals, insurance companies and attorneys. At the same time, health problems are growing so rapidly that most people will be sick much of the time.

Eighty percent of the products
are made by people
who don't feel good.

Theodore Roosevelt
Conservationist and Twenty-sixth President
of the United States — 1858 to 1919

One of the biggest problems in shifting to a health care system based on prevention is that most people hold doctors in awe. And, most traditional doctors do not believe that delayed food allergies exist or understand preventive care.

When the principles underlying delayed allergies are adopted, national health care costs will go from over $800 billion to under $400 billion per year. This could put a third of the traditional doctors will be out of work. They could begin helping people that need doctors in undeveloped countries.

The solution to the health care emergency will not start until the monopoly held by traditional doctors is broken and people are free to choose the type of health care which works for them.

It is not hard to see why some traditional doctors are waging war against the more cost-effective approaches which also help people to become free from their symptoms. Each dollar spent on effective, alternative approaches takes hundreds of dollars away from doctors who over-prescribe drugs, surgery and traditional allergy injections. The economic and physical health of the nation is being damaged unnecessarily.

This problem exists throughout the country and is caused by traditional doctors from different specialties, not just "board-certified" allergists. In a report done by Bill Moyers for PBS titled *Who Owns Our Government?,* he pointed out that the American Medical Association financed the campaigns of both the Republican and Democratic candidates, so no matter who wins the election, traditional doctors maintain their monopoly over health care.

Traditional doctors try to justify their actions by claiming that they protect the doctor-patient relationship and guarantee quality health care while keeping costs down. In fact, traditional doctors stay in control of people's thinking about health care and block knowledge about effective ways to prevent health problems. This causes health care to be low in quality and high in cost.

*The Republicans and Democrats are
converging into a single party:
the Power Party.
There are more than 4000 PAKs
representing special interest groups
in America — doctors, car dealers
you name it. They all want something
and pay millions to get it.
It's nothing more than legalized bribery.*

Ralph Nader
Consumer Advocate and Author

One reason the cytotoxic test is attacked is that it reveals there are delayed allergic reactions to chemicals. There is now overwhelming evidence that chemicals damage some people at very low levels because of delayed allergic reactions.

A 1992 study that demonstrates the existence of delayed chemical allergies was done by Kathleen Rodgers, an immunotoxicologist at the University of Southern California's School of Medicine. The study demonstrates that exposures to the pesticide Malathion causes the mouse immune system cells to react even though the exposures are 700 times lower than the toxic level. Malathion and similar pesticides are regularly sprayed on our foods, in our yards and on our homes by helicopters.

The doctor who led the attack on the cytotoxic test and the existence of delayed food and chemical allergies is Abba Terr, MD. The foundation of his professional reputation is his published studies of patients who were suffering from chemical allergies and had been so diagnosed by chemical allergy specialists. Dr. Terr claimed that their health ailments were caused by mental problems and that chemical allergies do not exist.

Dr. Terr received most of his patients from health insurance companies who were looking for a doctor to help them avoid reimbursing their policy holders. Without testing, he decided in every case that the patients did not have chemical allergies. He got the insurance reimbursements denied even though chemical allergy specialists had confirmed the diagnosis and the people were free from most of their symptoms when they avoided the chemicals that had caused reactions on their allergy tests.

Dr. Terr also decided that the patients' problems were psychological and often referred them to psychiatrists, including his wife, for talk therapy

and mind-altering drugs. These drugs are made from chemicals which often cause additional problems for these previously-verified chemical allergy patients. This is in addition to the regular, long-lasting, serious side effects of the drugs.

Dr. Terr is very influential throughout the country and is often relied on by the press, government agencies and insurance companies. His professional credibility is based on his theory that delayed food and chemical allergies do not exist and that the cytotoxic test or any other test which demonstrates they do are false. He feels that the symptoms are caused by defective thinking of the patients and thus are psychological. This is also the current position of the American Academy of Allergy and Immunology and of several allergy organizations it has created.

The National Academy of Sciences is the major scientific organization in the United States and is world renowned. It recently completed an extensive study on whether delayed chemical allergies exist. These reactions are also called multiple chemical sensitivities. Its National Research Institute concluded in the report titled *Biologic Markers in Immunotoxicology* that the symptoms are caused by damaging physical reactions to chemicals and are not psychological.

The report singled out Dr. Terr for special mention by referring to his published study on 50 patients whom he had helped deprive of their insurance benefits by claiming they did not have chemical allergies. On page 135 the report states, "Terr's conclusions are a poorly supported opinion expressed by one who has evaluated patients on behalf of a workers' compensation appeals board."

The National Academy of Sciences report should be a turning point now that Dr. Terr's work has been exposed and his beliefs and those of other traditional allergists have been discredited. However, politicians they have supported are still under their influence, so that little progress is likely without public pressure.

Although Dr. Terr has no formal training in environmental medicine, he travels around the country testifying against people who have been diagnosed by environmental medical specialists as having delayed chemical allergies. Because of the overwhelming body of evidence available, people who lost their insurance benefits due to Dr. Terr's testimonies should be located and their benefits be reinstated. The damage also should be reversed wherever he influenced government regulators and the press regarding cytotoxic testing and the existence of food and chemical allergies.

The facts remain: delayed allergies exist and the white blood cell test for discovering delayed food and chemical allergies has been proven effective and safe while reducing health care costs. There is extensive evidence that many people have been helped and no evidence that anyone has been harmed.

The white blood cell test is used after the doctor has diagnosed the health problem. The test is then used to select the optimum foods for the person. Because white blood cell testing is not used for diagnosis of disease, there is no need for it to be approved by any government agency.

The traditional allergists who said it was impossible to test for delayed food allergies by using a person's white blood cells have been proven wrong. Unfortunately, they have not yet acknowledged their mistake. They still control a large part of the medical establishment and the government bureaucracy.

The opposition to new, better approaches often lasts until those in power retire or die. Most of the doctors who are resisting the awareness of delayed food and chemical allergies and white blood cell testing are elderly. The use of these scientific discoveries is growing.

Personal History

When I began studying ways to maximize health and longevity in 1969, there were few books or medical articles that were reliable when the health problem was a chronic or degenerative disease. Clinical ecology and environmental medicine were not being taught in any medical school (and still are not). One actually had to spend time with the researchers who were doing the work. I spent several years studying the different approaches of the scientists and doctors, while working with associates to improve white blood cell testing.

During 1974 and 1975, I did a comprehensive study of Dr. Theron Randolph's program for helping people with a broad range of chronic physical and mental problems. With his awareness of delayed food and chemical allergies, he was able to identify the allergic factors, and when they were removed, the patients' health quickly

improved. When the items were reintroduced, symptoms rapidly returned. I followed a group of 34 patients for one month. Their starting symptoms covered a broad range of chronic physical and mental health problems. After a week of fasting and three weeks of testing, all 34 patients had discovered the foods and chemicals which caused their health problems and were feeling much better.

During 1976 and 1977, I did a study of the approach Nathan Pritikin had begun to use to help people with degenerative diseases such as heart disease, diabetes, stroke and cancer. The use of a very low fat, very low cholesterol, low protein and high complex carbohydrate diet often freed them of their poor circulation caused symptoms and began to reverse their degenerative diseases.

The approaches to health Dr. Randolph and Nathan Pritikin developed are similar in three important aspects: they are both based on eating health building foods and avoiding drugs and surgeries. Both have a sound scientific basis. However, the approaches are very different in that Dr. Randolph did not address the importance of the balance of macronutrients, and Nathan Pritikin paid little attention to the importance of delayed food allergies. Because each approach is a part of the foundation of any effective preventive care program, I began assisting them in their campaigns to improve the awareness of health care professionals and the public. The consulting work I did for them enabled me to see first hand the immense value of their work. I later discovered the potential of combining their separate breakthroughs.

In 1976, I tried a unique combination of approaches on myself. This new program so dramatically improved my health that I decided to change my career and began sharing these new breakthroughs in health and longevity. This included an improved white blood cell test for delayed food allergies. Those who followed the program became free of most of their health problems and became supporters of The Quality Longevity Program.

In addition to helping people become free of their delayed food allergies and reducing chemical exposures, I shared the importance of a diet very low in fat and cholesterol, moderate in protein and high in complex carbohydrates.

This approach was first made popular by

Nathan Pritikin. When this is combined with non-allergic foods, specialized supplements, aerobic exercise and reduced total calories, the results were beyond my highest expectations. When these different health breakthroughs are brought together there is a synergistic effect — the results are greater than the sum of the parts.

I brought Dr. Randolph and Nathan Pritikin together for a day in the hope each would begin to use the other's research, and help people to become free of chronic and degenerative diseases at the same time. Each was so focused on his own area that neither enlarged his program.

In 1978, I gave my first public presentation at the Esalen Institute explaining a unique combination of the new scientific health discoveries. I then presented several one-day workshops in California for doctors and people interested in improving their health. This started a rapid growth in the use of the cytotoxic test and increased the overall awareness of delayed food and chemical allergies.

I combined the effective parts of these nutritional approaches and several other health breakthroughs for the first time and published them in *Quality Longevity* in 1980.

At the beginning of 1981, the future for a more accurate, non-damaging and inexpensive white blood cell test for delayed food and chemical allergies looked bright. There had been numerous magazine articles explaining the importance of this new understanding of allergies which included case histories of people who had turned their health around by using their test results and counseling.

Even the American Medical Association saw no problems with white blood cell testing for allergies and issued the cytotoxic test an insurance code to facilitate payment. Most insurance companies stood behind their clients claims for reimbursement for the cytotoxic test.

The medical establishment had no idea how widely the test was going to be used to help people become free of a broad range of ailments. A few years later, traditional allergists and some traditional doctors began losing their patients who had the white blood cell test and no longer had to keep going to them. Traditional doctors mounted a multifaceted campaign to end the availability of the test.

By 1981, my associates and I had made several more improvements in the cytotoxic test so that the results more closely disclosed what was happening inside the body. In order to calibrate the antigen levels, we started with the levels recommended by the developers of the cytotoxic test, William Bryan, MD and his wife, Marian Bryan. We found that the original levels were too weak to reveal many of a person's delayed food and chemical allergies. Using a process of testing and follow-up and then re-testing, we were able to calibrate each item's antigen level to a point where people would become free of their symptoms by using the results of one improved cytotoxic test.

The Bryans had recommended in their medical articles that this research be done, but because of the time and expense it had not been successfully accomplished. We worked on this project for five years, during which time we helped numerous people become free of their symptoms.

We also had patients who had taken our test, fast on clean water in a clean environment for a week so they became free of delayed food and chemical allergy-caused symptoms. We then had them food-and-chemical challenge test for a month, one item at a time for a total of three a day, to receive an indication which foods were causing their non-IgE food and chemical allergy symptoms. We used this information to better calibrate our test.

We opened Medical Service Center to provide doctors and their patients with the improved cytotoxic test and accurate, individualized nutritional counseling. During the mid-1980's, we helped more than 8,000 people of all ages and health levels become free from their health problems, enjoy a higher level of well being and reduce their health care costs.

The overwhelming majority of these people we tested and counseled experienced significant improvements in their health. The people were of all ages and had a broad range of health problems. Two follow-up surveys showed that nine out of ten people who received our improved cytotoxic test, read *Quality Longevity* and took advantage of our counseling, became free of most of their symptoms.

The Quality Longevity Program works very

well for people who want to become free of something they are addicted to. Without food addictions causing problems, other addictions can be more readily overcome.

This approach to health care has been used successfully to improve people's health and reduce their medical costs while providing the best of preventive care. This is accomplished without causing harmful side effects.

We tried to find people who had no delayed food allergies by testing world-class athletes who had no known health problems. We found that these individuals had far fewer reactions than the average person. However, everyone we tested had reactions to some foods. The athletes found that their performance improved when they avoided their allergic foods. Some of the athletes who were tested and then changed their way of eating went on to set new world records and win medals in the 1984 Olympics.

It was a great breakthrough when the awareness that germs cause infections began helping peoples' health. The major infectious ailments of that time were practically eliminated. This same level of breakthrough is available to us today when we convince the medical establishment to start helping people with delayed food and chemical allergies. Another level of improvement is available when fat, protein and cholesterol are consumed in proper amounts.

Almost all of the people who came to Medical Service Center for testing had been to several traditional doctors, spent large amounts of money and had been unable to become free of their health problems by using traditional medical methods.

Most of our clients who were receiving traditional allergy injections were still suffering. After they received our improved white blood cell test and followed their individualized programs, nearly all became free of their symptoms and no longer needed their traditional allergy injections. Those who needed specialized neutralization therapy were able to have it done rapidly and with reduced discomfort, while saving time and money.

A survey of the people who came into Medical Service Center found that their average health care expenditures had averaged over $5,400 during the previous year. After using The Quality Longevity

Program their medical costs dropped dramatically.

We invited the University of California at Irvine to participate with us in a study to measure how effective The Quality Longevity Program is at improving peoples' health and reducing health care costs. After meeting with Chancellor Daniel Aldrich, he gave the dean of the medical school a letter recommending a study be done of the successes Medical Service Center was having.

The dean was also interested in researching delayed food allergies and presented our proposal to the medical professors. The dean told me they rejected the idea because what we were suggesting contradicted much of what they were teaching medical students, and they were worried about the political ramifications.

The traditional medical establishment claims it practices preventive care, and most of the public believes this. The medical establishment tells women to practice preventive care by having a mammogram. Mammograms are important, but they are diagnostic medicine, not preventive care. Practicing true preventive care means recommending a very low fat diet and recommending foods which do not kill your white blood cells.

On my travels,
I saw few die of hunger;
Of eating, a hundred thousand.

Benjamin Franklin
Scientist, Author and A Founding Father
of the United States — 1706 to 1790

Preventive care is so foreign to most medical doctors that they are continually trying to discredit doctors who use this approach. Medical doctors receive only superficial training in nutrition and no training in the advanced concepts that explain how foods affect the body. This helps to explain why more doctors are not aware of how better to help people and why it is difficult to find white blood cell testing.

There will be no real solution to the health care problem so long as traditional medical doctors dominate the health care industry, the pharmaceutical industry, the health insurance industry and the related government agencies.

Traditional medical doctors give federal politicians $15 million dollars each year to prevent competition. An unknown amount is given to state politicians. So long as government employees and the public are under the control of, and stay in awe of, traditional medical doctors and their methods, there will be little awareness that testing for and treating delayed food and chemical allergies are essential parts of preventive care. Any treatment program which does not include the best prevention program is incomplete at best.

The California Medical Association, in conjunction with the American Academy of Allergy and Immunology, launched a campaign to misinform the public and damage our reputation. It did this by writing inaccurate articles and sending misleading information to insurance companies, the press and government agencies.

One government agency which received this information was the Medical Board of California. It then filed a lawsuit against Medical Service Center and its staff designed to intimidate, discredit and close us down.

The suit made unfounded claims, including a claim that the cytotoxic test had no value for helping people. It tried to support this claim by having traditional allergists testify that there were no peer-reviewed medical articles supporting the cytotoxic test. However, as shown in this report, several peer-reviewed articles existed and prove the exact opposite. By 1985, the studies and articles supporting the principle of the cytotoxic test had grown to an overwhelming 53 for and 6 against. The evidence has continued to grow — by 1991 it was 60 for and 6 against. In medical journals it was 52 to 6.

Later, it was discovered the traditional allergists who testified against Medical Service Center were the same ones who originally pressured the Medical Board of California to file the lawsuit. These allergists, led by Dr. Terr, were paid large sums of money to testify in the case and were given accolades by their trade groups (medical associations) for removing the competition.

The Medical Board of California filed its lawsuit even though it was unable to find any people whose health had been damaged by having gone to Medical Service Center. There were several other reasons the case should never have been filed. The Center had previously been inspected in the first part of 1982 by the California Department of Health Service — Food and Drug Branch. This group is the state equivalent of the federal Food and Drug Administration (FDA). The California Food and Drug people found that white blood cell testing for delayed food allergies did not violate any California regulations.

Medical Service Center was also inspected by the federal FDA in 1985 and found to be in compliance with federal regulations. The Medical Board of California was not deterred from its attack by the facts. It was being pressured by the California Medical Association, and traditional allergists. It is important to remember that the California Medical Association is a private support group designed to protect the image and income of its members. It is not designed to help patients become well or promote preventive care or effective treatment. Medical associations are actually trade unions and lack objectivity. The California Medical Association is the most powerful, traditional and aggressively backward of any state medical association.

The complaining group consisted of traditional allergists who were losing their patients to Medical Service Center. However, people who took the improved cytotoxic test and used the related counseling were pleased because they were becoming free of their symptoms and were no longer spending large amounts of money and time on visits to traditional allergists.

The traditional allergists continually complained that centers doing cytotoxic testing were making huge amounts of money and they argued that patients should go to traditional allergists and get "proper" care. This thinly-veiled complaint simply means that the traditional allergists wanted the money instead of it going to centers using preventive care.

Throughout history, no one has become wealthy promoting preventive care. Medical Service Center belonged to an association of food-allergy testing centers. No center made more than moderate profits and all ended up losing money. However, traditional allergists who promote prescription drugs, surgery and allergy injections are still making huge amounts of money and most patients are still suffering.

For the state to have a valid lawsuit, its attorneys had to prove that people had been harmed. When the state's attorney was asked by the judge what harm was being done by Medical Service Center, his only reply was that people had wasted their money and their money should have gone to traditional allergists. At that point the case should have been thrown out of court and a public apology should have been made to Medical Service Center and its staff.

The Medical Board of California tried to obtain a court injunction to close Medical Service Center without having a trial. It failed. In an attempt to put Medical Service Center out of business on a technicality, it obtained a requirement to have Medical Service Center apply to another state agency for a laboratory license. This was an obvious conflict of interest because the licensing arm of the state would then block the Medical Board of California's strategy if it granted the license. This is the equivalent of forcing a wife to testify against her husband; thus, an honest license procedure was very unlikely.

Medical Service Center requested and received a written agreement from the licensing department that it would not deny a license because of any question about the value of cytotoxic testing. The licensing department also agreed it had no legal right to deny a license because of the type of testing being done. In addition, the California Department of Health Services licensing department had previously agreed in writing that a laboratory license was not required for white blood cell testing when used for nutritional counseling.

After the Department of Health Service's inspector finished her comprehensive inspection of our center, she stated in front of five witnesses that we had passed the inspection for receiving a laboratory license. However, when we received written notice two weeks later, the Department of Health Service said we had failed because the cytotoxic test had no value: "The efficacy...has not been established." This was in direct violation of the State of California's written agreement with Medical Service Center and state law. Supporting state documents are on file.

The Medical Board of California was not worried about losing its case because it had filed it using a special State statute which took

away our right to a jury trial.

The case dragged on at great expense to Medical Service Center and to taxpayers. The traditional allergists and State prosecutor continued to send false and derogatory information to the news media in order to win their case in the press. These continued attacks reduced the income of Medical Service Center and thus our ability to defend ourselves and defend people's right to choose effective preventive care using cytotoxic testing.

Medical Service Center was badly damaged by negative "Position Statements" of the California Medical Association because insurance companies used them to renege on their agreements to reimburse their policy holders who were Medical Service Center's current and potential clients. This caused our income to drop dramatically. This financial damage and the cost of defending ourselves hurt us severely. Even though many suffering people wanted our help, we were forced to close in 1987. The California Medical Association withdrew its related negative "Position Statements" in 1991, but by then it was too late to help us.

The case never made it to trial. Unethical industry and government tactics often enable them to win cases against those providing preventive care when they do not have a case which would hold up in court. Using threats and negative press releases also forces others out of business. By 1985, the other centers providing cytotoxic testing had closed.

Government agencies should not have the power to decide which type of health care is the best. Agencies invariably support the status quo and attack new approaches. This happens because the traditional approaches are backed by an established industry with power and political influence. This is the fundamental nature of bureaucracies. Progress in health care has been crippled for decades because bureaucratic agencies are not capable of deciding what type of health care you should choose.

However, government agencies do need the power and responsibility to inform the public based on independent outcomes research. This would include warning labels on products, like those now found on cigarettes and certified raw cows' milk. Warnings on medical procedures would include recommendations for safer, more effective approaches. An example would be to require a signed consent from a patient before coronary bypass surgery could be done. The consent form would explain how the correct diet approach is almost always more effective and does not have the expense and deadly complications of surgery and drugs.

This approach would educate the public about the government's beliefs without removing their right to make decisions about their own health care. This approach would also enable government agencies to become effective at protecting citizens' health, and it would save taxpayers' money.

In the future you will be able to tell which types of doctors know the truth about preventive care. The doctor's health and their patient's health will be much better than the average, and both will be living much longer. Today you can be sure that traditional doctors do not understand preventive care. Their health and longevity, just like the average American's, is poor compared to other developed nations.

Americans were so sickly in 1992 that over 800 billion dollars was spent on traditional medical procedures. In addition, the Surgeon General reported that 68 percent of the population was dying from dietary-caused diseases. The full potential for great health and longevity will not be known until a large group of people uses the principles which are the foundation of The Quality Longevity Program.

Those who tell you that Americans have the best health care in the world do not know what they are talking about. Health care levels should be measured by infant mortality rates, the number of times people have to go to the doctor per decade, how much money has to be spent on health care, the health of children and adults, and the population's average longevity. By all these indicators and more, Americans are in serious trouble.

The only areas where we are "best" are the numbers of fancy test machines we have, the numbers of dangerous surgeries we do and the numbers of symptom-producing drugs we have.

Health Pioneers

I am deeply indebted to many people for their generous sharing of information and support. Of great importance are the contributions of Theron Randolph, MD. His four major discoveries are: first, most people with chronic symptoms have non-IgE, delayed food and chemical allergies; second, people can be tested for food and chemical allergies by fasting and then re-exposing them;

third, delayed food and chemical allergies often become physical addictions; and fourth, many serious mental problems are caused by delayed food and chemical allergies.

These four discoveries are so important that if Nobel Prizes were given for new discoveries in preventive care and environmental medicine, Dr. Randolph would have received more than one.

Nathan Pritikin should have received a Nobel Prize for the first demonstration in a published medical study that artery plaques can be reduced by diet alone. He also started the major public and medical awareness that degenerative diseases are best treated by proper diet and can be prevented the same way.

The changes in people's health and well being that have been brought about by aerobic exercise should bring Kenneth Cooper, MD, a Nobel Prize.

When you look at the Nobel Prizes presented in medicine over the past decades for ideas later shown to be false and damaging, such as the lobotomy, you can see that the Nobel Awards Committee needs help.

Credit should be given to the other pioneers for their contributions and for stopping the traditional allergists from totally monopolizing the field of allergy. Understanding the importance of testing and treating delayed food and chemical allergies can help state and federal officials become free of the influence of traditional allergists and the medical-drug complex.

Each one of us adds a little to our understanding of nature, and from all the facts arises a certain grandeur.

Aristotle
Greek Philosopher — 384 to 322 BC

The Future

The foundation is now in place for a major improvement in people's health. First, the positive scientific studies in this report confirm the value of white blood cell testing, and the negative studies are exposed as inaccurate. Second, delayed allergy-caused health problems are epidemic and growing despite record sums of money being spent for medical care. Third, health awareness in the United States and other modern countries has grown to such a high degree that traditional allergists and others are having trouble suppressing awareness. Fourth, the traditional medical establishment is beginning to understand the value of white blood cell testing and beginning to see the importance of helping people with delayed food and chemical allergies.

When you combine the desire of people to be free of their health problems and the desire of people, businesses, governments and insurance companies to reduce the overwhelming medical costs, you can see there is an outstanding opportunity for a change in the approach to health care that is founded on removing the cause of symptoms instead of treating symptoms.

Most people spend their lives hoping for a cure for the major diseases. Something better is already here — prevention.

This approach to health care has changed my life. It dramatically improved my health, the health of my friends and the health of people who asked for information. This new awareness also gave me an opportunity for a challenging new career and the opportunity to make a lasting and important difference in the world. I invite you to take advantage of this approach for great health and longer life.

With your awareness and support, the health problems in this country and those around the world can be dramatically reduced.

In the future, people in government must become aware of the motives of the traditional medical establishment. Today, government prosecutors rely on the traditional medical associations to decide what is proper in health care. They do not understand that these associations are actually trade groups that function like labor unions. The traditional medical associations control what is printed in their traditional medical journals and who is selected for government jobs and as university professors. To ask these people what is the whole truth about health care is like asking the trucking union if airplanes should be able to carry packages. There are non-traditional associations of doctors which have extensive scientific evidence to support their belief in preventive care.

New Research

Since 1976, there has been an ongoing research program to develop a new white blood cell test. The test needed to have all the advantages of the cytotoxic test, plus the latest concepts and improvements, without any of the past problems. Also, the test needed to be readily performable in the doctor's office. In 1988 a new procedure called the Prime Test™ was developed which satisfied these needs.

The Prime Test utilizes past improvements while taking advantage of a new design. This modern white blood cell test solves the problems involved with the cytotoxic test, other white blood cell tests and the antibody tests. Rather than disclosing only one type of allergic reaction, the Prime Test simultaneously discloses several different types of reactions.

The Prime Test has been used for several years throughout the United States and in Europe. Doctors are observing outstanding improvements in the health of their patients. The test is designed to give results which parallel the information gained from fasting and food-challenge testing or provocative neutralization testing, without their associated problems and costs.

Doctors who are interested in practicing preventive care and want to remove causes instead of only treating symptoms, now have a test available which does not miss damaging reactions. The Prime Test is economical and can be reliably performed by the doctor's staff.

If you would like to know more about delayed food and chemical allergies or want more information on the Prime Test, contact Advanced Health Center at 34146 Selva Road, Suite 200, Monarch Beach, California, 92629. Phone (714) 661-4001.

Ethical manufacturers of non-toxic, quality products who give physicians and the public honest information about their products should be permitted to carry out their research and commercial activities.

Marshall Mandell, MD
Pioneer in field of
Delayed Food Allergies and Author

Chapter 12
Famous and Infamous Health Programs

One of the first writers to have a significant impact on nutrition and health was Paul Bragg. In the early 1900's, he began writing books and speaking about the importance of eating organically-grown vegetables and of exercise. He opened the first health food store in 1914.

I met him in 1973 when he was 92 years old. He was more robust and dynamic than most men in their twenties. He was not familiar with delayed food allergies, but developed an interesting technique for dealing with them. He would fast one day a week, drinking only clean water. Thus, without realizing what he was accomplishing, one day a week he had no delayed food allergy exposures.

He would also fast for a full week every three months. That enabled him to experience the withdrawal from food allergies and what it was like to be free of reactions. He experimented with different foods and tried to discover which ones worked for him. Primarily he ate fresh vegetables and occasionally some fish.

When he was 16 he contracted tuberculosis and went to a health spa in Switzerland where he recovered on fresh foods, clean air and exercise. He did not have the information on how damaging dairy products are that is available today, and ate goats' milk yogurt. However, many of Bragg's ideas were helpful, and famous people from all walks of life credited their health improvements to his advice. He continued enrolling people into eating better and exercising until he died at the age of 95.

Another influential author was Adelle Davis. She wrote a number of books which had a big influence during the 1960's. She taught the importance of eating health building foods and that the Standard American Diet was a disaster. Unfortunately, there was not enough scientific research available to guide her, and many of her diet recommendations were as bad as those underlying the Standard American Diet.

Adelle Davis did not understand delayed food allergies and thought eating yogurt every day was good for health. She was probably allergic and addicted to some of the foods she ate repetitiously such as dairy products and wheat. She may have mistaken her craving for a food as a valid sign that the food was good for her and everyone else. This is a common mistake made by diet authors. She smoked cigarettes, often over-ate, and had a weight problem. In her day, it was difficult to learn about delayed food allergies, food addictions and related health problems. Also, she did not know about the problems caused by fat levels above 10 percent of total calories, and died of cancer when she was 70.

Adelle Davis is to be commended for helping many people to begin thinking about the foods they eat. If she were writing her books today, they would probably be very different from what she wrote long ago. It is sad so many people are still following her obsolete advice.

Another person who had a major impact on the public's thinking about health and what to eat was Walter Alvarez, MD. He worked at the famous Mayo Clinic and his articles on health appeared in newspapers throughout the country.

While at the clinic, Dr. Alvarez wrote a nationally syndicated article disclosing that his thinking was confused on Mondays and that he was very tired throughout that day. He discovered the cause was a delayed reaction to the chicken he ate every Sunday night. No chicken and he was fine on Mondays. He tested this reaction for a long time until he finally concluded he had some type of allergic reaction to chicken. He believed this type of reaction could be a common cause of many health problems and that the medical community should emphasize the importance of food allergies.

After Dr. Alvarez's article was published, his fellow doctors at the Mayo Clinic thought he had made a big mistake. They figured it was a great opportunity to get rid of their popular rival who had so many unconventional ideas.

The next morning they entered his office and told him that his supervisor wanted to see him. They told him he was going to be fired for having written such a ridiculous article. They marched him down the hall toward his supervisor's office. Fortunately, Dr. Mayo happened to see them in the hall and congratulated Dr. Alvarez for having discovered the cause of his problem. Dr. Mayo said he also had been suffering from the same symptom for years.

Dr. Alvarez was not fired, and for a while the Mayo Clinic had two doctors with some

131

understanding of delayed food allergies. Drs. Alvarez and Mayo are long gone, as is the awareness of delayed food allergies at the Mayo Clinic. Dr. Alvarez outlived his fellow doctors and died at 94.

One of the most influential medical doctors in the United States today is Dean Adell, MD. He is on national radio and television every weekday and has an audience of over two million people. He gives good medical advice in some areas and has the courage to take controversial positions. After reviewing the scientific evidence, he is openly against circumcising male infants. He is outspoken in support of the government's controlling illegal drugs by making them legal, taxing them and then using the money to educate the public about the damage caused by addictions and drugs.

Dr. Adell's medical training left him without an understanding of nutrition and how foods cause degenerative or chronic ailments. He mistakenly tells people who call in concerned because their blood cholesterol is over 150 to stop worrying.

Dr. Adell promotes preventive care but keeps shooting himself in the foot by attacking Clinical Ecology. He does not realize that he is ridiculing a fundamental part of prevention. He is open to scientifically-proven approaches, so there is hope he will read the medical studies and attend medical conventions presented by the American Academy of Environmental Medicine. If he understood about delayed food allergies, he would change much of his advice.

Another very influential author was Paavo Airola. He was born in Finland and studied several different nutrition-based health approaches in Europe. He taught that eating differently from the traditional diet was essential for good health.

Airola explained the importance of eating a low protein diet. He taught that the diet should contain 10 percent protein. This was during the 1960's: the heyday for high fat, high protein, high cholesterol and low carbohydrate diets.

Airola had a large following and wrote several popular books. Unfortunately, it was not until shortly before he died that he discovered that delayed food allergies are a major cause of health problems. Airola had already written his books by the time he became aware of food allergies. Fortunately, he wrote about his new awareness of delayed food allergies in *Let's Live* magazine shortly before he died.

Many current readers of his books are not aware of the understanding he obtained shortly before he died, and they are still following the advice in his books. His books suggest repetitious eating of cereal grains, nuts, yeast and a number of other foods which cause food allergy reactions. Like many of the writers who followed after him, he did not know about the problems caused by vegetable oil and food allergies when he wrote his books.

It would be hard to find writers who have promoted more erroneous approaches than Dirk Pearson and Sandy Shaw. Their primary source of information is studies supporting the use of supplements to solve nearly every health problem. They believe that when you take hundreds of supplements you can eat whatever you want and be healthy.

The danger of this approach is obvious once you know the causes of the different ailments. Many people have been caught up by this magic-bullet approach. It is easy to like this approach because it is similar to the medical/drug/surgery approach to solving health problems while letting you hold on to your old damaging habits.

Pearson's and Shaw's full recommendations could create an annual bill for supplements exceeding $10,000 a year. They pride themselves on taking their different supplements and eating two or three desserts after their meals of high-fat, high-cholesterol, high-sugar and allergy-causing foods. They claim they have no health problems.

Pearson writes about his lifetime of health problems. Unknown to him, his type of symptoms are caused primarily by delayed food and chemical allergies. He claims that he is cured by taking his heavy load of supplements.

By taking large doses of different supplements, you can mask some of the symptoms of food allergies. However, the underlying damage goes on. His magic-bullet approach is unsound and causes health problems.

For over sixty years, there has been a health-promoting group living in this country most people have never heard about. They are called Natural Hygienists, and their approach is based on eating the foods that humans ate before 12,000 years ago. Thus, they eat no cereal grains or dairy products and eat mostly vegetables and large quantities of nuts and seeds. There are some people who are helped by this approach.

Natural Hygienists do not believe delayed

food allergies and food addictions exist. They try to ignore them and recommend people go on a forty-day fast; no food, only clean water. This is the hard way to avoid food allergies.

The Natural Hygienists often have trouble feeding people after the fast because they unknowingly give them foods they are allergic to. Some of these people become severely ill and a number have had to be rescued by food-allergy specialists.

Herbert Shelton was the driving force behind this movement and he helped people become aware of health problems caused by dairy products. However, without understanding delayed food allergies and the 10–10–80 balance, Natural Hygienists have trouble helping others or themselves.

One of the Natural Hygienists' theories was written in a pamphlet by Herbert Shelton called "Food Combining Made Easy." The pamphlet is full of ideas about which foods combine properly with other foods.

There is some value to this idea. When you eat fruit, eat it by itself. Thus, do not mix fruit with vegetables or meat. Most fruit is high in simple sugars that impair the digestion of other foods. The idea that you cannot eat vegetables and fish together is not supported by scientific studies. One can summarize the helpful ideas underlying food combining by saying, "Eat fruit by itself and never eat dairy products."

During the 1980's, Shelton's pamphlet was expanded into a book called *Fit For Life* by Harvey and Marilyn Diamond. The book sold well because it promotes another magic-bullet approach: eat foods in the "right" combination, and you can eat almost anything you want, and all your health problems will go away, and you will lose weight.

Diamond had no awareness of delayed food allergies when he wrote his book. Medical Service Center's staff tried to share the science of delayed food allergies and addictions with him in 1985. However, he rejected the possibility that he had missed a major element of healthy nutrition and did not enlarge his approach.

Diamond did not know about yeast infections caused by the yeast called Candida Albicans. He also did not know that eating fruit makes yeast infections worse and claimed that all-fruit meals were the best way to eat. High fruit diets are actually high sugar diets.

The book, *Fit or Fat,* by Covert Bailey, has helped many people improve their health because of well-written advice about using exercise to elevate your metabolism. He warns against fasting because he has seen many people have trouble achieving health after they have fasted.

Any book or person who recommends eating the same food day after day is making a fundamental mistake because repetitious consumption is one of the causes of delayed food allergies. Another way to become allergic to a food is to eat a food that is not natural for humans. That is why so many people are allergic to dairy products and cereal grains. These foods were not eaten until a few thousand years ago, and they do not work well for us now.

The Macrobiotic Diet Program has some positive aspects to it, such as not allowing any dairy products. However, it is fundamentally flawed. This approach grew out of a religious-like belief and is not based on science.

Macrobiotic theory states that everyone should eat brown rice at every meal. This leads to a diet which has more than 50 percent of its calories coming from brown rice. Rice is a cereal grain and thus not a natural food for humans. When one eats rice repetitiously, there is a high probability of becoming allergic to it.

The allergy-causing substances exist throughout the cereal grain; however, they are concentrated in the outer coating, called the bran. Eating a cereal grain with its bran coating increases the probability and severity of allergies.

The oil in brown rice becomes rancid within a week of its being hulled if the bran is cracked. Even when soft rubber wheels are used in hulling, around 10 percent of the brown rice is damaged and becomes rancid and health wrecking. The orientals have known what they were doing for the last few thousand years by removing the bran coating from their brown rice to make it into white rice. The lost nutrients and fiber from the bran are fully covered by eating fresh vegetables.

Many people who follow the Macrobiotic rules find their health slowly deteriorating. Because of very persuasive books promoting this diet and the addictive nature of rice, people have difficulty becoming free of Macrobiotics.

The original rules for beginning a Macrobiotic diet told the person to eat only brown rice for 10 days. This caused many people to become severely allergic and addicted to rice. Most people can fast on clean water for 10 days without obvious health problems. However, when people ate only brown rice for 10 days, many became sick and a few died. This brown-rice-only idea almost ended the Macrobiotics movement, and has been dropped.

Macrobiotics originally had another idea which had to be believed on faith. The founder said you should eat foods common to your part of the world. This implies the human body's nutritional requirements change around the world. There is no scientific evidence to support this myth.

When people eat local foods, they have health problems if those foods do not have the 10–10–80 balance of macronutrients. The original Eskimo diet had 25 percent fat, 40 percent protein, 35 percent carbohydrates and high cholesterol. By 45 years old their arteries were severely clogged, and their bones were demineralized. When Eskimos traveled, the middle-aged would break bones and thus could not keep up and had to be left behind to die. Therefore, there were almost no old Eskimos.

The Macrobiotic diet helps some people in the beginning because it allows no dairy products, is low in wheat, fat, cholesterol and protein and is high in complex carbohydrates. However, with a health profile and a delayed-allergy blood test for people who have been on the Macrobiotic diet for a few months, one often finds they are not very healthy and have become allergic to rice.

If you have been on Macrobiotics and have trouble believing this, try going off all rice and other cereal grains for seven days. Most people experience some withdrawal symptoms when they go off rice and then a clearing from their symptoms around day five. On day seven, have a breakfast of only brown rice. After re-exposure, most have a delayed allergic reaction to the rice and re-experience some of their symptoms. They will have discovered which of their health problems are caused by brown rice and how damaging delayed food allergies are. Macrobiotics and other diets high in cereal grains do not work in the long run.

Many current leaders of Macrobiotics have acknowledged the previous mistakes and are writing about how common delayed food allergies are.

There is a common, though mistaken, belief that people can tell what vitamins or minerals they are deficient in. However, if you are zinc deficient, for example, you will not automatically seek out foods high in zinc. If you find yourself craving a food, it is likely that you are addicted to it, not because you need it. When you have been tested to see what foods you are allergic to and then stay off them for a week, you break the addictive cycle. Then you can begin to tell what foods are good for you. Otherwise, your body tells you only what you crave and are addicted to, not what you need.

One of the first popular books on diet with a scientific foundation was *Live Longer Now* by Jon Leonard, J. L. Hofer and Nathan Pritikin. This 1974 book was not widely read and did not have a large impact; however, it clearly explains the value of the 10–10–80 balance of macronutrients.

When *Live Longer Now* was written, it was unpopular with many writers who had already written health or nutrition books, because their books were shown to have a major defect. This happened again in 1980 when Theron Randolph, MD, wrote *An Alternative Approach to Allergies*. Traditional allergists are still trying to suppress Dr. Randolph's research on delayed food and chemical allergies because his book explains why traditional allergists are, at best, ineffective, and, at worst, dangerous to the people who go to them.

Dr. Randolph and people using his scientifically verified approaches are not popular with traditional allergists because their scientific research makes traditional allergists look foolish. There have been a few valuable books written in the last few years which explain the importance of delayed food allergies. Unfortunately, none incorporated the importance of a low-fat, moderate-protein, high-complex-carbohydrate diet.

The reason why most people on typical delayed food allergy programs do not become significantly better is because they were not accurately tested for food allergies and they were eating too much fat and protein. Testing by fasting and then food-challenging usually makes people more reactive to foods. It also causes them to become allergic to additional foods because the challenge method of eating a meal of just one food overloads the body and increases the chances of becoming allergic to the food being tested.

When people eat foods and take supplements they are not allergic to and eat health building levels of fats, proteins and carbohydrates, they have a good chance of becoming free and staying free of symptoms and enjoying a long, healthy life.

Through the years, there has been a continual flood of books on how to lose weight. Most of them have been based on a faulty understanding of human nutrition and the inner workings of the body. These obsolete books are based on eating a high protein, high fat, low carbohydrate diet.

The protein we eat is broken down into amino acids. The by-product of this process is increased blood acids and several chemicals which damage our bodies. These chemicals are flushed out by water, through our kidneys. The acidity is buffered by exercise and minerals from the bones and tissues.

People on high protein diets believe they are losing fat, but they are primarily losing water and vital minerals. Thus, people lose weight rapidly, but also lose their health. They are also filling up their fat cells with fat from the diet. When they go back to their old eating habits, they gain the water back and find they are heavier than before.

The Stillman Diet, the Atkins Diet and many others are dangerously high in protein, cholesterol and fat, which cause degenerative diseases and lead to an early death.

Dr. Atkins has added a little carbohydrate to his original approach; however, it is very hard for some people to change their minds once they write a book. Atkins' dietary protein and fat recommendations remain dangerously high. However, he is to be acknowledged for helping his patients with delayed food allergies and for speaking out against the many errors of traditional medicine.

The original approach for treating hypoglycemia, or low blood sugar, was a high-fat, high-protein diet. People where supposed to eat six times a day. Dr. John Tintera put this diet together and led the hypoglycemia movement until his unfortunate death from a massive heart attack. He followed his own nutritional advice and died young at 59. Modern diet recommendations for hypoglycemia include the 10–10–80 balance of macronutrients and avoiding delayed food allergies which upset blood sugar levels.

The health supporting diet for hypoglycemia is free of the foods you are allergic to so that you do not upset your blood sugar and blood insulin levels. The diet should also be high in complex carbohydrates so your blood sugar levels do not drop. You then have energy slowly entering your system throughout the day as the complex carbohydrates are gradually broken down by your digestive tract.

Once you understand how your body works, you see that there is not one type of diet for one disease and another diet for a different disease. The best diet for all diseases is the one that is free of foods and chemicals you are allergic to, and free of excess fat, protein, sugar and cholesterol.

One of the pioneers in nutrition was Max Gerson, MD. He put together a diet which required people to drink vegetable juices and avoid a number of foods in the hope of curing cancer. It is interesting that many people became free of their cancer following the Gerson Program. If you study his program, it is not hard to see why. His original diet was totally free of dairy products and consisted almost entirely of vegetables. The diet is quite close to the 10–10–80 balance of macronutrients. He is to be credited for helping many people and for increasing the awareness that diet is a major part of any cancer cure.

A damaging approach to diet and health came about from a misunderstanding involving the thyroid gland. The thyroid gland is upset by allergic reactions to foods, becoming stimulated or depressed, causing hyperactivity in some people and chronic fatigue in others.

Unfortunately, Dr. Broda Barnes decided that health problems were caused by some type of defect with nearly everyone's thyroid gland and that most people needed to take thyroid medication. It is hard to believe today, but he believed you could take thyroid gland extract and then eat a high fat, high-protein, high-cholesterol diet and not have to worry about heart disease, cancer or most other ailments.

When I debated Dr. Barnes on a radio talk show, I pointed out that there is no group of people anywhere in the world who eat the high-fat, high-protein diet he suggests and avoid severe heart disease. He avoided my statement. I then pointed out that when people with abnormally high thyroid levels eat the foods he recommended they still died of heart disease, cancer or other degenerative disease. He replied by saying something humorous.

Dr. Barnes was very charismatic, with a quick wit, and many people to this day still believe what he wrote and thus take thyroid drugs and continue to clog their arteries with each high-fat meal. Thyroid medication works as a stimulant, similar to caffeine, and thus covers up many serious health problems.

When Dr. Barnes' wife came down with cancer, he had her go on a low-fat, low-protein and high-complex-carbohydrate diet (the Gerson Program). It was too late — she died from cancer of the pancreas. He also suffered from his own advice: he became senile and died from a stroke.

Through the years a few people have promoted the idea that people with different "body types" should eat different foods. All "body types" who do not use the 10–10–80 balance develop clogged arteries and people who eat foods which kill their white blood cells develop chronic ailments.

There is no medication, no pill, no herb, no stress-relieving approach, no homeopathic technique, no vitamin, no supplement of any type, that can undo the damage caused by eating damaging foods. It would be like putting dirty water into your car's gas tank and thinking you could then add a fuel additive to make it run fine.

The misinformation goes on and on because people are still looking for a magic health bullet or pill. They want to keep eating the foods they love, not realizing that often the love is actually a physical addiction, caused by a delayed allergic reaction.

An important contribution to health has been made by Roy Walford, MD. He has written two books which explain the importance of eating fewer calories: *Maximum Life Span* and *The 120-Year Diet*. The scientific studies presented demonstrate the importance of eating fewer calories. Dr. Walford recommends 1500 calories a day or less depending on size and activity rather than the Standard American Diet of 2400 calories or more.

Dr. Walford does acknowledge the value of Nathan Pritikin's work and feels the 10–10–80 balance of macronutrients is a good way to eat fewer calories. Unfortunately, he did not understand the science underlying the balance and makes dangerous recommendations for fat levels of not more than 20 percent and protein levels of 24 percent of calories. His cholesterol recommendations are the traditional deadly 300 milligrams per day instead of 80 milligrams per day.

I shared information about delayed food allergies with Dr. Walford in 1982. He could not imagine that he had missed such a major part of the health picture and rejected the existence of delayed food allergies.

Eating fewer calories adds to longevity and helps people who want to lose weight. This is another reason to avoid fat and stay free of foods that cause over-eating because of food addiction.

Several authors have written popular books that have been very influential, only later to discover they missed the important awareness of delayed food allergies. This happened to Jane Brody, who wrote one of the best-selling diet books of the 1980's called *Jane Brody's Nutrition Book*. After millions of her books had been sold, she discovered the importance of delayed food allergies. In July, 1990, she wrote a good article in *The Saturday Evening Post* titled "Food Sensitivity: The Mystery Ailment." Unfortunately, her new awareness of delayed food allergies was not in her earlier books.

There have been several extensive studies done by the traditional medical establishment in conjunction with the government to determine whether their diet recommendations of 30–15–55, with up to 300 milligrams of cholesterol a day, have helped people to live longer. One, called "Mr. FITS," lasted several years, involved thousands of people and cost over $100 million of your tax money.

All of the studies confirm that the standard diet recommendations are of no help in extending life expectancy. This is true because the diet recommendations of the American Heart Association, the American Cancer Society and the federal government are close to the Standard American Diet, with its excessive fat, protein and cholesterol. They also have no testing program or counseling for people with delayed food allergies.

With all the scientific evidence available since 1974 supporting the 10–10–80 balance of macronutrients, you would think that most professional writers would be up to speed. Not so. A book from Harvard Medical School was published 12 years after Nathan Pritikin's first book and is titled, *Your Good Health*. The book is written by three doctors: Bennett, Goldfinger and Johnson. The writers demonstrated no understanding of the importance of consuming under 80 milligrams of cholesterol a day. This level is adequately below your saturation level of 200 milligrams. These doctors say, "The amount of cholesterol in the diet has a relatively small effect on the levels of cholesterol in the blood. Eggs are the only significant direct source of cholesterol in the American diet."

They also give advice about cholesterol in the blood, "...a level of 200 mg/dl is about as high as anyone would want." The scientific studies showing the danger of these recommendations are explained on pages 48, 55, 56 and 57. The charts on pages 60 and 61 show that you want your blood cholesterol level to stay under 150 mg/dl.

These Harvard doctors recommend lowering your cholesterol "by reducing dietary fat to around 30% of calories." Several medical studies have shown that this is not low enough to make a difference. However, eating 30 percent of your calories in fat is a major cause of cancer. See pages 58 and 59.

The writers of this health-damaging book are very influential and powerful. William Bennett, MD, is the editor of the *Harvard Medical School Health Letter*. Stephen Goldfinger, MD, is Associate Dean of Continuing Medical Education at Harvard. Timothy Johnson, MD, is Medical Editor for the American Broadcasting Corporation. All three are also professors of medicine at Harvard Medical School. Have sympathy for their students and the people the students will eventually try to help.

You can see how much trouble we are in: this dangerous advice is coming from one of America's leading medical schools. This is not a new problem for Harvard. Its department of nutrition is highly subsidized by food producers, and they influence what is taught. The previous head of the department, Jean Mayer, MD, claimed that all carbohydrates are the same in the way they affect the body — if this were true it would mean eating carrots is the same as eating white sugar.

The type of thinking that causes a problem is not the type of thinking that will solve the problem.

Albert Einstein
Physicist — 1879 to 1955

When Harvard Medical School professors do not understand the fundamentals of treating and avoiding degenerative diseases, you can be sure traditional doctors do not understand the more technically-complex field of delayed food and chemical allergies. Do not trust a traditional doctor when you need to become free of food-caused diseases.

There have been a number of very successful books based on the 10–10–80 balance of macronutrients. After Jon Leonard's and Nathan Pritikin's first book, *Live Longer Now,* they individually wrote several follow-up books. Then came the books by Julian Whitaker, MD, *Reversing Heart Disease* and *Reversing Diabetes*; Robert Haas's book, *Eat to Succeed*; and the books by John McDougall, MD, including *The McDougall Plan for Super Health and Life-Long Weight Loss.*

Unfortunately, these books missed the importance of delayed food and chemical allergies. They cause health problems because they claim that high cereal grain diets support health. Most also claim non-fat dairy products are safe to eat.

Because none of these books explains the importance of delayed food allergies, people have trouble staying on their 10–10–80 diets. They are allergic and addicted to some of the foods and this makes their chronic ailments worse. It makes no sense to avoid damaging foods which cause degenerative ailments while eating allergy-causing foods which cause severe chronic ailments.

I was doing consulting work during the late 1970's for Nathan Pritikin. A call came into his center from a friend of the tennis champion, Arthur Ashe. Ashe started having pain in his chest when he exercised. His doctors were recommending coronary by-pass surgery, and his friend was looking for a better approach. Nathan explained that several people who had gone through his program had originally been scheduled for by-pass surgery but after going on his program they no longer needed surgery and were symptom-free.

Arthur Ashe's friend asked how long Ashe would need to stay on The Pritikin Program. Pritikin answered, "as long as he wants to stay free of his symptoms." Unfortunately, the friend was looking for a magic bullet which would allow Ashe to go back to his old eating habits.

The rest is history. Ashe had coronary by-pass surgery and was so weakened he had to quit professional tennis. After a couple of years of being on the American Heart Association's diet, his heart was in trouble again. This is a common problem. He decided to have the surgery again. Ashe announced in 1992 that he had contracted AIDS from an HIV-infected blood transfusion during his second surgery in 1983. Ironically, had Ashe received good advice and properly changed his diet, the diet would have helped him improve his tennis and he would not have died from AIDS.

Coronary bypass surgery is very dangerous, even if one decides in advance not to allow the doctors to use a blood transfusion. The body is permanently weakened from the surgery. To keep the altered heart circulation from quickly clogging up after the surgery, one must go on a diet based on the 10–10–80 balance of macronutrients — the same balance of macronutrients that would have avoided the surgery in the first place.

Some of the books from the past explain an important piece of the health puzzle while missing other important pieces. Dr. Randolph was not aware of the importance of the 10–10–80 balance of macronutrients and the value of vitamin and mineral supplements when he wrote his books and articles.

Nathan Pritikin knew that traditional medicine and the government were wrong regarding their fat and cholesterol recommendations. Unfortunately, he trusted their vitamin and mineral recommendations. However, he knew people had delayed food allergies and when he was getting started he sent some of his clients to St. Louis for cytotoxic testing when they were having trouble on his program.

I put together a conference in 1978 for Nathan Pritikin and Dr. Randolph with about 40 other doctors who understood the value of helping people by removing their delayed food and chemical allergies. The meeting was at the Pritikin Center in Santa Barbara. I hoped they would understand the value of each others' discoveries. However, neither Pritikin nor Randolph broadened their programs.

Kenneth Cooper, MD, knew that traditional medical recommendations for exercise were wrong when he started the aerobics movement, but he continued to trust the traditional diet recommendations of up to 30 percent fat and 300 milligrams of cholesterol a day. There is deadly difference between 30–12–58 and the 10–10–80 balance of macronutrients. Also, Cooper does not understand the importance of food and chemical allergies.

Conclusion

The recommendations of the traditional medical/drug/government complex are incorrect regarding preventive care. This is also true for many of their ways of treating disease.

One reason some traditional allergists are not treating people properly is money. When you have an appointment with a traditional allergist, you are often asked questions for ten minutes and then you are given a prescription for a drug and a bill averaging $70. You are told to come back for skin testing and then allergy injections. The staff takes care of these procedures, leaving the doctor time to enroll more patients and run a production line operation.

When you go to a doctor practicing preventive care, you give an extensive history to a person who knows what questions to ask. You are then tested to find out what is happening inside your body and what foods are compatible for you. After your results are ready, you receive in-depth counseling on how to avoid the causes of ailments. This takes hours of the doctor's and his staff's time.

The initial cost is sometimes higher with the preventive care approach. However, you do not have to keep going back to the doctor, and you spend much less money on health care from then on. Traditional doctors and drug companies need to keep you coming back regularly to keep their incomes high and stay in control of how health care is practiced.

The solution to the health care crisis is to deregulate health care so that preventive-care specialists can compete with traditional doctors and the drug industry.

The approach which works is to avoid foods to which you are allergic and to avoid foods which cause degenerative disease. When correct supplements along with aerobic and strength exercise are added, there is the opportunity for great health.

In 1980, these scientifically valid principles came together for the first time in *Quality Longevity*. Some food-allergy specialists hesitate to use part of the Quality Longevity Program because they do not want to avoid high-fat, high-protein, high-cholesterol foods in addition to allergy-causing foods.

Degenerative disease specialists recommend the 10–10–80 balance but some have trouble appreciating the Quality Longevity Program because they do not want to give up the low-fat foods that often cause allergy problems. However, the awareness continues to grow. More people are eating foods they are not allergic to, along with eating the health building balance of fats, proteins and carbohydrates. These people are enjoying the best of both worlds.

It is important to make changes as soon as new approaches are shown to be correct. Do not wait until the current authorities change their minds or you will spend years suffering and lose many enjoyable years of your life. There are no negative side-effects caused by using The Quality Longevity Program. The evidence shows you will have significantly improved health, spend far less on medical care and have many joy-filled years.

Wisdom is knowing what to do.
Knowledge is knowing how to do it.
Success is doing it.

Chapter 13

Helpful Information and Sample Forms

The information in this chapter will give you added insights
and help you integrate the new information you have gained.

*Let nothing that can be treated by diet
be treated by any other means.*

Maimonides
Hebrew Physician to the Egyptian Royal Family — 1135 to 1204 AD

Components of Nutrition

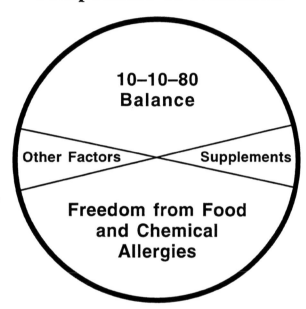

Components of Health

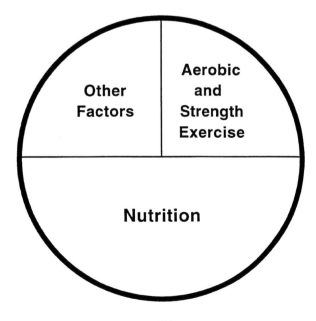

Types of Major Ailments and Optimum Health Approaches

Surgery	**Drugs**	**Allergy Free Life-style**	**10–10–80 Balance**
is needed for repairing some	are needed to be free of some	is needed to be free of and treat	is needed to be free of and treat
Injuries	**Infectious Diseases**	**Chronic Diseases**	**Degenerative Diseases**

There are insurmountable differences in the way injuries and infections should be treated compared to chronic and degenerative diseases. Chronic and degenerative diseases should be treated by using preventive care. The traditional medical establishment still relies on drugs and surgery for all four types of ailments, and thus the low level of people's health continues to decline.

The best way to solve the problem of accidental injuries is to avoid the accident. However, if one does happen, modern medicine has developed surgical procedures which can accomplish dramatic results.

The major improvements in fighting ailments caused by infection have come about by removing the causes through improved sanitation over the last 100 years. However, if an infectious disease does develop, the proper drug for a tested and verified infection can be a life-saver.

Modern medicine continues to have failures when it uses surgery and drugs to remove the symptoms of chronic diseases. When the delayed allergies that are causing the symptoms are removed, the symptoms go away. When surgery is used, vital organs are often damaged or lost. When drugs are used, patients often develop damaging reactions and addictions to the drugs. Surgery, drugs and allergy injections leave the patient weaker and delay healing.

Modern medicine is also having a high failure rate by using expensive surgery and powerful drugs on degenerative diseases. No amount or type of medicine will ever be able to overcome the effects of eating meals with excessive fat, protein, sugar and cholesterol.

We can avoid cell-killing allergic reactions by being tested and then eating foods compatible with our unique bodies. We can avoid lipotoxic or fat-poisoning reactions by using the 10–10–80 balance of macronutrients, thus avoiding foods which are damaging to everyone.

In summery, we can be free of accidental injuries by being careful at home, at work and by driving carefully while wearing our seat belts. We can be free of infection by avoiding germs and keeping our immune systems strong. We can become free of both chronic and degenerative diseases by eating compatible foods.

...if you know how to look and learn, then the door is there and the key is in your hand.

Krishnamurti
Teacher, Philosopher and Author — 1895 to 1986

Testing Menu

Name _____   Date _____

After finishing day 4, return to day 1. Use organically grown foods whenever possible. Weights are for foods as purchased.

Day	Snack	Breakfast	Snack	Lunch	Snack	Dinner
1 and 5						
2 and 6						
3 and 7						
4 and 8						

Personalized Supplements

Day 1 _____

2 _____

3 _____

4 _____

Emotional Symptoms Caused by Delayed Food and Chemical Allergies

The following information covers a broad range of emotional or mental symptoms caused by delayed food and chemical allergies. This understanding was begun by Theron Randolph, MD, after 30 years of research and clinical experience. The accuracy and value of this approach for helping patients has been confirmed by doctors and scientists from around the world. When used by psychiatrists, their approach changes from using drugs, surgery and talk therapy to removing the cause of upset brain chemistry, and then counseling which includes the awareness of delayed allergic reactions.

When doctors do not understand that delayed allergic reactions cause physical and mental symptoms, they claim the physical symptoms are caused by mental problems. Understanding that delayed allergic reactions cause both enables people to get well.

The following is from a 13-page medical paper by Theron G. Randolph, MD, titled "Specific Adaptation" published in the *Annals of Allergy*, Volume 40, May 1978.

Directions: start at zero (0) and read up for stimulated reactions and read down for depressed reactions.

Plus 4	Manic with or without convulsions	Distraught, excited, agitated, enraged and panicky. Circuitous or one-track thoughts, muscle twitching and jerking of extremities, convulsive seizures and altered consciousness may develop.
Plus 3	Hypomanic, Toxic, Anxious and Egocentric	Aggressive, loquacious, clumsy (ataxic), anxious, fearful and apprehensive; alternating chills and flushing, ravenous hunger, excessive thirst. Giggling or pathological laughter may occur.
Plus 2	Hyperactive, Irritable, Hungry and Thirsty	Tense, jittery, hopped-up, talkative, argumentative, sensitive, overly responsive, self-centered, hungry and thirsty; flushing, sweating and chilling may occur as well as insomnia, alcoholism and obesity.
Plus 1	Stimulated but relatively symptom-free	Active, alert, lively, responsive and enthusiastic with unimpaired ambition, energy, initiative and wit. Considerate of the views and actions of others. This usually comes to be regarded as "normal" behavior.
Even 0	Behavior on an even keel as in homeostasis	Children expect this from their parents and teachers. Parents expect this from their children. We all expect this from our associates. [When people do not get what they expect they often blame the person by mistake.]
Minus 1	Localized allergic manifestations	Running or stuffy nose, clearing throat, coughing, wheezing (asthma), itching (eczema and hives), gas, diarrhea, constipation (colitis), urgency and frequency of urination and various eye and ear syndromes.
Minus 2	Systemic allergic manifestations	Tired, dopey, somnolent, mildly depressed, edematous with painful syndromes (headache, neckache, backache, neuralgia, myalgia, myositis, arthralgia, arthritis, arteritis, chest pain) and cardiovascular effects.*
Minus 3	Brain-fag, mild Depression and Disturbed thinking	Confused, indecisive, moody, sad, sullen, withdrawn or apathetic. Emotional instability and impaired attention, concentration, comprehension and thought processes (aphasia, mental lapse and blackouts).
Minus 4	Severe Depression with or without Altered Consciousness	Nonresponsive, lethargic, stuporous, disoriented, melancholic, incontinent, regressive thinking, paranoid orientation, delusions, hallucinations, sometimes amnesia and coma.

* Cardiovascular manifestations, including rapid or irregular pulse, hypertension, phlebitis, anemia and bruising tendencies may occur at any level. See the diagram at the top of the next page. It shows how the above reactions often run their course.

How Reactions Are Often Experienced

Symptoms cover the full range of severity and time. Some show up clearly during a meal, others cause mild stimulation during the meal and leave a person needing a nap an hour later. Sometimes the stimulation lasts for a day or two, then leads to a week of dullness and three weeks of fuzzy thinking.

Being stimulated may reach any level, plus 1 through plus 4, before merging with a similar withdrawal stage. Start at 0 and go clockwise. Reactions can follow the curves clockwise or they can go counterclockwise, starting depressed and becoming stimulated. Republished by permission of Theron G. Randolph, MD.

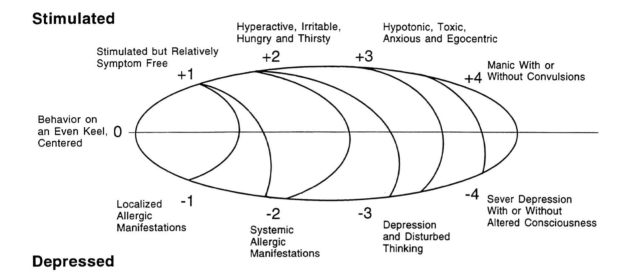

Stimulated

Stimulated but Relatively Symptom Free

Behavior on an Even Keel, Centered

Hyperactive, Irritable, Hungry and Thirsty

Hypotonic, Toxic, Anxious and Egocentric

Manic With or Without Convulsions

Localized Allergic Manifestations

Systemic Allergic Manifestations

Depression and Disturbed Thinking

Sever Depression With or Without Altered Consciousness

Depressed

Example of Food Challenge Testing

Repeat once for a total of eight days.
Use organically grown foods when possible.

Name _John Adams_   **Date** _4/10/85_

Day	Breakfast	Snack	Lunch	Snack	Dinner
1 and 5	potato - 16 oz	pear - 1 or 2	carrots - 14 oz	cabbage - 6 oz	zucchini squash - 16 oz
2 and 6	broccoli - 18 oz	papaya - 1	string beans - 14 oz	celery - 6 oz	butternut squash - 20 oz
3 and 7	tomato - 18 oz	orange - 1 or 2	lentil - 4 oz (dry weight)	cucumber - 6 oz	halibut - 4 oz
4 and 8	yellow necked squash - 20 oz	blueberries - 4 oz	peas - 18 oz	parsnips - 6 oz	cauliflower - 18 oz
		(fresh or frozen)			

Food Testing Log

NAME: DAY: DATE: /   /   PAGE:

Rate symptoms: 1 - slight	2 - mild	3 - moderate	4 - severe.		
Other	Other	Pulse	Time	**MEAL**	**Change**
					+
				Start	−
				Finish	
				20 after	
				40 after	
				60 after	
				80 after	
				MEAL	**Change**
					+
				Start	−
				Finish	
				20 after	
				40 after	
				60 after	
				80 after	
				MEAL	**Change**
					+
				Start	−
				Finish	
				20 after	
				40 after	
				60 after	
				80 after	

Example of a Food Testing Log

NAME: *John Adams*   DAY: *Monday*   DATE: *8/24/80*   PAGE: *4*

Other	Other	Pulse	Time	MEAL	*string bean - 20 oz.*		Change
							+ 6
		64	7:10 am	Start	*Feeling fine, slept well, no ear ringing, hungry*		−
		68	7:40	Finish	*Fine, no change*		
		70	8:00	20 after	*same*		
		68	8:20	40 after	*same*		
		66	8:40	60 after	*Fine — have energy — may have cleared, will retest in 5 days*		
				MEAL	*corn - 4 oz. corn meal*		Change
							+ 20
		68	12:00	Start	*Feeling fine — hungry*		−
		74	12:30	Finish	*Feel OK, slightly stimulated*		
		79	12:50	20 after	*Restless, full but want more to eat "hungry," right ear ringing-2*		
		88	1:10	40 after	*Angry — hands and feet cold, headache-3*		
		86	1:30	60 after	*Tired*		
		84	1:50	80 after	*Took a nap, still don't feel good, did not clear on corn*		
				MEAL	*cod-4 oz., poached in water (spring)*		Change
							+
		74	8:00 pm	Start	*Fair, not hungry, right ear ringing still-2, headache-1*		− 16
		76	8:20	Finish	*Same*		
		68	8:40	20 after	*Same*		
		60	9:00	40 after	*Joints ache — may be delayed reaction from corn or a reaction from cod, will retest in 1 week*		
		58	9:20	60 after	*Tired — ear ring 2, headache 1*		

Rate symptoms: 1 - slight   2 - mild   3 - moderate   4 - severe.

The above Challenge Testing technique is helpful for double checking the foods your Prime Test reported as compatible, or for follow-up testing. If you did not react to a food you have avoided for a significant length of time, the Prime Test will show that food to be non-reactive if it is not a fixed reactor. However, you may start reacting to the food after eating it again. This may happen at the first or second, or at some later meal.

Be sure to check each food carefully so none gets back into your diet and causes problems.

You can also test foods not on your Prime Test by using the above Challenge Test. Challange Testing works only moderately well if you are free of symptoms and have been eating your compatable foods.

This type of Challenge Test was used in the past after a five-day to ten-day fast on just water and in a specially cleaned environment. It required medical supervision and took a month to test for 70 foods. There were health problems created by this fasting and challange approach and it cost over $15,000.

People must avoid all their food and chemical allergies for about a week before the Challenge Test will work with any reliability to discover allergies. This is why traditional allergists are not able to test successfully by telling suffering patients to try eating a food and then seeing how they feel.

Comparing Natural Foods for Humans with the American and Other Diets

Natural Foods for Humans	Ounces	Calories	Fat %	Protein %	Protein Grams	Carbohydrate %	Cholesterol Milligrams	Vitamin C Milligrams	Calcium Milligrams	Iron Milligrams	Magnesium Milligrams	Zinc Milligrams
Carrots	35	404	4	7	11	89	0	80	370	7	189	1.3
Beets	35	302	3	9	11	88	0	100	160	7	123	3.0
Broccoli	17	168	7	28	15	65	0	550	500	5	90	1.1
Trout	2	55	19	81	12	0	40	0	9	1	16	.4
Squash	35	160	4	13	10	83	0	220	280	4	122	2.0
Apples	17	290	9	1	1	90	0	20	35	1	35	.1
Peas in pod	17	278	5	16	17	79	0	135	130	10	62	11.0
One Day Total	158	1657	6%	13%	77gr	81%	40 mg	1105 mg	1496 mg	34 mg	644 mg	18.8 mg
Standard American Diet		3300	36%	12%	99gr	52%	500	20 to 300	500 to 3000	8 to 20	100 to 400	2 to 10
Traditional Medicine and Government Recommendations			Up to 30%	12%	37gr	58%	Up to 300	60	800 to 1500	10 to 18	350	15
Pritikin, McDougall, Ornish			5 to 10%	10%	37gr	80%	0 to 80	60 to 90	300 to 1000	10 to 60	350	15
Whitaker, Lovendale			5 to 10%	10%	37gr	80%	0 to 80	2000 to 8000	300 to 800	10 to 50	600 to 1600	15 to 40

The above food values are from the United States Department of Agriculture Handbook No 8. Recommendations are for moderately active 150 pound males. Calculations are made with actual values for converting grams to calories, not approximations. Rev. I/95

This chart helps explain the 10–10–80 principle and enables people to stop worrying about weather they are eating enough protein.

Human beings evolved on a diet which averaged more than 1000 milligrams of vitamin C a day. When we eat foods which have no vitamin C, such as cereal grains and dried beans, we are likely to end up consuming far less than 1000 milligrams a day. In addition, allergies increase our need for vitamin C. Therefore, it is helpful to take additional vitamin C each morning before breakfast and again before dinner. Find a type compatible with your body.

Ester-C works well for most people. We receive all the calcium we need from foods as grown, and thus there is no nutritional need for dairy products.

It is possible to have a deficiency of some minerals because allergic exposures cause an acid increase in the body which is neutralized by drawing important minerals out of our bones and organs. Moderate to high-protein diets also cause an acid increase and mineral loss. If you have been having allergic reactions or have been eating the typical amount of protein, you will need to replenish your minerals.

Mineral supplements should be based on your body's unique requirements. Changing the body's mineral levels takes time. When you take vitamins or minerals, be sure they are free of binders or fillers.

Eating fewer calories has been shown to reduce ailments and extend life expectancy in animal studies. Therefore, depending on your height and activity levels, you can be healthy eating between 1200 and 2800 calories a day. All the evidence indicates you will feel better and live longer. There are special supplements and digestive aids your counselor can help you with.

White Blood Cell Testing and Counseling for Delayed Food and Chemical Allergies: A Follow-up Study

Jeffrey R. Prager, D.D.S.

Background

I went through Medical Service Center's food-allergy testing and counseling program and experienced a marked improvement in my health. I offered to conduct a study to see what percentage of its clients had benefited from its type of white blood cell test and specialized counseling. The results cover the highlights of a follow-up study conducted from the first of January through March, 1985.

Results

I interviewed 47 of its clients. Of these, 96 percent reported their health was improved. The distribution was: 71 percent reported their health was significantly improved, 25 percent reported their health was slightly improved and 4 percent reported no change.

The following common symptoms were relieved by the testing and counseling program:

fatigue	sinus problems
overweight	mucus problems
headaches	abdominal distress
joint pain	insomnia
muscle pain	moodiness
skin problems	anxiety
scalp disorders	depression

Additional benefits that were reported by some individuals in the study:

increased ability to concentrate
increased desire to exercise
decreased asthma severity

Conclusion

This program is a non-damaging approach for identifying delayed food and chemical allergies and for removing the underlying cause of numerous health problems. Those who carefully followed the program experienced the best results. The success reports from the clients were impressive. None of the clients reported negative side effects. Only 4 percent reported no change. With 96 percent of the people experiencing health improvements, there is clear evidence the white-blood-cell testing and counseling program is effective.

More than 90 percent of the clients interviewed were satisfied with the program and enjoyed sharing their new understanding of health with their friends. This study demonstrates that white-blood-cell testing and specialized counseling programs could dramatically improve the health of people throughout the country.

The above study was followed by a larger one done by Medical Service Center's staff. The second survey showed a success rate of 91 percent. Several additional physical and emotional symptoms were relieved. Some symptoms were completely relieved and others were reduced to minimal levels.

Over a six-year period, more than 8000 people were tested and counseled by Medical Service Center. The overwhelming majority was helped and no one was harmed. Many people reported that their medical bills were dramatically reduced after they started The Quality Longevity Program.

Traditional allergists claim delayed food allergies do not exist and try to restrict the availability of white blood cell testing and the related counseling.

How to Prepare for Your Prime Test

48 HOURS PRIOR TO HAVING YOUR BLOOD DRAWN

1. Avoid cortisone, hydrocortisone, cortisone type medications, cortisone derivatives and steroid medications of all types for at least 48 hours before your blood is drawn. This includes skin creams that contain any cortisone such as Cortaid and Hytone. Avoid nose sprays with cortisone such as Vancenase. If possible, avoid cortisone and steroid type medications for a week prior to your test. These medications reduce allergic reactions temporarily; however, they often cause the allergic reactions to become worse in the future. These drugs weaken the white blood cells and make it difficult to perform the Prime Test. Let the doctor's office know the last time you had a cortisone or steroid exposure so, if necessary, the laboratory technician can reduce the problem while performing your test.

2. It is also important to avoid anti-histamines and decongestants for 48 hours before your test. These include decongestants like Neo-Synephrine and the bronchodilator, Alupent. If you think you may have some problem avoiding your medications for 48 hours or more, talk with the doctor for special instructions.

3. Continue to eat the foods you have been eating, unless advised differently.

10 TO 16 HOURS PRIOR TO HAVING YOUR BLOOD DRAWN

1. Do not consume any food or liquid other than high quality bottled or filtered water. Avoid water from opaque or translucent (foggy) plastic bottles. Clear plastic bottles are acceptable and glass ones are better. Filtered water must go through a reverse osmosis filter and an activated charcoal filter to be acceptable.

2. Avoid all drugs and medications unless your doctor advises you differently. Be sure to discuss your medications with the doctor.

3. Avoid cigarette smoke, colognes and perfumes. Avoid other chemicals as best you can.

THE MORNING OF YOUR TEST

1. Do not brush your teeth. Most tooth brushes have tooth paste in them and most tooth pastes are full of chemicals.

2. Avoid lipstick and all cosmetics, most have several chemicals in them.

3. Do not exercise.

4. Drink eight ounces of quality bottled or filtered water during the morning before you give your blood sample.

5. Do not smoke.

6. If you come down with a cold or flu before your test date, it is best to reschedule your test.

7. Remember to keep your arm straight for five minutes after you have had your blood drawn to reduce the chance of bruising. In other words, do not bend your arm over the cotton.

IMPORTANT INFORMATION

1. Read at least the first five chapters of the book *Quality Longevity* carefully so you will be ready for your counseling and benefit fully from the information. Your health will improve faster if you finish the book as soon as you can.

2. Payment is due at the time your blood sample is given.

Petition for Change

The petition on page 149 can help politicians in state and federal governments to make the necessary changes in health care. Make copies and sign one and have those who feel as you do join with you. Send additional copies to your aware friends to sign and have signed by their friends to help create the necessary changes.

Send signed copies to representatives and key people in government. Also send copies for follow up to the Quality Longevity Research Institute at 34146 Selva Road, Suite 200, Monarch Beach, California, 92629.

Petition to the President, the United States Congress and State and Local Governments

The signers of this petition believe that dramatically improved health and longevity are now possible at significantly reduced cost for all Americans by rapidly making major improvements in the health care system.

Much of the current discussion on health care is focused on containing the cost of treating people after they become ill. However, the most effective way to reduce cost is to reduce illness by using preventive care. We believe that by emphasizing prevention rather than treatment of illness, we can achieve a much healthier population at a cost far below the current level.

A drastic reduction in illness will occur when people take an active role in maintaining and improving their own health. To do this, they need the latest, most useful, scientifically valid information. The government's role should be to educate every American by disseminating preventive care information through all the media.

We advocate the following government actions:

1. Promote the free flow of information about preventive care, with special emphasis on exercise and nutrition, including the role of delayed food allergies. The government needs to educate the public about industry groups that promote health damaging foods, pesticides, chemicals, prescription drugs and unnecessary medical procedures. This approach is being used with tobacco and alcohol and should be extended to other health-wrecking items.

2. Establish national goals for health and medical care. These would include a dramatic reduction in coronary bypass surgeries and other operations for heart disease that can now be treated by diet. Reduce the incidence of breast, prostate and colon cancer by an education program that shows the cause-and-effect relationship between diet and these cancers. Also included would be an education program to inform the public about the many common ailments caused by delayed food and chemical allergies.

3. Design financial incentives to encourage people to improve their own health.

4. Stop the government-supported monopoly in health care by allowing people the freedom to select the approach that works for them.

With the current medical approach, the cost of extending health care to everyone in our country will be overwhelming. There is now an opportunity to cover this added cost and have money left over by shifting the emphasis to preventive care.

The rapid implementation of these principles will stop the massive escalation of health care costs. The principles will result in a happier, more productive people who are responsible for their health and know how to achieve and maintain it.

Name Printed	Address	Phone Number
Name Signed		( )
Name Printed	Address	Phone Number
Name Signed		( )
Name Printed	Address	Phone Number
Name Signed		( )
Name Printed	Address	Phone Number
Name Signed		( )
Name Printed	Address	Phone Number
Name Signed		( )
Name Printed	Address	Phone Number
Name Signed		( )

Send signed copies to the Quality Longevity Research Institute at 34146 Selva Road, Suite 200, Monarch Beach, California, 92629. They will be delivered to the President, with copies going to the United States Congress and state and local governments.

The Results of Removing Delayed Food Allergies

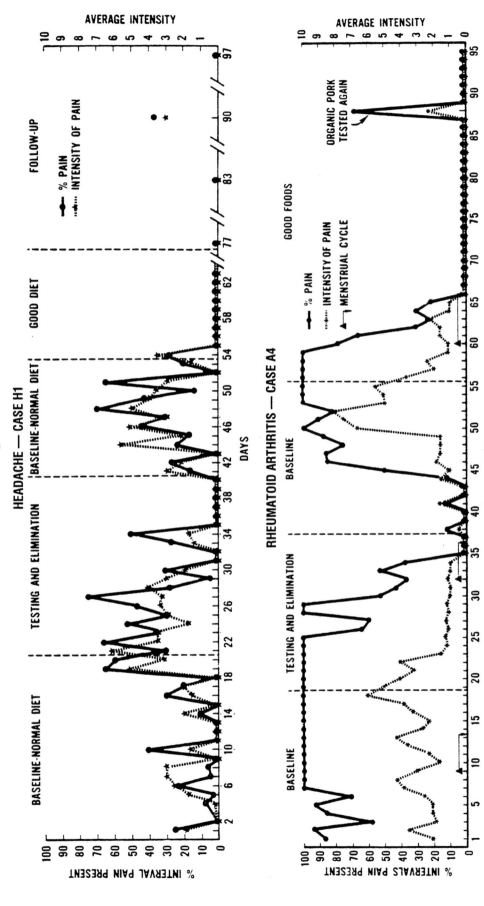

The above charts are from a controlled study on delayed food allergies. The type of testing used was trial-and-error. The people were fed one food at a time, for a total of three foods per day for several weeks. The "good diet" consisted of foods which did not cause symptoms, without regard to fat, protein or carbohydrate content.

After the people discovered and avoided the foods which caused their delayed food allergy

reactions, their symptoms went away. The symptoms came back when the damaging foods were eaten again. No other approach can turn symptoms on and off as shown, because no other approach removes the cause.

The above individuals became free of headaches and rheumatoid arthritis by avoiding delayed allergic reactions. This is impossible according to traditional medicine, even though it has no idea what the underlying cause of these

ailments is. Traditional treatments are addicting, health damaging drugs or damaging surgeries.

Other ailments which were part of this study were insomnia, depression, compulsive eating, obesity and diminished mental acuity. Symptoms were significantly reduced or eliminated.

These studies were completed in 1982 by Dan R. O'Banion, PhD and presented at that year's annual meeting of the American Academy of Environmental Medicine.

Typical Cycles of Chronic Ailments

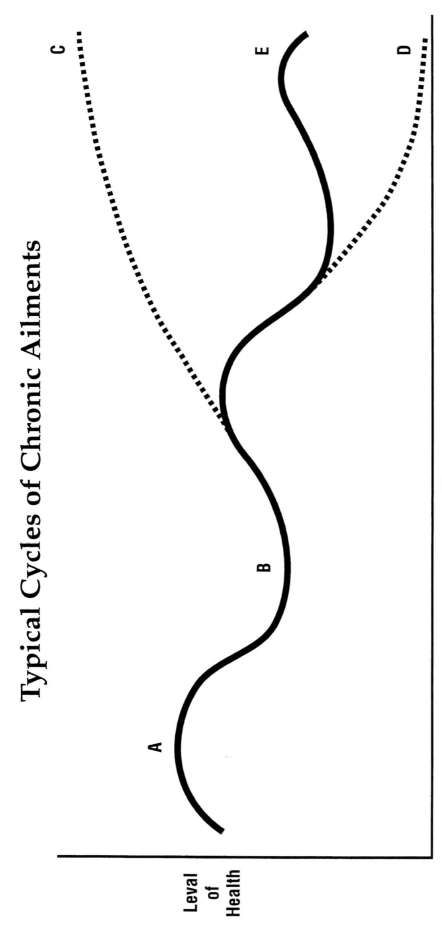

Leval of Health

Time

This graph shows the typical downward progression of health which most people experience. If you do nothing different than follow the traditional medical approaches, your health will unevenly progress downward as you become older. This cyclical regression is shown by the curve from **A** to **E**. You may not notice the decline because of the roller coaster-like progression. If you make improvements in your life style at point **A**, you may become discouraged because your health may go down before it goes up. Positive changes may not show up for several days or weeks. However, if you follow through, you will more rapidly have high level health, as represented by point **C**.

If you make the wrong types of changes at point **B**, you may be happy at first but end up with poor health at point **D**, and not know the cause unless you are aware of the cyclical nature of the chronic ailments which are caused by delayed food and chemical allergies.

The cycles vary greatly depending on the person. One person's health may go up and down over a week and another's over years.

If you make the right choices, you will achieve higher levels of health than the average and enjoy life much more and much longer. It is not too late to decide to have great health, and with the information now available you can achieve it. The sooner you start, the higher the level of health you will be able to enjoy. Learn what great health is like before you decide it takes too much effort.

The Path to Great Health

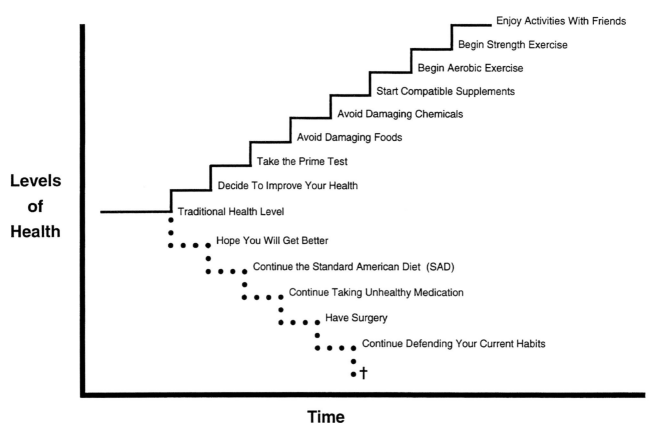

Longevity Curves

The Quality Longevity Program moves the life span curve to the right (thick line). The potential is for the average person to live over 20 years longer and for many people to live over 100 years.

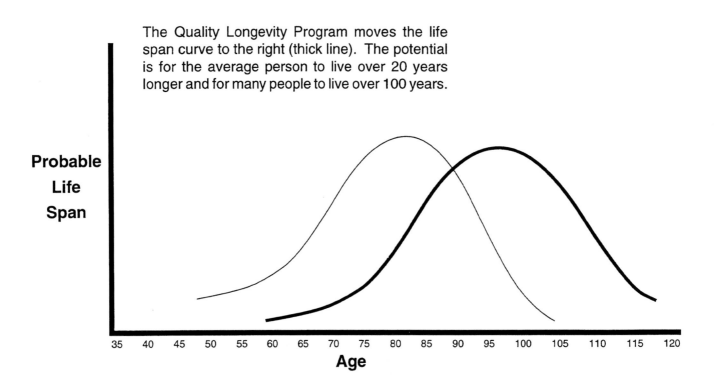

Chapter 14
Added Insights Into The Items Tested

The more you know about the foods, chemicals and other items tested for, the better you will be able to use the Prime Test results and put together a health building menu.

Many foods cause small problems, some cause big problems. By putting together meals with lots of variety that are compatible with your immune system and are not inherently damaging, you can build and maintain great health.

You may recall eating one of the following foods and getting sick even though your Prime Test indicated it did not cause allergic reactions for you. This happens when you avoid a food you are allergic to and your body has time to reduce the elevated levels of immune complexes (the components food break down to) and IgG antibodies. Thus, your blood will indicate that you are not allergic to the item. However, after one, two, or three exposures, you may get a reaction again. The Prime Test reflects the delayed allergic reactions in your body at the time of your test. It is important to combine your history with your test results and then double check your test results.

There are times when reactions will show up on the Prime Test even though the person has never eaten the food. This can happen for a couple of reasons. One is that the molecules of one food closely resemble the molecules of another food the person is allergic to, and the white blood cells mistake it for the allergic food. Sometimes people find they get a reaction the first time they eat a food which was an allergic reactor on their test. A second way you can get a reaction to a food you have never eaten is if your mother was allergic to it and you have inherited a delayed allergy from her. Delayed food allergies are different from airborne allergies and can be passed from mothers to infants.

The foods are listed in the same order as they appear in *Clinical Ecology,* the medical textbook on delayed food and chemical allergies. Panel D gives a cross section of the foods available and covers half of the items on Panel G.

Panel D

1 – **negative control** has no antigens in the chamber and shows the level of dead white blood cells in the person's blood. This chamber is also used to tell, before the test is done, if the individual has a high number of dead white blood cells because of using cortisone creams or other cortisone medications, or if there is some other problem.

The laboratory technician will see what percentage of the white cells are dead before a reaction starts, giving insight into what is happening in the person's body. This becomes the base line for reading the test chambers that have food or chemicals in them. Thus, when the technician looks at the carrot chamber and sees that eight percent of the white blood cells are dead, he already knows that eight percent are dead on the control, and thus knows that there has been no allergic reaction.

2 – **positive control** shows what the cells look like when a major reaction takes place and most of the white blood cells are dead.

Vegetable Products

3 – **yeast** is a very common allergy-causing item. This test covers both brewer's yeast and baker's yeast. Mushrooms, like yeast, are in the fungus family and have yeast underneath their crowns. Thus, if you have a reaction to yeast, be cautious of mushrooms.

Cereal grains (items 4 through 11) are a large part of the diet; however, they provide nothing that is not better supplied by fresh vegetables. This includes fat, protein, complex carbohydrates, vitamins, minerals, fiber, etc.

Cereal grains are usually considered to be complex carbohydrates if they are whole grains and simple carbohydrates if they are refined. However, over 95 percent of a cereal grain is the same whether it is refined or not. The only difference is the thin outer coating and germ are removed to make refined cereal grains.

Because cereal grains, both whole and refined, have to be cooked thoroughly before they are safe to eat, they are absorbed by the body almost as rapidly as white sugar and thus cause health problems even if you are not allergic to them.

The cereal grains are tested in their whole form and are organically grown, as are all the foods on the test panel, with a few exceptions. One example: there are no organically grown sharks.

4 – **barley** is included because it is a common item in the American and European diets. Barley malt is used to help yeast grow when making bread; thus, people get a far more repetitious exposure to barley than they realize.

Barley has 2 percent fat, 8 percent protein and 90 percent carbohydrate.

5 – **wheat** is one of the most repetitiously eaten foods. It causes several different types of health problems for humans. It has gluten in it which, in many people, breaks down the wall of the small intestine and thereby adds to food allergies because undigested food enters the blood. This means that, even if a person is not allergic to wheat, it can be disruptive to the digestive tract and leave it with open sores and damage, which can cause improper assimilation of foods.

You may already have found you are very allergic to wheat and have been avoiding it for some time. If your Prime Test does not show a reaction, it is not a sure indication that wheat will not cause allergy symptoms for you. Occasionally, the test will miss a food if you have not eaten it for a while. The test reflects the state of your body at the time you gave your blood sample.

You need to combine your experiences of food reactions with the results of your Prime Test and be guided by your doctor and health consultant.

Wheat has 5 percent fat, 13 percent protein and 82 percent carbohydrate.

6 – **rye** is in some breads and alcoholic beverages. Rye is so closely related to wheat it can be interbred with it; the cross is called triticale. On the Prime Test form, wheat and rye are tied together by a vertical line to the left of their boxes to indicate their close relationship. People who are allergic to wheat find they are much healthier if they also avoid rye.

A mold sometimes grows on rye which causes hallucinations. The mold is artificially copied to make the drug, LSD. Other cereal grains develop similar molds.

Rye has 4 percent fat, 11 percent protein and 85 percent carbohydrate.

7 – **oats** are not usually consumed repetitiously. Recently, it has become more popular because oat bran helps lower blood cholesterol levels.

Oats are not a very common cause of allergic symptoms. Wild rice is usually thought to be closely related to rice, but it is in the same subfamily as oats.

Oats have 16 percent fat, 13 percent protein and 71 percent carbohydrate.

8 – **rice** is a major allergy-causing food in the orient, where it is eaten very repetitiously. Because rice has become more popular in America and Europe, it is now a common allergy-causing food. The allergy-causing part in the rice is concentrated in the bran coating; thus, eating brown rice increases the chances of developing rice allergies and for them to become more severe. This may be one of the reasons orientals knew not to eat brown rice. If people are allergic to rice they need to avoid all forms of it.

Rice has 4 percent fat, 7 percent protein and 89 percent carbohydrate.

9 – **millet** is not in many foods and is one of the least-reactive cereal grains on the panel.

Millet has 6 percent fat, 10 percent protein and 84 percent carbohydrate.

10 – **sugar cane** is in the cereal grain family and is very common in the diet. The allergic reactivity to sugar cane is not so common as many people think. However, many people think they are allergic to it because the ingestion of any simple sugar causes the white blood cells to become weakened and fragile. This causes reactions to allergy-causing foods and chemicals to be more severe.

Sometimes people can have a combination of reactions if they are allergic to sugar cane and also have a reaction to the foods they eat with it.

Sugar cane has 0 percent fat, 0 percent protein and 100 percent simple carbohydrate.

11 – **corn** is a major cause of food allergy symptoms. Corn is often eaten by itself and combined with many other foods as corn starch, corn sugar, high fructose corn sugar, dextrose, glucose, invert sugar and corn oil. People who are very allergic to corn may not be able to consume regular vitamin C supplements because they are made from corn and have corn starch fillers in them.

Corn is called "maize" in most areas of the world, except the United States. The rest of the world uses the word "corn" to designate all cereal grains.

Corn has 9 percent fat, 7 percent protein and 84 percent carbohydrate.

12 – coconut is also widely used and many people are allergic to it. It is used is in soaps and in shampoos as sodium laurel sulfate. Repetitious exposure and allergic reactions to coconut are much more common than most people realize.

Coconut has 86 percent fat, 3 percent protein and 11 percent carbohydrate.

13 – pineapple is a food to be eaten with caution. Its skin contains an enzyme that can damage the digestive tract.

Pineapple is usually contaminated with pesticides. In Hawaii, cows that were fed pineapple sprouts became so contaminated with pesticides that their milk had to be thrown out because it also was full of pesticides.

You may not show up reactive to pineapple on your Prime Tests but find yourself sick after eating it because you react to one of the pesticides used on pineapple.

Pineapple has 3 percent fat, 3 percent protein and 94 percent carbohydrate, mostly simple carbohydrate.

14 – asparagus can be purchased frozen throughout the year, It is a good complex carbohydrate food but is difficult to find organically grown.

About 70 percent of the population has an inherited enzyme reaction that is indicated by an unusual odor in their urine after eating asparagus.

Asparagus has 8 percent fat, 27 percent protein and 65 percent complex carbohydrate.

15 – onion is often used to add flavor, is fairly common in the diet and has become a fairly common allergic reactor. It is low in nutrients and adds little to the intake of vitamins or minerals.

Onion has 2 percent fat, 11 percent protein and 87 percent complex carbohydrate.

16 – garlic is added to many foods for its distinct flavor. It, like onion, is thought to have several medicinal qualities. However, the ailments it is supposed to reduce go away when people stop eating foods they are allergic to and use the 10–10–80 balance of macronutrients. If you are allergic to garlic, even trace amounts of it in your food will keep you sick.

Garlic has 1 percent fat, 12 percent protein and 87 percent complex carbohydrate.

17 – banana can be a health-building fruit, and is available organically grown. Regular bananas are usually contaminated with pesticides. The fact that bananas are gassed to ripen them is not a problem because the gas used is the same one produced by the bananas to ripen them naturally. Bananas are a good food to use as snacks and can be taken with you to have something to eat when traveling.

Banana has 2 percent fat, 4 percent protein and 94 percent carbohydrate, some complex and some simple carbohydrate.

18 – vanilla is a commonly used flavoring that few people are allergic to. In its liquid form, it often contains alcohol and other ingredients that may cause problems.

19 – black pepper is a common allergic reactor because of its wide usage. Black pepper can not be broken down by the digestive tract. The sharp pepper particles go through the digestive tract, cutting up the lining of the small and large intestine. Anything which damages these linings can help increase the incidence of food allergies.

One reason black pepper and wheat must be avoided is to diminish the chances of developing new allergic reactions. Even if you are not allergic to black pepper, it is best to avoid it.

20 – buckwheat is not related to wheat and is not a cereal grain. It is in the same family as rhubarb. Buckwheat often works for people who are allergic to cereal grains.

Buckwheat has 6 percent fat, 12 percent protein and 82 percent carbohydrate.

21 – beet includes beet and beet sugar and the sugar is often consumed repetitiously. Most people do not eat beets very often but unknowingly are eating it as beet sugar so it often shows up as an allergy-causing food.

Beet has 3 percent fat, 10 percent protein and 87 percent carbohydrate.

22 – spinach is not a very common allergy-causing food. However, it is high in oxalic acid, which blocks assimilation of minerals, thus it should not be eaten very often.

Spinach has 11 percent fat, 32 percent protein and 57 percent complex carbohydrate.

23 – avocado is common in the diet. However, it is not a frequent allergy-causing food.

Avocado, like almost all nuts, is dangerously high in fat. It has 82 percent fat, 4 percent protein and 14 percent carbohydrate.

24 – cabbage is a health-building food. It has an ingredient in it which reduces the chances of developing colon cancer.

Cabbage has 7 percent fat, 13 percent protein and 80 percent complex carbohydrate.

25 – brussels sprouts like almost all fresh vegetables, are high in fiber. They also have many of the same good characteristics as cabbage.

Brussels sprouts have 9 percent fat, 28 percent protein and 63 percent complex carbohydrate.

26 – broccoli is one of the richest sources of vitamins and minerals and has many of the same good characteristics as cabbage.

Broccoli has 9 percent fat, 28 percent protein and 63 percent complex carbohydrate.

27 – cauliflower has many of the same good characteristics as kale, cabbage, brussels sprouts and broccoli. These foods are high in protein so do not over do.

Cauliflower has 9 percent fat, 28 percent protein and 63 percent complex carbohydrate.

28 – mustard is a common flavoring. Few people are allergic to it.

The first four items in this food family: cabbage, brussels sprouts, broccoli and cauliflower, are all closely related. If you are allergic to one, you need to be careful and not overly consume the others. You do not need to avoid the others, but be cautious because you are somewhat susceptible to foods in this family.

29 – strawberry is a tasty fruit and makes a delightful snack. However, its carbohydrate is mostly simple sugar, so do not overeat.

Unfortunately, strawberries are heavily sprayed with pesticides, so you may get an allergic reaction when you eat them, even though strawberries did not react on your Prime Test. Allergic reactions to pesticides and other chemicals are common.

Strawberries have 11 percent fat, 6 percent protein and 83 percent simple.

30 – apple is very commonly consumed and often given in large amounts to young children as apple juice. A high percentage of children and adults are allergic to apples because of repetitious consumption of apple juice. An apple a day can make you very allergic to apples and keep doctors very wealthy.

Apple juice is a very concentrated form of simple carbohydrate and causes sugar overload.

If you are not allergic to apples, eat them fresh and organically grown. This is more often possible today, because the apple-growth-control chemical called Alar has been outlawed.

Apples have 9 percent fat, 1 percent protein and 90 percent carbohydrate, mostly simple.

31 – pear is not often consumed repetitiously and, therefore, causes allergic symptoms less often than apples.

Pears have 5 percent fat, 5 percent protein and 90 percent carbohydrate, mostly simple.

32 – plum is the fruit from which prunes are made. It is much better to eat plums, because the dried prunes become a concentrated sugar like other dried fruits. Dried fruits develop a yeast coating on them during the drying process.

Plums and prunes contain an inflammation-causing chemical which breaks down the lining of the small and large intestines. In response to this chemical, the body rushes the fruit out of your body, and it is this damaging reaction that causes the laxative effect.

Plums have 1 percent fat, 2 percent protein and 97 percent carbohydrate, mostly simple.

33 – almond often causes allergic reactions..

Almonds have 76 percent fat, 11 percent protein and 13 percent carbohydrate.

With one exception, nuts range from 68 to 87 percent fat. Frequently nut and seed oils have turned rancid by the time you buy them.

One nut which tastes good and is not high in fat is the chestnut. Chestnuts have 6 percent fat, 5 percent protein and 89 percent carbohydrate.

Nuts are a common allergy-causing food. Cashews are one of the most reactive; they are related to poison oak and poison ivy. About 70 percent of us are allergic to poison oak and poison ivy.

34 – peach is a good snack food if you are not allergic to it.

It has 2 percent fat, 5 percent protein and 93 percent carbohydrate, mostly simple.

35 – apricot is a great source of beta-carotene.

It has 3 percent fat, 7 percent protein and 90 percent carbohydrate, mostly simple.

36 – nectarine is less often an allergy-causing fruit than peach.

It has 1 percent fat, 3 percent protein and 97 percent carbohydrate, mostly simple.

The next food family is legume (items 37 through 51). Most of these foods are low in fat, very high in protein and high in complex carbohydrates. Two exceptions in this otherwise health-building family are peanuts and soy. Both are high in fat and cause other health problems.

The fat and complex carbohydrate content of most beans promotes health. However, the protein content is very high, and this can damage your health if you eat too many beans along with other high protein foods.

Legumes can be purchased year round and are usually available organically grown. They have a wide range of interesting flavors and, when properly cooked, can be a good addition to the diet. There are many more legumes than are listed on this test panel. Additional types of beans can be challenge tested by the individual, one type per meal, to see if they are compatible.

37 – carob can be used in place of chocolate, helping some people get free of their addiction to chocolate.

Carob has 3 percent fat, 4 percent protein and 93 percent carbohydrate.

38 – lentil is a very flavorful bean. In the past, lentils have been a large part of the European diet. The religious observance of Lent was named after lentils because at that time of year people usually had only lentils left to eat.

Lentils have 2 percent fat, 25 percent protein and 73 percent complex carbohydrate.

39 – split pea is in the same subfamily as lentil, so if you react to one, be careful of the other.

Split peas grow naturally as a half round pea and are not a green pea that has been split in half by a little man.

Split peas have 2 percent fat, 24 percent protein and 74 percent complex carbohydrate.

40 – peanut is one of the inherently damaging members of the legume family.

Peanuts cause more allergy problems than any other legume. These allergies often progress into addictions. It is not uncommon to see people try to eat a few peanuts, then go on to stuff themselves with them and then eat a big dinner without understanding what caused them to lose control. How often do people feel ill after a plane flight and never guess that their symptoms might have been caused by the "free" peanuts?

Remember, there is something unique about the type of fat in peanuts. When combined with cholesterol, all vegetable oils build blockages in the arteries of test animals at the same rate, except peanut oil. Peanut oil has been shown to build blockages in arteries faster than any other oils.

Peanuts are often contaminated with a mold which excretes aflatoxin. A few parts per million of aflatoxin causes liver cancer. In the United States, less than one percent of the people get liver cancer, but in a remote area of Africa where moldy peanut consumption is much higher, 24 percent of the population dies of liver cancer.

There is nothing health-building about peanuts, yet parents keep feeding peanut butter to their children, thinking they are helping their health.

Peanuts have 70 percent fat, 16 percent protein and 14 percent complex carbohydrate.

41 – kidney bean has many positive characteristics. Kidney beans digest slowly and thus provide energy over a long period of time and are readily available organically grown.

One problem with kidney beans and other beans in its subfamily is they contain an enzyme which causes flatulence (rectal gas). Soaking them overnight and discarding the water before cooking them in new water reduces this disconcerting but non-harmful problem. Other beans in this subfamily, called vulgaris, are: pinto, navy, black, calico, red, pink, bush, string and great northern.

Kidney beans have 4 percent fat, 23 percent protein and 73 percent complex carbohydrate.

42 – **pinto bean** is used in Mexican refried beans.

It has 3 percent fat, 23 percent protein and 74 percent complex carbohydrate.

43 – **string bean** is one of the few beans we are able to eat fresh. Although this bean is in the vulgaris subfamily, it does not cause gas to any significant degree.

String beans have 7 percent fat, 16 percent protein and 77 percent complex carbohydrate.

44 – **navy bean** (haricot bean) is small, white and commonly used in soups. This bean is also readily available organically grown and makes a tasty side dish.

Navy beans have 4 percent fat, 23 percent protein and 73 percent complex carbohydrate.

45 – **lima bean** is available frozen and dry and has a unique flavor which is enjoyable to most people after some practice.

Lima beans have 4 percent fat, 20 percent protein and 76 percent complex carbohydrate.

46 – **mung bean** is a very small green bean with great flavor when cooked like other beans. However, this bean is usually eaten sprouted and is the common bean sprout.

Mung beans have 5 percent fat, 27 percent protein and 68 percent complex carbohydrate.

47 – **pea** is one of the most common legumes and is usually eaten thawed, after being frozen.

Peas have 5 percent fat, 26 percent protein and 69 percent complex carbohydrate.

48 – **chick pea** (garbanzo bean) is widely eaten in the United States, Europe, India and the middle east. It is large and takes longer to cook — two hours instead of one — and should be soaked overnight.

Chick peas have 11 percent fat, 20 percent protein and 69 percent complex carbohydrate.

49 – **blackeyed pea** (cowpea) is flavorful but hard to find organically grown. It is available fresh, frozen and dried.

Blackeyed peas have 4 percent fat, 23 percent protein and 73 percent complex carbohydrate.

50 – **soybean** is commonly eaten after having been thoroughly processed. It contains a damaging enzyme which must be processed out or it can not be digested by humans. This marginal food item is often a cause of delayed allergic symptoms and is damagingly high in fat.

Soybeans have 37 percent fat, 29 percent protein and 34 percent complex carbohydrate. Soy bean oil is one of the cheapest oils and is often used in salad dressings.

51 – **alfalfa sprouts** are a nutritious addition to meals. They are now much more common in the American diet because of the popularity of salad bars. They start as very small beans, called seeds, and must be eaten very fresh to be health building.

*You can't keep from getting older,
but you don't have to get old.*

George Burns
Almost a 100 year old comedian.

52 – **lemon** is widely used as a drink, and as flavoring on fish and salads. If you are allergic to lemons it is a also good idea to avoid their close cousin, limes.

Lemons have 7 percent fat, 7 percent protein and 86 percent carbohydrate, mostly simple carbohydrates.

53 – **orange** is often repetitiously consumed as orange juice and has become a common cause of food allergy symptoms. Orange juice is naturally high in simple carbohydrate. This makes the white blood cells sick so they cannot effectively do their job of eating viruses, bacteria and cancer cells. Remember to give people with colds lots of water instead of orange juice or any other sugar laden drink. High sugar consumption is another reason why today's children are so sickly. Spending bankrupting amounts of money on traditional medical approaches does not reverse the damage caused by eating improperly.

Oranges have 3 percent fat, 7 percent protein and 90 percent carbohydrate, mostly simple carbohydrate.

54 – **grapefruit** is the least reactive of this family and is often available organically grown.

Grapefruits have 2 percent fat, 4 percent protein and 94 percent carbohydrate, mostly simple carbohydrate.

55 – grape often causes delayed food allergies. Grape juice is used as the sugar in many beverages for children. Adults have some other uses for grapes — they are commonly used to make alcoholic beverages such as wine, champagne, brandy and cognac. Many people notice a damaging reaction more clearly when they drink red wine, which is white wine that has had the red coloring of the grape skin added back after fermenting. There is more of the allergy-causing substance in the skin; however, if you react to grapes, you need to avoid all types of wine.

You also need to avoid wine if you are allergic to yeast, because wine is actually grape sugar converted into alcohol by yeast. Yeast eats the grape sugar and then excretes alcohol as a waste product. To get free from drinking alcohol it is helpful to think of it as yeast urine.

Alcohol is an inherently damaging liquid, whether it is made from grapes or cereal grains. Alcohol, upon contact, damages the lining of the tongue, esophagus and stomach. It is very abrasive to delicate tissue and leaves open sores along the digestive tract for undigested food particles to get into the blood.

Alcohol causes a number of other health problems and is metagenetic (causes birth defects) in very small amounts. If a mother drinks when she is pregnant, her child is likely to suffer for a lifetime. Men and women who drink alcohol have children who have increased allergy problems. One of the reasons delayed food and chemical allergies are much more common today is the long term effect of Prohibition, (the now defunct law against drinking). As an act of defiance, more people started drinking, especially women. Alcohol damages the fetus by damaging its immune system.

Drinking wine or other alcoholic beverage before a meal is said to "improve" the appetite. This happens because cravings start if the person being allergic and physically addicted to grapes, brewer's yeast or some of the added chemicals.

As you travel around the world, it is amazing to see how much of the land is used for growing wine grapes. Wine manufacturing consumes vast amounts of national resources: land, water, fertilizers, pesticides, labor and capital. The end result is diminished health.

Grapes have 4 percent fat, 3 percent protein and 93 percent carbohydrate, mostly simple carbohydrate.

56 – chocolate is made from husked, roasted and ground cacao seeds. Cocoa powder is the same as chocolate but with much of the fat removed. They often cause delayed allergic symptoms, and most people become physically addicted to them if they consume them repetitiously.

Consuming addictive foods and beverages often brings on the cravings for even more addictive items. When you eat meals which have foods in them that you are allergic and addicted to, notice how much you want something with chocolate in it after the meal. Once you understand this relationship, you will have a major part of the solution to children's and adult's ever-increasing drug problems.

Cacao seeds are grown in South America and are heavily contaminated with chemicals and pesticides. Cockroaches and other insects love them and chocolate is full of their excrement and body parts.

Chocolate was "discovered" by the Spanish explorers who came to the new world. It is one of the new-world foods which has caused multiple health problems. After Cortes captured Montezuma, the last Aztec king, Cortes agreed to let him go if he gave him Mexico's gold. Montezuma agreed, but after getting the gold, Cortes killed him anyway. Before Montezuma died, he put a curse on the European explorers and all their descendants for all time. (Maybe the ailments we get after eating chocolate are the real Montezuma's revenge.)

After eating chocolate, the king of Spain decided it was an aphrodisiac and could be eaten only by him and his friends. Chocolate was kept a secret from everyone else for the next 100 years.

If you have been carefully avoiding chocolate because you find you are physically addicted to it, you may not show a reaction on your Prime Test because you have been avoiding it. You may still get a reaction when you eat it, so combine your Prime Test results with your experience of eating the food.

Chocolate has 74 percent fat, 6 percent protein and 20 percent carbohydrate. Cocoa powder is chocolate with some of the fat taken out. It has 44 percent fat, 13 percent protein and 43 percent carbohydrate.

57 – **tea** is green-leaf tea and contains a caffeine-like chemical. Green tea is made into black tea by fermentation, meaning yeast was involved. Tea is a significant allergy reactor for people in England. It does not cause allergic reactions so commonly in America, but the incidence is increasing as people break their addiction to coffee. Tea has many damaging side effects, such as its stimulant effect which hides your real state of exhaustion and poor health. Tea also contains tannic acid which tans the delicate tissue in the mouth, throat and larynx. Tea often becomes physically addicting.

Caffeine and caffeine-like chemicals are very powerful stimulant drugs, and if someone tried to bring them on the market today, they would not pass *properly* done safety tests.

58 – **papaya** is an interesting and unusual fruit. There are two major versions of it: Hawaiian and South American. Hawaiian are about the size of a grapefruit and South American are much larger. As with all fruit, you want to be careful not to eat too much of it or eat it too often because it is mostly made up of simple carbohydrates.

Another problem with papayas is that it is hard to find them organically grown and they are often heavily sprayed with pesticides. This high level came about because the government set the "acceptable" level by estimating that the average adult ate two papayas per year. If you eat them more often, or a child eats them, or you are allergic to the pesticides used, you may find that papayas do not work for you. This reason for pesticide overuse exists for many other foods.

Papayas have 2 percent fat, 5 percent protein and 93 percent carbohydrate, mostly simple carbohydrate.

59 – **carrot** is a good source of vitamins and minerals. It is a root vegetable, also known as a tuber.

Carrots are usually available organically grown. However, they have a natural pesticide in them to protect them from bugs when they are growing. It is best to avoid eating them in very large amounts at any one time. This is true of many other fruits and vegetables.

It is best to eat carrots raw, steamed or lightly cooked. It is never best to eat any food juiced because the first important step in digesting a carbohydrate food is to work your saliva, with its digestive enzymes, into the food with your teeth, as you carefully chew it. Juicing also releases the simple carbohydrates in fruit too rapidly for your body to handle them.

Carrots are a health-building food because they are a good source of complex carbohydrate, without much simple carbohydrate. Carrots are low in fat and protein.

Carrots have 4 percent fat, 7 percent protein and 89 percent carbohydrate, mostly complex carbohydrate.

60 – **celery** is a commonly eaten food. It is important not to eat celery if it has been bruised. In recent tests, the bruised part of celery develops a chemical which has been shown to cause cancer.

No studies have shown that people who drink celery juice or eat cooked celery have a higher cancer rate. However, heavy consumption of celery, either juiced or cooked, should be avoided until the necessary research is done.

This family includes parsnip and caraway seeds. You can test them on your own by having a small meal of parsnips or by putting caraway seeds on a food you have confirmed to be healthy for you.

Celery has 5 percent fat, 13 percent protein and 82 percent carbohydrate, mostly complex carbohydrate.

61 – **blueberry** can usually be purchased frozen throughout the year without added sugar and fresh occasionally.

Blueberries have 7 percent fat, 4 percent

protein and 89 percent carbohydrate, mostly simple carbohydrate.

62 – cranberry is a rather tart fruit when eaten alone. Cranberries have come into increased consumption because of their good taste when combined with corn sugars or other sugars. Be careful — most cranberry juice is actually a high-sugar drink.

Cranberries have a chemical in them which makes it difficult for bacteria in the bladder and urethra to attach to the surrounding tissue. This dramatically reduces infection, because the bacteria are passed out of the body. The ailment caused by this infection is often called cystitis and is a common complaint for women. Be careful, because most of the cranberry juices on the market have few cranberries and lots of sugar. Sugar weakens the white blood cells' ability to attack bacteria, viruses and yeast throughout the body.

Cranberries have 13 percent fat, 3 percent protein and 84 percent carbohydrate, mostly simple carbohydrates.

63 – olive is eaten by itself and is used to make olive oil. Olives go through extensive processing because they are so bitter they cannot be eaten.

Health claims are made for olive oil and it may be somewhat less damaging than other oils; however, it's value is insignificant compared to no added oil. Olive oil helps to cause cardiovascular disease, type 2 diabetes, several types of cancer and other ailments.

It has 90 percent fat, 3 percent protein and 7 percent carbohydrate. Olive oil 100 percent fat.

The next group (64 through 71) is the nightshade family. It has allergy-causing foods for some people but for others, the foods work well.

Some people claim the nightshade family is always damaging. This happens because they get terrible arthritis when they eat potatoes or tomatoes and then write books claiming they have found the cause of arthritis. However, once people understand that delayed allergies exist, they realize these are allergic reactions for some, but not for everyone.

This entire family is made up of items that were discovered in the Americas and are referred to as "new world" foods.

64 – potato is a commonly eaten food and is consumed in many different forms. It is a good source of complex carbohydrate if it is steamed or boiled — not baked. When potatoes are baked, most of their carbohydrates are converted to sugar because of the high temperature involved.

Potatoes have a chemical in them called solanin which is damaging to everyone. This toxin becomes more concentrated as the potato ages. It can be seen as a greenish color under the skin. When you see this, do not eat the potato.

Potato skins contain molds, yeast, pesticides and sometimes aflatoxin. Never eat the skin on russet potatoes and clean or peel red and white potatoes. It works fine to peel a russet and then bake it, if you want an occasional baked potato.

Potatoes have 1 percent fat, 8 percent protein and 91 percent carbohydrate.

65 – tomato works well for some people if they are not allergic to them.

There is a little-known substance in tomatoes called lectins. Lectins cause inflammation in the body similar to allergic reactions. Therefore, many people do better if they avoid tomatoes. A few other foods have lectins but tomatoes are the highest. People with type O blood are damaged more by lectins than people with other types of blood.

Tomatoes have 8 percent fat, 13 percent protein and 79 percent carbohydrate.

66 – tobacco has been shown helpful for killing insects. And whether smoked in cigarettes, pipes or cigars, chewed or taken as snuff, tobacco has been shown to damage everyone's health. This includes other people's smoke, known as side stream smoke. Be very careful not to breathe other people's smoke, especially when you are trying to break an addiction to tobacco. Other people's smoke can get you re-addicted. Your cravings are reactivated for tobacco or anything else you are addicted to. Promote non-smoking wherever possible.

67 – chilli pepper is a common spice used in many types of cooking, especially Mexican. Many people find that their digestive tracts become inflamed when they eat hot spices even if they are not allergic to them.

68 – bell pepper is also known as a green or red bell pepper. In fact, red bell peppers are green ones that have finished ripening. Red bell peppers have much more flavor and nutrients, particularly vitamin C.

They are excellent snack foods and should be purchased without a wax or oil coating and washed before eating to help remove pesticides.

Bell peppers have 3 percent fat, 4 percent protein and 93 percent carbohydrate.

69 – yellow sweet potato is a good source of complex carbohydrate. It is important to peel, slice and steam rather than bake sweet potatoes, because baking turns most of it into a rapidly assimilated, simple carbohydrate.

Yellow sweet potatoes have 8 percent fat, 13 percent protein and 79 percent complex carbohydrate.

70 – "yam" is actually a maroon sweet potato, not an actual yam. In the American markets there are no actual yams. True yams are grown in South America and are the color of potatoes, except they are longer and have little flavor.

It is important to prepare and cook "yams" like yellow sweet potatoes.

"Yams" have 8 percent fat, 13 percent protein and 79 percent complex carbohydrate.

71 – sesame is very common in the American diet because it is often used on top of bread. For some people it is a major allergy reactor. Sesame seeds are high in fat and become rancid very easily.

Sesame seeds have 77 percent fat, 11 percent protein and 12 percent carbohydrate.

72 – coffee is one of the most damaging, allergy-causing and addictive items there is.

The stimulating impact of caffeine masks symptoms of chronic fatigue, which is not discovered until people stop taking this or other stimulant drugs.

Most people are surprised at how enjoyable life is without taking a powerful stimulant drug. Stimulants leave people tense and off center, a condition they often reverse in the evening with a powerful depressant drug — alcohol.

The caffeine taken out of coffee to make decaffeinated coffee is added to "soft" drinks to begin the addiction process in children and wreck their health.

Some people who have broken their addiction to alcohol, legal and illegal drugs, and coffee, claim their coffee withdrawal symptoms were the worst. There are several damaging chemicals in coffee, thus decaffeinated coffee is still damaging and addictive. Decaffeinated coffee still contains about three percent of its original caffeine.

73 – cucumber is a good snack food and a health-building addition to meals. By shopping around, you can find several different types of cucumbers.

Cucumbers have 6 percent fat, 10 percent protein and 84 percent carbohydrate.

74 – winter squash has many different varieties. There is acorn, spaghetti, turban, banana and butternut squash, plus many more. Winter squash have hard skins and big seeds — neither should be eaten.

Winter squash average 5 percent fat, 7 percent protein and 88 percent complex carbohydrate.

Pumpkin is also a winter squash but is rarely consumed except in pumpkin pie. Most fresh pumpkin has little flavor and is usually eaten with lots of sugar and spice.

75 – summer squash has many different varieties. Zucchini is the most common, but yellow crook neck and scallop squash are also readily available, often organically grown. Summer squash are eaten with their skins on and seeds in.

Summer squash average 6 percent fat, 16 percent protein and 78 percent complex carbohydrate.

76 – cantaloupe is a common member of the melon family. Other members are honeydew, casaba and yellow. These seasonal foods are best eaten by themselves because they need to be digested rapidly or they will cause digestive problems for many people.

Melons average 4 percent fat, 8 percent protein and 88 percent simple carbohydrate.

77 – watermelon is in a different part of the family than the other melons. It causes severe allergic symptoms for some people.

Watermelons have 6 percent fat, 6 percent

protein and 88 percent simple carbohydrate.

78 – lettuce shows up as an allergic reactor for some people because of repetitious consumption. Some people who can eat head lettuce and green lettuce cannot eat red-tip lettuce or some other lettuce. If you do find you are allergic to the head lettuce that is used in the Prime Test, experiment with the other lettuces and you may find some are healthy for you.

Lettuce averages 10 percent fat, 16 percent protein and 74 percent carbohydrate.

79 – safflower oil is occasionally used for cooking. It is high in poly-unsaturated oil and widely promoted because it does not break down as easily when used for cooking.

Like all other oils, it is 100 percent fat. Adding a small amount to an otherwise health-building meal will significantly increase the fat content of the meal and cause numerous diseases.

Vegetable oils are actually harder for your body to clean out of your circulation than are animal fats. It is important to remember that after a meal, it takes about nine hours for your body to clean vegetable oils out of your circulation, but animal fats are cleaned out in about six hours. When these fats are circulating with your red blood cells, the red blood cells cannot deliver oxygen very well to all the rest of the cells of your body. This makes your cells sickly.

In every group of people from all around the world, it has been shown that those who eat diets moderate or high in vegetable oils have high rates of cancer. This includes olive oil. The optimal level of fat in the diet is the level found naturally in most fresh vegetables — which is about 10 percent fat.

Animal Products

Many studies have been done which clearly show that most ocean or freshwater-derived meat is contaminated with pollution and/or preservative chemicals. One insightful study was published in *Consumers Reports* in 1993 and disclosed that most fish in the markets and restaurants were contaminated and often mis-labeled.

Fish and all other animal products need to be thoroughly cooked to kill parasites that are in them. If the parasites get into your body, your health will be continually reduced.

The government passed a law that wetting fish in the market to make them look fresh was illegal. The year was 78 BC and the government was Imperial Rome. Problems with fish quality are not new and have gotten worse.

80 – shrimp are a questionable food even if you are not allergic to them. They usually live in polluted water and accumulate the water's toxins in their bodies.
Shrimp spoil easily after they are caught and are often soaked in preserving chemicals. These chemicals can cause allergic reactions and do not solve the problem of rotting meat.

Shrimp have 8 percent fat, 85 percent protein and 7 percent carbohydrate.

81 – lobster is not very commonly eaten. It has the same pollution problems as shrimp and is also very high in protein. Thus, eating much lobster can cause the body to lose minerals because high protein foods leach minerals out of the body.

Lobster has 19 percent fat, 79 percent protein and 2 percent carbohydrate.

82 – crab suffers from the same problems as other shellfish.

Crab has 19 percent fat, 79 percent protein and 2 percent carbohydrate.

83 – salmon is one of the few fish which is high in fat. The meat is red because salmon eat shrimp whose skeletons have a red pigment that colors the salmon meat.

Salmon has 56 percent fat, 44 percent protein and 0 percent carbohydrate.

Like all red meat and poultry, fish averages around 70 milligrams of cholesterol per three and a half ounces. Thus, if you eat a similar amount of fish as you did red meat, your blood cholesterol levels will not go down and you will not become free of heart disease.

84 – cod is lower in fat than salmon; thus, it is dangerously high in protein. When you eat fish, eat very small portions, under three ounces. Do not eat fish every day or you will rip the minerals out of your body.

On the west coast of the United States, many people eat what they think is red snapper but is actually rock cod. So if cod does not cause problems for you, west coast "red snapper" is an acceptable fish for you. Real red snapper is caught off Florida's coast and is very different in appearance and taste. It is rarely obtainable on the west coast.

Cod has 2 percent fat, 98 percent protein and 0 percent carbohydrate.

85 – **bass** has the same problems as most fish, and like most ocean fish, it lives in contaminated water, eats other fish that are contaminated and thereby accumulates the pollution.

Bass has 12 percent fat, 88 percent protein and 0 percent carbohydrate.

86 – **tuna** causes several serious health problems. Years ago, tuna was so plentiful that it was inexpensive and thus eaten repetitiously. Many people are allergic to tuna.

Contrary to some of the studies done by the government, mercury and lead levels in most tuna are dangerously high. It turned out the government's testing equipment was contaminated so the government did not see an increase from a "non-contaminated" tuna to the test sample. When follow-up testing was carefully done at a university, most tuna was found to have health-wrecking levels of mercury and lead in it.

One lady had her amalgam (silver with mercury) fillings replaced with gold or composite material because her mercury test showed high levels of mercury fumes in her mouth. She then had her mouth tested again. She flunked the test and was angry to find she still had mercury fumes in her mouth. She then discovered that the tuna she had eaten an hour before her test was still releasing mercury fumes in her mouth. After washing out the microscopic amounts of tuna left in her mouth, she passed the test.

Tuna is very high on the ocean's food chain and is usually contaminated with mercury and thus needs to be avoided. This is also true of swordfish.

Tuna has 6 percent fat, 94 percent protein and 0 percent carbohydrate.

87 – **halibut** is a bottom-feeding ocean fish and sometimes has high levels of contaminants.

Halibut has 11 percent fat, 89 percent protein and 0 percent carbohydrate.

88 – **sole** is closely related to flatfish, flounder and sanddab. These fish are bottom feeders and are often contaminated by ocean pollution and chemicals used in processing.

Sole has 4 percent fat, 96 percent protein and 0 percent carbohydrate.

Some fish can be obtained from clean waters. However, in processing they often have antibiotic solutions put on them along with other chemicals to reduce spoiling. So select your fish with care from a reliable fish market.

Most fish are a very concentrated source of protein. A piece of fish the same size as a steak will actually overload you with about three times as much protein. This happens because steaks are around 75 percent fat and 25 percent protein. Because fish averages over 80 percent protein, a large serving of fish can seriously diminish your body's reserves of vital minerals.

89 – **chicken** is often contaminated with salmonella bacteria and growth hormones. Be sure to cook it thoroughly and do not use the knives, forks or cutting surfaces used to prepare chickens to prepare any other foods until all utensils and surfaces have been carefully cleaned. Otherwise, health building vegetables can pick up the bacteria from the meat and carry it into your body.

Chicken breasts are lower in fat than red meat but are damagingly high in protein. Chicken meat has the same amount of cholesterol as fish and red meat — about 70 milligrams for each three and a half ounce portion.

Chicken breast meat has 18 percent fat, 82 percent protein and 0 percent carbohydrate. Leg meat has 33 percent fat, 67 percent protein and 0 percent carbohydrate.

90 – **chicken egg** is one of the most allergy-causing foods, in part, because of repetitious consumption.

Each egg yolk is extremely high in cholesterol no matter how you measure it or raise the chicken: it has over 200 milligrams of cholesterol. That is about the same as three pounds of beef or any other animal product.

It is important to remember that the human body becomes saturated at about 200 milligrams of cholesterol a day. When you hear of studies which claim eating five or ten eggs a day did not increase the cholesterol in people's blood, it was because they are saturated at about 200 milligrams a day. Thus, any increased cholesterol intake from the additional eggs did not get absorbed, so the added intake of cholesterol did not raise their blood cholesterol levels.

To get your blood levels of cholesterol level down rapidly, you need to eat 0 to 30 milligrams of cholesterol a day until your blood cholesterol level is under 150, and then stay under 80 milligrams a day.

Recent studies have shown that about 24 percent of eggs in the market are contaminated with salmonella bacteria. Eggs have an enzyme which blocks the assimilation of the B vitamin, riboflavin. Cooking eggs thoroughly kills the bacteria and deactivates their enzymes.

Chicken egg has 64 percent fat, 34 percent protein and 2 percent carbohydrate. Because eggs are high in protein they help to rip the minerals out of the body.

Eggs add nothing that is needed in the human diet, and most of their contents are very damaging.

Man lives on one quarter of what he eats.
On the other three quarters, lives his doctor.

Translated from the hieroglyphics
on an Egyptian Pyramid — 3800 BC

91 – turkey is usually less contaminated than chicken, but still needs to be purchased with great care. It is lower in fat than red meat, but is a concentrated source of protein. Thus, it should be eaten in very small portions; otherwise, it will cause a mineral depletion in your body while damaging your liver and kidneys.

Turkey breast meat is 20 percent fat, 80 percent protein and 0 percent carbohydrate. The leg meat is 37 percent fat, 63 percent protein and 0 percent carbohydrate.

92 – pork is very high on the food chain and is often contaminated with chemical fertilizers and pesticides which accumulate in the meat. Pigs are often given antibiotics to keep them

from dying before they are slaughtered. These and other drugs end up in your body, causing a broad range of health problems.

Pork must be cooked thoroughly to kill parasites that may be in the meat. If the parasites get into your body, your health will be continually reduced.

Pork, is 70 percent fat, 30 percent protein and 0 percent carbohydrate. Even very lean pork gets over 46 percent of its calories from fat, and the remainder is protein.

93 – beef has similar problems as pork, and is often contaminated with salmonella bacteria.

Beef has an additional problem: it has been consumed so repetitiously that it is often an allergy-causing food. Beef and milk are closely related and almost everybody notices that they feel better and are healthier when they avoid them both entirely.

Beef and veal average over 50 percent fat, under 50 percent protein and 0 percent carbohydrate. Beef has 70 milligrams of cholesterol per three and a half ounces, and veal has 90.

94 – cows' milk and other dairy products are some of the most damaging items you can eat. This includes butter, cheese, yogurt, whey, lactose, etc.

Dairy products are often given to young children under the age of two. They cannot digest or assimilate them well and get started on a life of health problems.

We often inherit our dairy allergies from our mothers because they were told to drink lots of milk when they were pregnant. Dairy products are a major cause of foods allergies, heart disease and cancer.

Dairy products are one of the most addicting of all the foods. The first response to going off of them is to have withdrawal symptoms. People often feel worse for 3 to 14 days and then feel better for the rest of their lives. Read the chapter on dairy products again for more insights into the advantages of staying free of all dairy products.

Do not be surprised if you keep going in and out of withdrawal if you do not break free of them entirely. Just a little butter on your vegetables will keep you addicted and sick.

Many people have been told they are

lactose intolerant because their doctor did not know how to test for delayed food allergies. True lactose intolerance is uncommon in Caucasians.

Cows' milk is 47 percent fat, 23 percent protein and 30 percent simple carbohydrate. The simple carbohydrate is the milk sugar called lactose. Low fat milk, called 2 percent milk, when calculated correctly, gets over 30 percent of its calories from fat.

Non-fat milk is almost free of fat, having only 2 percent of its total calories from fat. However, it then becomes high in protein, 42 percent, and is 56 percent sugar.

Butter gets 99 percent of its total calories from fat, .5 percent protein and .5 percent simple carbohydrate. It has similar allergy-causing problems as other dairy products, but is often slower-reacting because it is more slowly digested due to its high fat content.

The manufacturing of butter concentrates the pesticides and other pollutants eaten by the cow, including the antibiotics. If you refine butter further by cooking it, you turn it into a product called ghee, which causes the same health problems as butter except it will not go rancid as rapidly. Ghee is 100 percent fat.

Butter and ghee have much more cholesterol than the same amount of water-free milk. Dry milk has 85 milligrams of cholesterol per three and a half ounces, where as butter and ghee have 250.

Margarine causes many health problems. It also dramatically increases the fat content of natural vegetable meals, so they go from 10 percent fat to over 30 percent fat.

Margarine has high levels of trans fats in it, and they cause cancer at an even higher rate than do un-hydrogenated vegetable oils. It makes no sense to become free of allergies and then switch to something like margarine. Adding either butter or margarine damages health. To have a healthy life you need to avoid them both.

If you react to cows' milk, you need stay free of all products made with anything that comes from cows' milk. Read labels carefully, including the product sheets you can get from the pharmacist when you are being told to take a prescription drug.

Prescription drugs sometimes have lactose or whey in them. Avoid all dairy products and everything that has any dairy product in it as though your health depends on it. It does.

*If you want to keep getting
what you're getting,
keep doing what you're doing.*

95 – **lamb** does not commonly cause allergic symptoms like beef and pork.

Lamb is not as contaminated with pesticides because it is not fed the same levels of pollution as beef and pork are. Do not eat it repetitiously and if you do eat lamb, eat it in very small quantities only if you are not allergic to it.

Lamb has 59 percent fat, 41 percent protein and 0 percent carbohydrate. Even lean cuts have 33 percent fat and 67 percent protein.

Other Allergens

96 – **honey** is a simple carbohydrate and damages your body like an equal amount of white sugar. White sugar is manufactured in big factories and honey is manufactured in little factories — the health consequences are the same.

Bees take pollen into their bodies and break it down from a complex carbohydrate to a simple carbohydrate. This causes a reaction in your body like white sugar does. It paralyzes and weakens the white blood cells and reduces their ability to kill viruses, bacteria and cancer cells.

There are different types of honey, both raw and pasteurized. Pasteurized honey is cooked to kill the organisms in it so its shelf life will be extended.

Some batches of honey are contaminated with microscopic amounts of botulism. This can be fatal to young children; therefore, honey should not be given to them.

It is possible to have severe, fast acting allergic reactions to honey because it has traces of pollen in it. These IgE type reactions have been shown to kill people on rare occasions. Sometimes it is the pollen itself, sometimes it is the saliva from the bees which people are allergic to.

The idea of eating bee pollen for health has some inherent difficulties. If you become allergic to pollen by eating it repetitiously, you can become allergic to the pollens in the air and be sick much of the time.

Chemical Allergens

97 – **B-complex vitamins** are synthetic in most vitamin tablets and are made by two companies for almost all pill manufacturers. Each B vitamin is made from a different chemical and people are often allergic to some of the B vitamins and not others. Test them one at a time to find the ones that are compatible.

98 – **BHT** is a common preservative used to stop products from becoming rancid. A very similar preservative is BHA and should also be avoided if you react to BHT.

99 – **sodium bisulfite** used to be a common preservative used on foods in salad bars. Because 13 people died from acute allergic reaction to it, its use was restricted to shrimp and a few other food items. This safety restriction was slow in coming because traditional allergists refused to believe people could have an allergic reaction if there were no proteins present.

Sodium bisulfite is a natural by-product of wine making. It has been shown to cause severe allergic reactions even though it does not show up on traditional allergy tests. However, it often shows up on the Prime Test.

100 – **formaldehyde** is commonly part of synthetic fabrics, and occasionally put in cotton. Wash clothes a couple of times before you wear them. It is best to buy organically grown cotton clothes. Furniture, plywood and chipboard are often made with glue containing formaldehyde: shop carefully.

101 – **aspirin** is one of the most commonly used over-the-counter drugs. One of the ways it works is by breaking up platelet aggregation in the body. Platelet aggregation is just one of the results of delayed allergic reactions.

Each 5 grain tablet of aspirin causes one teaspoon of bleeding from the walls of the stomach. Children sometimes develop lasting brain damage.

Aspirin is commonly used to reduce arthritic pain, a disease often caused by delayed allergic reactions.

Nobody gets a headache or any other pain because they have an aspirin deficiency.

The chances of a second heart attack have been shown to be reduced for people who take a small amount of aspirin each day. When platelet aggregation is reduced, circulation is improved and thus delayed allergic reactions may play a small part in heart disease. It is better to avoid food and chemical allergies than take aspirin. However, small doses of aspirin may be helpful for those at high risk of having a heart attack, at least until their new diet reverses their risk factors. In one study, the effective amount was less than 10 percent of a typical 5 grain tablet.

One study did not use pure aspirin, but aspirin buffered with magnesium. It is known that increasing magnesium intake helps to reduce high calcium levels, and high calcium levels increase the chances of a heart attack. Thus, some of the benefit may have been from reduced calcium in the blood.

Two studies done on aspirin have shown that the taking of aspirin to reduce heart disease significantly increased the incidence of stroke.

No aspirin studies have been done on people following the 10–10–80 program. People who have been using this diet principle long enough do not have heart attacks.

102 – **Tylenol** is a common replacement for aspirin and is believed to have serious side effects. If you eat your compatible foods you do not have much need for pain killers.

Be careful of Ibuprofen. Although it is widely used as a pain killer, 70,000 people have been hospitalized because of complications. Some complications are severe and over 7,000 people have died.

How many of those people could have been saved if they had known their pain was caused by delayed food allergies? Taking drugs to treat symptoms often causes new symptoms and the old symptoms become worse.

103 – **saccharin** is a common artificial sweetener which often causes delayed allergic reactions.

It is often addictive and has been shown to cause cancer in animal tests.

104 – Equal like NutraSweet, is an artificial sweetener which contains aspartame and causes allergy problems for many people, as well as other health problems. Even though two un-refuted studies showed aspartame caused brain cancers in test animals, the FDA approved it in 1983 because of pressure from fast/junk food companies. According to the National Cancer Institute, the frequency of brain cancers has risen dramatically since 1983. In addition, aspartame is 10 percent wood alcohol, which damages the eyes and breaks down into formaldehyde — a known carcinogen.

105 – MSG is the abbreviation for monosodium glutamate. It inflames the nerve endings in the taste buds and thereby tricks you into believing a food has better flavor than it does. After damaging the nerve endings in your mouth, it travels throughout your body causing havoc, until it hits your brain cells and causes serious problems.

Check labels closely, avoid products like Accent and most Chinese restaurants that use MSG. Even the better Chinese restaurants that ban MSG entirely, occasionally have it in their meals because food items imported from China sometimes have it in them without the restaurant's knowledge. MSG is hidden in additives like "hydrolyzed vegetable protein."

106 – food coloring causes delayed food allergies occasionally and can be a serious problem. However, it is nowhere near the problem dairy products, wheat or a dozen other foods are.

107 – petroleum by-products are one of the most common delayed allergy reactors. It is important to reduce it to the lowest possible level. We are exposed to it from many sources: car exhaust, smog, diesel fumes, the fumes from burnt natural gas (gas stoves, furnaces and water heaters), jet exhaust, and the out-gassing from most soft plastics. Many people have to move from their smoggy neighborhoods in order to become well.

The Prime Test discloses delayed allergic reactions and as most airborne reactions are the acute IgE type, they do not show up on this test.

Airborne Allergens

108 – dust is occasionally involved in delayed allergic reactions, but is commonly involved in acute IgE allergic reactions. The allergic-reacting substance is not dust but the excrement from dust mites which live wherever people do. Dust mites do not eat dust; they eat dead, flaked off, human skin.

The idea promoted by traditional allergists to humidify air turned out to be a disaster. Dust mites multiply so much more rapidly in moist environments that they put to shame the most romantic rabbits.

Traditional allergists try to stop people from reacting to dust mite droppings by injecting the excrement into them twice a week. Allergy shots and cortisone drugs are the main tools of traditional allergists and they claim their approach should be the only one available. Most people are less effected by airborne allergens when they are eating their compatible foods because their allergic load is so reduced.

109 – mold is a common delayed allergic reactor and should be reduced wherever possible. Low humidity helps to reduce mold.

110 – pollen mix is a combination of grass and tree pollen and can help explain why symptoms vary during different times of the year.

Items Not On The D Panel

Canola oil is being promoted as a health building fat. It may be a little less damaging than other oils but is no where as good as no added oil.

Take vitamins with caution. You need to select a type of vitamin C which is as free of corn as possible. Highly purified forms of vitamin C do not have corn starch in them. Ester-C is the least allergy causing for most people.

Use the information in this chapter to better understand the foods you are eating and chemicals you are exposed to. The more knowledge you have, the more powerful you will be at improving your health.

Most people find it helpful to test for more items than are on the Panel D. Panel G tests for 220 items.

Life is made up of problems.
The satisfaction from solving
problems is what makes
life so rewarding.

Chapter 15
Fine Tuning and Complementary Therapies

There are some valuable steps you can take to improve your health once you have established the correct health foundation. This foundation is made up of eating foods which are compatible with your white blood cells and compatible with your body's ability to use fat, protein and carbohydrate.

It is important to remember that these steps need to be taken after you have the foundation working for you. If you start the fine tuning and complementary therapies before you improve your way of eating, the other therapies will just be treating symptoms and will only mask your problems temporarily. You can end up in trouble again, sometimes with even bigger problems.

Many of these complementary therapies have been tried on their own with some success. However, without the foundation in place, successes do not last because they are built on quicksand. Once you are eating the foods best suited to your body, these secondary approaches can have powerful and lasting benefits.

These complementary therapies can be viewed as steps up a staircase to great health — steps to be taken one at a time as energies permit. Choose the timing and sequence of steps your health requires. Your health counselor can help you work out which therapies are most important for you.

Some of the following therapies are very helpful, some offer little and some offer no help, depending on the person. People with serious health problems often find fine tuning and complementary therapies valuable in obtaining good health, and eventually great health.

Aerobics and Lymph

Aerobic exercise is absolutely necessary to obtain and maintain good health. Aerobic exercise happens when you raise your pulse rate above 100 beats per minute for 15 minutes. This opens your capillaries while toning and conditioning your body. As your health improves, the pulse-rate target goes higher and the time increases. Start your exercising gradually.

The lymph system has channels throughout your body, but has no pump to circulate and clean out the waste that accumulates there. The lymph channels are where the remnants of your dead white blood cells go. Other broken-down tissues also end up in your lymph ducts.

Exercise causes the large muscles to contract; thus, they work like a pump which cleans out the lymph system. Do aerobic exercise four or more days a week — your body needs all the help it can get.

To facilitate the cleansing of the lymph channels in the legs and body, it is beneficial to turn yourself upside down and let gravity work for you. Lie on your back with your legs up the wall. For more powerful cleaning (if you do not have high blood pressure, eye vessel damage, etc.) hang upside down. This is more effective following aerobic exercise.

Antigravity boots and other inversion devices make hanging upside down easy and enjoyable. For a catalogue of helpful items call Gravity Plus at (800) 383-8056 or (619) 454-1626.

Body Work

Massage relieves tension and helps the lymph system. Lymphatic massage is particularly beneficial because it helps to clean out the lymph ducts. Find a massage practitioner who is good at lymphatic massage and see the benefits. Learn about massage and find a friend to trade massages with.

A technique known as Cranial Sacral Massage involves adjustment of the plates that make up the skull. Some people have experienced health benefits by having this done. More research is needed to better understand why this is helpful.

Other types of body work which are helpful include deep tissue work, Rolfing and Heller Work.

Minerals

For all the organs and systems in your body to work properly, they need the right levels of minerals. Food allergies and eating moderate to high levels of protein create high acid levels in the body, causing a broad range of essential minerals to be leached out of your body. To find out what your body's mineral levels are, have an accurate hair mineral analysis done. Then take your individualized mineral supplements to support your immune system and numerous other body functions.

It can take months to get your trace mineral levels built up to where they belong. Do not be surprised if it takes a while to become fully healthy. The stomach needs to have an adequate level of hydrochloric acid in order to assimilate minerals supplied by foods and supplements.

Vitamins

Vitamins are also essential for your body to work right. On a diet very high in fresh vegetables, you receive an abundance of vitamins, minerals and fiber. However, if we eat cereal grains (which have no vitamin C) or processed and cooked foods, we need supplements. And, to accelerate healing and make up for past deficiencies, it is helpful to supplement accurately. There are few problems caused from taking vitamins, except if you are allergic to the chemicals or foods they are made from. It is possible to overdose on vitamin A, D, E and B_6 but occurrences are very rare. Your health counselor is best able to advise you on your particular needs.

Essential Fatty Acids

To be fully healthy throughout our lives we need mothers' milk when we are infants. It has omega-6 fatty acid. Later in life, we can get this essential nutrient by taking evening primrose oil, borage oil, black current seed oil or flaxseed oil. Omega-3 fatty acid is also important and can be supplemented by taking flaxseed oil or fish oil. Low fat diets help us to utilize fatty acid supplements. To reduce their rancidity, regular vegetable oils are treated to remove their essential fatty acids.

Other Supplements

There are many helpful supplements to take besides vitamins and minerals. As with vitamins and minerals, you have to select supplements carefully so that you will not have allergic reactions to them and reverse some of the progress you have made. Do not fall into the trap of taking something with the hope it will let you eat a damaging food without harm. Using the magic-bullet approach shoots you in the foot, even if the bullet is a blank, because you are diverted from changing the way you eat and exercise.

One supplement which is well tolerated and helps the body to rebuild is Co-Enzyme Q_{10}. This supplement supports your cells' basic enzyme system that they use for repair. After getting your health foundation working for you, try taking 100 milligrams a day and see how you feel.

Toxic Metals

It is important for your overall health to remove toxic metals from your body. Your hair analysis often, but not always, discloses your levels of toxic metals. The level in your hair depends on whether the toxic metals are locked in your tissues or

circulating in your blood. If they are in your blood they will be picked up by the roots of your hair as it grows, and are measurable in a hair mineral test.

Amalgam fillings are made of silver and mercury. Even trace amounts of mercury are toxic to your white blood cells, brain cells and most of the other cells in your body.

The mercury from amalgam fillings out-gases when you chew and it is then absorbed into your body. It often does not show up on regular blood tests because the mercury is locked inside your body's cells or is elevated only after chewing.

Going to the dentist is never pleasant; however, having your amalgam fillings removed is not as unpleasant as it sounds because the dentist is drilling out the old metal, not your sensitive teeth. If you have amalgam fillings (sometimes called silver fillings) it is important to replace them with gold or composite material.

When you have them removed, be sure the dentist puts a small oxygen cup over your nose so that you breath pure oxygen while the dentist is working in your mouth. Wherever possible have the dentist use a rubber dam around the tooth being worked on. These two precautions keep you from inhaling or ingesting mercury gas while the old fillings are being removed.

A follow-up to having the amalgam fillings removed from your mouth is a special therapy designed to remove mercury from your body's cells. This type of therapy is not the traditional EDTA type used to clean out other toxic minerals. The effective procedures for mercury removal are called DMPS and DMSA therapy. People with low levels of mercury in their blood before the treatments get high levels of mercury in their urine after their treatments because these therapies released mercury from their cells.

Root Canals

Many people still have teeth that should have been removed because of extensive cavities. Instead of removing a tooth, the dentist took the nerve out of its channel and plugged it up with a foreign materiel to save what was left of the tooth. When the nerve is taken out, the tooth's supporting blood vessels are also removed and then the white blood cells cannot clean out the tooth because throughout the tooth there are microscopic tubes which get bacteria in them. These bacteria continue to release toxins into the body as long as you have a tooth with a root canal.

An important book to read about root-canal problems and solutions is by George Meinig, DDS. He was a nationally renowned expert on how to do root canals, and is now the nationally renowned irritant to dentists who still do root canals. His book is titled *Root Canal Cover-up* and can be ordered by calling (805) 646-2865.

Gums

Another problem which commonly affects people with delayed food allergies is periodontal disease — the breakdown of the gums around the teeth. This allows food and bacteria to get down the sides of the teeth and around their roots. This is the primary cause of tooth loss — not cavities.

Delayed food allergies cause damage throughout the body and this can often be seen in the gums. It is imperative you eat your compatible foods if you want to have healthy gums. If you already have periodontal disease, you need to go to a competent periodontist and have the type of teeth cleaning and support treatments they do which help stop the progression of periodontal disease.

Going to a periodontist twice a year can save your teeth and ability to chew your food. If you do not chew thoroughly it is hard to build your health.

Toxins

Some people still have symptoms when they are eating their compatible foods and avoiding allergy causing chemicals, because of chemical residues locked up in their bodies. Some of these residues are from prior medications, some are from pesticides, some are chemicals from or still in their home or work environment.

One method of removing these toxins from the tissues is the Hubbard Detox Therapy. This approach starts by using small (20 milligram) doses of the B vitamin called niacin. Niacin causes a flush by opening the capillaries. This shows up as tingling and a pink glow in the skin.

The niacin is followed by aerobic exercise on an exercise bicycle and then by taking a warm, but not hot, sauna. Hot saunas are too debilitating because you have to stay in the sauna for a long time for the therapy to work. This therapy must be done with the supervision of a properly trained health professional.

After doing this for a few days the amount of niacin, exercise and the length of time in the sauna are increased. After a few weeks, many people have profound experiences of improved health.

Most other detox therapies have you eating some herb to clean out your intestine, liver or gall bladder. However, if you eat right every day and get aerobic exercise, your body will have no trouble cleaning itself out. You also save money and avoid toxic reactions from the herbs. Most of the ailments which herbal detox therapies are supposed to cure are actually caused by delayed allergic reactions.

Parasites

Many people have intestinal parasites because they eat contaminated meat and water. These parasites can keep people at low levels of health even when they are eating properly.

There are only a few laboratories which do accurate stool testing for parasites. One that does is Great Smokies Diagnostic Laboratory in Asheville, North Carolina. Their phone number is (800) 522-4762 or (704) 253-0621.

There are now techniques for killing parasites without making people sick. One non-toxic treatments for killing parasites is made from grapefruit seeds.

Yeast Infections

A major problem which affects many people is yeast infections. There has been a dramatic increase in yeast infections because of the increasing numbers of people with delayed food allergies.

The most commonly written-about yeast is Candida Albicans. However, there are at least nine different yeasts which cause problems. It is not very helpful to be tested for Candida because the problem may be made worse by a combination of other yeasts. Even if you are tested for antibodies to Candida, the test does not disclose if you are currently having a problem or if you had a problem in the past and still have Candida antibodies. To complicate the yeast problem, almost everybody has some yeast in their body; it is elevated levels which causes problems.

White blood cells are what keep the level of yeast in the body under control. Diets with moderate to high amounts of simple carbohydrates (sugar) make yeast problems worse. Adding to the problem is the use of antibiotics and birth control pills.

Many herbs and medications have been tried to help the white blood cells reduce yeast levels. One effective treatment involves taking a prescription drug called Diflucan. It is important to eat correctly before and after becoming free of a high yeast level, or your yeast problem will come back. Avoid eating leftovers — yeast grows on them, even in the refrigerator. Acidophilus and bifidus help to replace yeast in the large intestine.

People are always blaming
their circumstances for what they are.
I don't believe in circumstances.
The people who get on in this world
are the people who get up and look for the
circumstances they want...

George Bernard Shaw
Dramatist, Essayist and Critic — 1856 to 1950

Enzymes

Many people who have had food allergies for years have reduced pancreatic function and thus cannot produce enough digestive enzymes to properly break down the foods they have eaten. They often start having delayed allergy reactions to foods found to be compatible on their Prime Test.

Most of the digestive enzymes we need to digest foods are made by our pancreas. An effective enzyme supplement is made from pork pancreas and is called pancreas compound tablets. By taking four uncoated tablets 40 minutes before a meal, many people start getting healthier and stop becoming allergic to the foods they are eating.

A good source for digestive enzymes is General Research Laboratories in California. Their phone number is (800) 421-1856 or (818) 349-9911.

Only the curious will learn
and only the resolute overcome
the obstacles to learning.
The quest quotient has always excited me more
than the intelligence quotient.

Eugene S. Wilson
American Attorney — 1879 to 1937

Cell Strength

One way to decrease allergic reactions is to strengthen the body's immune cells. There is a prescription drug called Sodium Cromolyn or Cromoglycate which helps do this without negative side effects for most people. Inhaling Cromolyn powder has become the standard treatment for people with asthma. It has replaced the use of cortisone, if the doctor has done his homework.

Besides being inhaled for asthma, Cromolyn powder can be used by people with delayed food allergies. It is dissolved in hot water and drunk half an hour before meals.

For Cromolyn to work, people need to avoid their major allergy-causing foods and chemicals, and then use it for added support. Cromolyn has been around for over 20 years, is rather expensive and you need a prescription. A good source is College Pharmacy. Their phone number is (800) 888-9358.

Inflammation

Our bodies reduce inflammation by producing a special liquid in the adrenal glands. It is common for the adrenal glands to become exhausted after years of eating the wrong foods and repetitious exposure to damaging chemicals.

A prescription medication can add this inflammation-reducer to the body and can be very helpful for people with delayed allergies. The medication is called adrenal cortical extract, known as ACE. It does not have any of the damaging side effects that all cortisone and steroid medications do.

ACE is the only known treatment for stopping the allergic inflammation caused by Poison Oak or Poison Ivy. For most people ACE is effective in reducing allergic inflammation.

Because of pressure from the manufacturers of cortisone drugs and harassment from traditional doctors who do not believe that delayed food and chemical allergies exist, the FDA took ACE off the market for several years. Now available again, it is often difficult to find because it is difficult to locate a doctor who will risk prescribing it.

Traditional Medicine

As damaging and incompetent as much of traditional medicine is at treating chronic and degenerative diseases, it does a few things very well. If you get in an automobile accident or fall off a ladder, traditional medicine usually provides competent emergency care, as long as you go to a good hospital and have a supportive and knowledgeable doctor on your team. This doctor may not believe in the importance of food allergies but can help with emergencies and infections.

You can tell that traditional doctors do not know what they are talking about when it comes to treating chronic symptoms, degenerative symptoms or preventive care — their average health is even worse than their patients.

You need to become your own expert on delayed food and chemical allergies.

Taking antibiotics for virus infections does not

work and damage your health. Antibiotics only kill bacteria, including the essential bacteria that enables your large intestine to work properly.

If you take antibiotics for a bacterial infection, wait two weeks after you stop taking the antibiotics and then take acidophilus and bifidus. This reestablishes the flora you need in your large intestine which were killed off when the antibiotics were attacking the bacterial infection in your body.

Provocative Neutralization

One approach for reducing allergic inflammation from unavoidable items, such as molds, airborne chemicals and an occasional food, is called Provocative Neutralization. The right microscopic dose of something to which you have a delayed allergic reaction often reduces some of the symptoms caused by the item. Although the scientific mechanism for this phenomenon has not been discovered, it can be helpful for some people. This technique finds a person's unique neutralizing dose of an item by trial and error injections. By giving themselves a sublingual drop of their neutralizing dose once or twice a week, they reduce some of the damage caused by their allergic reaction to that substance.

Provocative Neutralization has some problems. First, it is expensive and very time consuming to get your unique dose established. Second, your individual dose often changes and you have to keep having it rediscovered. Third, the testing is hard on your body and often leaves you sick and exhausted. Fourth, it only reduces some of the allergic damage from a particular exposure and lessens some of the symptoms. This is nowhere near as effective as avoiding the allergic reacting food. In one study, less than 20 percent of the people who used their white blood cell test results needed to be neutralized for any remaining symptoms.

Full-Spectrum Light

It is important to have our life-styles as close to how we evolved as possible. We evolved in an environment where we received, almost daily, the full spectrum of sunlight, including ultraviolet light, onto our bodies and into our eyes.

There has been increased public awareness of people who get very sickly in northern climates and only recover when they look at full-spectrum-florescent tubes for half an hour each day.

This therapy works because some of the optic nerve does not go to the brain to deliver visual pictures, but branches off and goes to our pineal gland, stimulating it to produce the hormone called melatonin. Melatonin is necessary for the brain, pituitary, adrenals, ovaries and testicles to work properly. The pituitary gland is the master gland for our entire endocrine system and thereby helps run our entire body, influencing growth, metabolism and maturing. Melatonin also regulates the body's sleep/wake cycles and other rhythms.

If you wear prescription or dark glasses all day or wear contact lenses that block ultraviolet light, you are losing the ultraviolet part of full-spectrum light. Ultraviolet light is essential for our endocrine system and many other parts of our bodies to work right. Oxygen-permeable hard contact lens materials that transmit ultraviolet light can be ordered by your eye doctor. Most soft lenses transmit ultraviolet light.

It is difficult to get prescription glasses or dark glasses that are ultraviolet transmitting. Avoid wearing dark glasses some of the time you are in the sun. If you can not wear contacts and have to wear regular glasses, take them off when you are outdoors for half an hour a day, several days a week.

People who do not eat dairy products nor too much protein and who live out in the sun all the time without dark glasses, usually do not get cataracts. An example is the natives in New Guinea. If they move into the city and start eating dairy products and too much meat, they start getting cataracts. Wearing dark glasses does not solve the cataract problem — a lifetime of proper diet does.

There are times when wearing dark glasses can be helpful because too much ultraviolet light can react with residue that develops in the cornea from eating dairy products and/or too much protein, and thus contribute to cataracts. Wear dark glasses above 5000 feet on sunny days and when the reflected light is bright. If you are outside in the sunlight most of the time and have eaten poorly for years, you may have residue in your lenses and need to wear dark glasses part of the time.

Half hour in the sun, several days a week, is enough to facilitate the functioning of most people's endocrine system if they are not wearing anything that filters out the ultraviolet light from their eyes. Enjoy the sun with respect.

The only thing that is really yours
is what you learn.

Hans Selye
Canadian stress researcher — 1907 to 1982

Herbs

There are a few herbs which appear to help the body to function better. The challenge is finding out which herbs work and taking them without becoming allergic to them. It is best to pick an herb that has the greatest chance of being helpful without causing damage. Try it for a short period of time to see if it brings you to a higher level of health and then stop taking it for a while to avoid becoming allergic to it.

One herb that may be helpful is Ginkgo Biloba. Another herb that helps some men with prostate problems is Saw Palmetto. There are many others that have exaggerated claims made for them and need to be approached with great caution after you have everything else working for you.

Numerous claims are made for herbal medicine. Because the Chinese have been using herbal medicine for five thousand years does not make the approach valid for every health problem.

When scientists actually studied the health of people in China, they saw that their good health related directly to their low fat, low protein, low cholesterol, high complex carbohydrate diet.

With a few exceptions, there is little evidence that the herbs sold by the ton to the hopeful buyers in China have value. When you look at the archaic religious beliefs that China's herbal medicine is based on, you see lack of scientific basis or controlled studies to see if the herb actually works. Examples are the beliefs that eating rhinoceros horns make men virile and eating tiger testicles make men potent. These fallacious beliefs are causing annihilation for the few remaining rhinoceros and tigers.

Back Problems and Muscle Tone

Back problems are one of the most common causes of severe and lasting pain. A major part of back problems is chronic muscle fatigue which causes the muscles to lose tone. Without the right foods and exercise, muscles slowly lose strength. Delayed food allergies are a major cause of chronic muscle fatigue and loss of muscle tone.

Healthy, toned back muscles hold the spine in alignment. When the muscles are healthy, the back functions properly and this keeps the discs between the vertebrae from rupturing.

Besides eating one's compatible foods, it is important to have a daily routine of exercises that tone the stomach and back muscles so that the back ceases to be a problem. Just doing the exercises by themselves does not solve back problems because the muscles do not respond well to the exercise if you are eating foods that cause the muscles to break down. Your back and posture are also helped by using the correct techniques for lifting items and using properly designed chairs and beds.

Muscle tone is important for the functioning of all parts of the body and toning and stretching exercises should be used in all areas of the body.

Chiropractic Adjustments

The top vertebra of the spine is called the atlas. The skull sits on the atlas. Some people have improved health by having this area positioned correctly by a specially trained chiropractor.

Other types of chiropractic adjustments are helpful if you have something out of alignment. However, the traditional adjustment of the neck has been shown to create additional neck problems. This happens because the spaces between the neck vertebrae are enlarged causing the neck to slip out of alignment more often.

Electromagnetic Fields

Some electrical appliances generate electromagnetic fields which have been shown to diminish — and in some cases significantly damage — health. If you live within a quarter of a mile of high voltage power lines, it is best to move. Do not sleep with an electric blanket on. If you have a water bed, connect the water bed heater to a timer so it heats throughout the day and is off when you are sleeping.

Be sure that there are no electrical circuits or appliances emitting electromagnetic fields around your head area while you are sleeping. Major emitters of electromagnetic fields are color televisions and computers — especially ones with color monitors. Health improves as you reduce the amount of time spent watching television and sitting in front of a computer.

Air Pollution

Carefully select the air you breathe. Live and work in an area where smog and other chemicals are minimal. Avoid indoor air pollution.

Everyone's health is damaged by having a gas stove indoors because the fumes that come from the top of the stove when the burners are on impregnate the air throughout the home and damage the immune system with a broad range on toxic gases even though you can not smell them. This is also true of the oven burners. Plus, the chemicals in the gas fumes in the oven impregnate the food being cooked. The gases include: carbon monoxide, ozone, nitric oxide and nitrogen dioxide.

Be careful of where you live and work because photo copiers and laser printers give off some of the same chemicals as do gas stoves. If you have a copier at home or work, be sure it is sealed off in its own room and the room is vented to the outside.

It is important to have the air in your home as clean as possible. Activated charcoal filters in the duct system or as part of the independent fan system are very helpful in taking the toxic gases out of the air. The particles are taken out of the air by improved negative ion generators such as the Airea. For a supplier in your area call Advanced Health Center at (714) 661-4001.

Acupuncture

A number of claims have been made for acupuncture. Often times they are hard to substantiate because allergy symptoms go up and down all by themselves whether you try any treatment for them or not. It is hard to tell whether acupuncture is helpful or whether the benefits are cyclical or placebo. It is important that acupuncture and all other therapies be tried on people after they are no longer eating the foods they are allergic to. (It works much better to remove a splinter than try to treat a wound that still has a splinter in it.)

Homeopathy

Homeopathy is a technique that tries to create symptoms that are the same as the ones you are already having by using extremely weak doses of a chemical. Sometimes the doses of the offending substances are so weak that none of the offending item is left in the solution.

If the symptoms are able to be created, it may be that the body's natural alarm mechanism is simply being exhausted so that nothing is felt when an allergy causing food or chemical is consumed.

Many people have looked for a valid explanation for how homeopathy works; however, so far, none has been discovered. This therapy should be tried as a last resort, if there are still symptoms after the person is not consuming items they are allergic to. The symptoms usually go away and there is nothing left to try and mimic with the homeopathic dose.

Enzyme Potentiated Therapy

Enzyme Potentiated Therapy involves a special combination of enzymes and antigens which are injected every three months to try and reduce the body's reactivity to those substances. Some people have experienced good results with this therapy and after eating properly for some time it might be tried if the person is still having significant symptoms.

Support Groups

To be successful at improving our life-style and changing the way we eat, it is essential to think clearly and to have the resolution and self confidence to continue taking the necessary steps up the staircase to great health. There are several organizations which put on workshops that greatly facilitate individual growth and self confidence. Growth and self confidence empowers people to eat their compatible foods and exercise. Low self esteem is a common reason people go back to eating their damaging foods after they learn what to avoid.

It is very helpful to do The Quality Longevity Program with someone. You get support by seeing other people's successes and sharing ways of making it easier. Join or start a support group with other people who have taken the Prime Test.

One support group that helps people with allergies is the Human Ecology Action League, known as HEAL. Their phone number is (404) 248-1898.

Always bear in mind
that your own resolution to succeed
is more important than any other one thing.

Abraham Lincoln
Sixteenth President of the United States— 1809 to 1865

Psychological Counseling

Support from a psychologist, psychiatrist or other counselor can be helpful when starting your health program. However, if the counselor does not understand how the emotions are upset by delayed food and chemical allergies, their advice will be based on old psychological beliefs and can be harmful. It does not work to blame your mother or father or any one else, including yourself, for your symptoms.

By eating your compatible foods and doing aerobic exercise in combination with the right type of counseling you will be empowered to solve your psychological and physical problems.

Summary

This chapter gives a brief outline of the complementary therapies to explore after you have your health foundation in place. Nothing replaces the need to eat foods that are compatible with your body. As new approaches come along they can be added to what is already working for you. However, nothing should be used as a magic bullet to replace eating and exercising properly.

New approaches are a threat to those who make their living using the old approaches. An example of this is the traditional allergists who convinced a couple of state agencies that white blood cell tests for delayed food allergies should not be allowed. To prohibit the best preventive care is the height of ignorance.

*Prohibition goes beyond the bounds of reason
in that it attempts to control
a man's appetite by legislation, and
makes a crime out of things that are not crimes.
It strikes a blow at the very principles
upon which our government was founded.*

Abraham Lincoln
Sixteenth President of the United States— 1809 to 1865

Conclusion

Much of the training medical doctors and chiropractors received is not relative to the actual cause of most of the common ailments. Do not be surprised if most health practitioners are critical of your new understanding of health. All people tend to be critical of those things they do not understand, especially if their professional standing and income is threatened.

*We are so concerned to flatter the majority
that we lose sight of how very often it is necessary,
in order to preserve freedom for the minority,
let alone for the individual,
to face the majority down.*

William F. Buckley, Jr.
American Conservative Author

As the level of people's health goes up, the need for doctors goes down. The minium goal is to have one doctor for every 500 people and the optimum is one for every 1000 people. America has the worst doctor to patient ratio of any nation in the world — one doctor for every 290 people. As the awareness of delayed allergies continues to expand, over half of the medical doctors and other health practitioners are going to find themselves unemployed if they do not learn to help people with delayed allergies.

Around 400 BC, Hippocrates spent much of his time working with patients who had numerous symptoms that he saw were related to the foods they were eating. It was not until the latter half of the twentieth century that Theron Randolph, MD, and those he inspired, discovered that the hidden cause of most chronic symptoms was delayed food and chemical allergies. With your help, this breakthrough can become the new standard for health care in the twenty first century.

In 1978, The Quality Longevity Program brought together, for the first time, the three major health breakthroughs in preventive care from the twentieth century. Each of these breakthroughs — the discovery of delayed food and chemical allergies, the discovery of the 10–10–80 balance of fats, proteins and carbohydrates, and the discovery of the aerobic effect — is of great importance for helping people become well. The simultaneous combination of all three creates a health benefit beyond the sum of the three — a synergistic effect.

Quality Longevity has given you the foundation that enables you to go to a higher level of health than was possible before. Once you have taken the Prime Test and have experienced being symptom free, you will know that you are moving along a path that will lead to great health, energy and longevity. All this will be accomplished without the continuing costs and negative side effects of drugs, surgeries, psychotherapy, allergy shots and repetitious trips to many different doctors.

If you start The Quality Longevity Program when you are young, you can prevent most ailments. Start later and you can get free of your symptoms and reverse most of the damage already done. Each year your body can become younger. It is your right to enjoy great health.

*Whatever you can do or dream you can,
begin it. Boldness has genius,
power and magic in it.
Begin it now.*

Goethe
German Philosopher, Poet Novelist, Author — 1749 to 1832

Quality Longevity

Shared Experiences

For more than ten years, I have been a laboratory technician at the leading health care centers in New York. As head of the allergy departments, I have used the better white-blood-cell tests for discovering delayed food and chemical allergies.

For the last seven years, the test that has continually provided the best results for patients and ease of use in the laboratory is the Prime Test.

I have been able to follow up with patients who had a broad range of symptoms before having the test. Their satisfaction with being free of symptoms is one of the reasons my work is so rewarding.

Cherith Matlosz, MLT
Physicians for Complementary Medicine, New York

Thank you for giving me the new understanding of health. Over the last eight years, I have seen numerous ways the new awareness of food allergies has improved my life and the lives of my friends.

It feels good to watch others improve their health after sharing with them about this health breakthrough.

I started off lucky. I grew up in the clean air of the countryside of Sweden. Some of the foods I was raised on were hard on my health, but I was free of most chemicals and had good genes.

I had no major health problems. However, I was delighted to discover that my health, energy and joy of life could get even higher.

As I travel around the world, I enjoy helping people find the path to great health.

Majlis Andersson
Santiago, Chile

I have been having symptoms my whole life and did not understand what was going on.

As a child I was hard to live with. I was tense and irritable. By the third grade I was having trouble in school. I was hyperactive and my doctor agreed with my fifth grade teacher that I needed a drug called Ritalin to calm me down. I took the drug for two years and got no help. I tried a preservative free diet and it helped a little but most of my school years were lost.

By the seventh grade I started smoking daily and drinking alcohol often. From age 15 until to my current age of 27, I have been using cocaine regularly. I am completely addicted.

A month ago I took the Prime Test and got the follow-up counseling. I stopped eating the foods I am allergic to and addicted to.

For the first time in my life, I have consistent self control. I am now free of cocaine and can see the real possibility of staying free of all drugs because I am free of the foods that caused my cravings and instability.

After looking back over my life and my experience of the last month, I see that delayed food allergies were making me hyperactive, tense and irritable. My illegal drugs reduced the discomfort caused by the symptoms of my food addictions. My attempts to stop these symptoms led to my drug addiction.

I have a new sense of well being, self confidence and self control in my life. I am now confident for the first time in my life that I am going to be able to stay free of addictive drugs because I am now free of the addictive foods that were underlying my addictive personality.

The Prime Test and The Quality Longevity Program should be tried by others who want to become free of their drug problems. Let me know how I can help get the word out.

Name withheld by request.

I have benefited again from The Quality Longevity Program. Ten years ago, I took your improved cytotoxic test and discovered I had food allergies. After avoiding my damaging foods, I had results which were nothing short of a miracle. I experienced wellness I had never had before. I felt wonderful and did not need any medications. Food is truly my best medicine.

I slowly began eating a few of my old damaging foods, thinking I could handle them. This proved to be a disaster!

It has taken me some time and suffering to rediscover that dairy products were making me sick.

When I removed my old damaging foods, including milk, yogurt and all other dairy products, all the awful aching I had in every joint and muscle left me. I am now feeling super again.

Being nearly 80 years old, I find health ever more precious. Thank you for doing the research and for The Quality Longevity Program.

Dorothy C. White
See first letter on back cover.

Shared Experiences

I have had weekly headaches most of my life. They started when I was a child. I am now in my 50's and have gone to several types of doctors through the years trying to find relief. I was told to try hormones and medications for my migraines. I followed their advice, but still had headaches and hated the way the drugs made me feel.

I then saw a nutritionist and tried extensive regimes of vitamins, minerals and dietary changes. I did get quite a bit of improvement, but I still had a couple of headaches a week.

I felt I was allergic to something I was eating, but could not discover more than one or two foods that were causing symptoms. I had heard of delayed food and chemical allergies but was not able to locate anyone who knew how to test for them. After I read about The Quality Longevity Program, I decided to try the Prime Test.

My test results and the follow-up program was very different from any other approach I had tried. I have been using my test results for the past four months. For the first time in years I have been free from headaches. The significant exceptions have been when I ate a food my Prime Test indicated was a problem.

I am very excited about my progress. I have not been hungry and have lost unwanted weight — 23 pounds. My energy levels are great.

I enjoy enrolling my friends in The Quality Longevity Program and watching their progress.
Carol W. Bailard
Santa Ana, California

The following are the highlights of a letter written on September 12, 1985 to Mark Lovendale when he was the Director of Medical Service Center. It was written by a medical doctor who was a leading medical authority in the California state government. He had tried the white blood cell testing for delayed food and chemical allergies and became free of his symptoms.

I enthusiastically support the work that you and your staff are doing and am looking forward to providing clinical evaluation and studies that will be of benefit in predicting behavioral changes as well as T cell pathology as a result of the AIDS virus.

What I have proposed and intend to accomplish utilizing the cytotoxic test is to provide a double blind study with controls as regards aberrations of behavior, particularly violence proneness and individual reactivity to industrial allergens as determined by the testing. Additionally, in a separate study, is that of assessing inmates diagnosed as having AIDS or AIDS Related Complex as they progress with the illness. Additionally, the effects of removal of proven allergens as a part or their treatment program will be evaluated.

As you may know, I have had some personal experience, all very positive, from the cytotoxic testing services provided by your facility. I am also aware that there is some controversy regarding cytotoxic testing compared to RAST testing and the old traditional skin test. I guess it is understandable in the face of something that is as new and challenging as your service. But I am dismayed to see the hesitancy that exists on the part of medicine to make vast use of this proven modality.

You and your staff are on the cutting edge of a new frontier in allergy testing that has great merit and I trust there will be no impediments thrown in your path to delay work and progress in this most significant area of need.
William A. Weathers, MD
Medical Director
California Medical Facility
Department of Corrections
Vacaville, California

While Dr. Weathers was working on helping prisoners with the new awareness of how delayed food and chemical allergies cause violent behavior in some people and how AIDS patients could be helped, other state officials were working on preventing this beneficial, non-damaging approach from being available to everyone.

The misguided state officials, and the traditional allergists that influenced them, got their way.

The studies recommended by Dr. Wethers are still waiting to be done.

The most expensive item
one can possess
is a closed mind.
Nothing will ever cost more.